Case Studies in Gastroenterology

Case Studies in Gastroenterology

Editor: Creed Moore

AMERICAN
MEDICAL PUBLISHERS
www.americanmedicalpublishers.com

AMERICAN
MEDICAL PUBLISHERS
www.americanmedicalpublishers.com

Cataloging-in-Publication Data

Case studies in gastroenterology / edited by Creed Moore.
p. cm.
Includes bibliographical references and index.
ISBN 979-8-88740-599-5
1. Gastroenterology. 2. Digestive organs--Diseases.
3. Digestive organs--Diseases--Treatment. I. Moore, Creed.
RC801 .G37 2023
616.33--dc23

American Medical Publishers,
41 Flatbush Avenue,
1st Floor, New York,
NY 11217, USA

ISBN 979-8-88740-599-5 (Hardback)

Contents

Preface

The main aim of this book is to educate learners and enhance their research focus by presenting diverse topics covering this vast field. This is an advanced book which compiles significant studies by distinguished experts in the area of analysis. This book addresses successive solutions to the challenges arising in the area of application, along with it; the book provides scope for future developments.

Gastroenterology is a branch of medicine which focused on the study, diagnosis and treatment of disorders related to the digestive system. The digestive system encompasses organs such as the esophagus, stomach, small intestine, large intestine, liver, gallbladder and pancreas. The field of gastroenterology is involved in the diagnosis and management of a wide range of disorders, such as the gastroesophageal reflux disease (GERD), peptic ulcers, inflammatory bowel disease, irritable bowel syndrome (IBS), and gastrointestinal cancers. These disorders can be diagnosed by studying the medical history, physical examination, and various diagnostic procedures. These procedures may include endoscopy, imaging studies, blood tests, and stool analysis. The treatment of these disorders may include lifestyle modifications, dietary changes, medications, minimally invasive procedures, or surgery. This book explores all the important aspects of gastroenterology in the present day scenario. It will serve as a valuable source of reference for graduate and postgraduate students.

It was a great honour to edit this book, though there were challenges, as it involved a lot of communication and networking between me and the editorial team. However, the end result was this all-inclusive book covering diverse themes in the field.

Finally, it is important to acknowledge the efforts of the contributors for their excellent chapters, through which a wide variety of issues have been addressed. I would also like to thank my colleagues for their valuable feedback during the making of this book.

Editor

1

Acute Esophageal Necrosis in a Septic Patient with a History of Cardiovascular Disease

Michael Coles, Victoria Madray, and Pearl Uy

Augusta University, 1120 15th Street, Augusta, Georgia 30912, USA

Correspondence should be addressed to Michael Coles; michaeljohncoles@gmail.com

Academic Editor: Gregory Kouraklis

Acute esophageal necrosis (AEN), or colloquially named "black esophagus," is a rare clinical condition often associated with ischemic injury to the esophagus secondary to splanchnic vasoconstriction during hypotensive episodes. We present a case of a 78-year-old man with extensive cardiovascular disease who was initially admitted for gallstone pancreatitis and possible cholangitis. His hospital course was complicated by possible sepsis secondary to aspiration pneumonia and hematemesis secondary to acute ischemic esophageal necrosis as noted on upper endoscopy. Interestingly, the patient only had a transient episode of hypotension (approximately 35 minutes) not requiring vasopressor support, which improved with fluid resuscitation, and endoscopic retrograde cholangiopancreatography (ERCP) done 3 days prior showed normal esophageal mucosa. Clinicians should be aware of the possibility of acute esophageal necrosis as a potential etiology of gastrointestinal (GI) bleed in patients with cardiovascular disease and sepsis.

1. Case Report

A 78-year-old Caucasian male with past medical history significant for coronary artery disease with multivessel coronary artery bypass grafting, paroxysmal atrial fibrillation on apixaban therapy, heart failure with reduced ejection fraction (~37%), chronic kidney disease stage III, and chronic abdominal aortic aneurysm (AAA) with graft repair in remote past was admitted and treated for gallstone pancreatitis and possible cholangitis. On hospital day 2, he produced 50 mL of coffee ground emesis and experienced a transient episode of hypotension to 70/50 mmHg, which improved with 1 L fluid bolus. The patient was treated empirically for aspiration pneumosepsis given hypotension and equivocal chest X-ray findings, but no organism was identified on culture data. Subsequent magnetic resonance imaging study showed filling defect of the common bile duct without dilation suspicious for cholangitis secondary to stone or sludge. A following endoscopic retrograde cholangiopancreatography (ERCP) showed duodenal diverticulum and erosive duodenitis; a common bile duct (CBD) stent was placed. On hospital day 4, a follow-up ERCP showed normal esophagus and no filling defect in the CBD, with persistent duodenitis. However, on hospital day 7, the patient complained of acute chest pain accompanied by 200 mL of bright red emesis. Of note, apixaban (5 mg twice daily) was restarted the night before, and INR was elevated at 2.5. The patient remained hemodynamically stable with a hemoglobin and hematocrit of 9.1 mg/dL and 27.4%, respectively, suggestive of hemostasis. However, his white blood cell count increased dramatically from 11,000 to 18,000/mm.[3]

Subsequent esophagogastroduodenoscopy (EGD) revealed circumferential black esophagus extending entirely from the proximal to distal esophagus (gastroesophageal (GE) junction noted at 40 cm from the incisors) and old blood in the gastric cavity, but no signs of active bleeding (Figures 1 and 2).

The images seen on endoscopy showed diffuse black discoloration, linear ulcers, and stark demarcation of involved and uninvolved mucosa at the gastroesophageal junction in the absence of toxin ingestion. A diagnosis of acute esophageal necrosis (AEN) was made, and the patient was continued on intravenous proton pump inhibitors

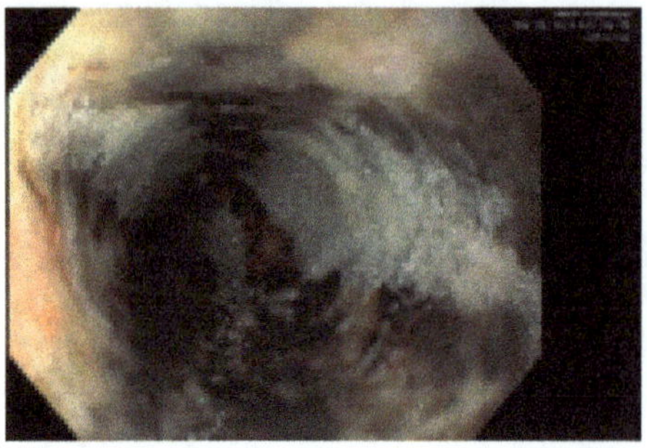

FIGURE 1: Diffuse black discoloration of the esophagus with linear ulcerated mucosa.

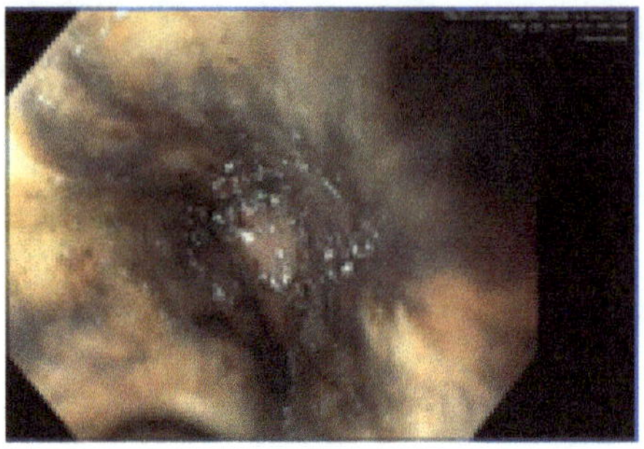

FIGURE 2: Circumferential black discoloration of the distal esophageal mucosa with clear demarcation with the uninvolved GE junction.

(PPI), antibiotics, and fluid hydration; apixaban was held. The rest of his hospitalization was unremarkable, and he was discharged to a long-term care facility. We intend to perform repeat endoscopy to confirm resolution of mucosal injury and rule out stricture formation.

2. Discussion

Acute esophageal necrosis (AEN) is rare with less than one hundred patient cases published in the literature and a prevalence of 0.2% [1]. Typically, AEN presents in critically ill patients with hemodynamic compromise such as cardiovascular disease or sepsis requiring intensive inotropic support [2]. The diagnosis of AEN can be made with endoscopic evidence of necrotic esophageal mucosa in the above-described clinical setting. Histologic evidence can confirm AEN but is unnecessary to make a diagnosis [3]. Our patient's hemodynamic stability despite panesophageal necrosis remains nebulous. Alternative diagnoses (pseudomenlanosis, acanthosis nigricans, and malignant melanoma) are possible and no tissue biopsy confirmed necrosis; however, the patient's symptom constellation and acuity of presentation were more consistent with AEN.

The etiology of AEN is multifactorial and largely thought to be due to an ischemic insult leading to decreased esophageal perfusion and impairment of the mucosal barrier of the esophagus. During episodes of hypotension or shock, the body's protective mechanism of splanchnic vasoconstriction results in decreased perfusion of visceral organs such as the esophagus, stomach, and intestines with loss of >90% of gastric blood flow [4]. The distal esophagus is most often involved in AEN, likely due to its decreased vascular supply in the face of a global hypoperfused state and vasoconstriction. A "two-hit" hypothesis theory has developed suggesting hypoperfusion increases opportunity for injury to the mucosa by a second entity such as toxins or acids that results in rapid onset of necrosis unless addressed and treated [1]. Therefore, a high level of suspicion for acute esophageal necrosis as a differential diagnosis for gastrointestinal bleed is imperative among patients with cardiovascular disease and sepsis given its high mortality rate of 32% and potential rapidity of onset requiring urgent treatment [1].

A notable feature in our case was the rapid necrosis secondary to one brief period of hypotension that hemodynamically responded to fluid administration. We propose that the extensive comorbid vascular disease present in our patient, especially the previous surgical treatment of AAA, resulted in ischemic necrosis of the distal esophagus consequent to limited hypotensive stress. The distal esophagus is normally perfused via the esophageal branch of the left gastric artery arising from the celiac trunk [1]. Although computed tomography angiography was not performed in our patient, esophageal vasculature supply proximal to the celiac trunk was also likely not well collateralized at baseline given the patient's vasculopathic manifestations elsewhere (coronary artery disease and chronic kidney disease). Already tenuous tissue perfusion was further compromised by a brief period of hypotension in the midst of sepsis possibly explaining panesophageal involvement.

AEN treatment aims to restore hemodynamic stability in hypotensive patients using fluids, blood transfusion, and PPI therapy [4, 5]. Patients should be nil-per-os due to risk of perforation of necrotic tissue with passage of food or tubing [4, 5]. After stabilization and treatment, repeat endoscopy can be utilized to confirm resolution of mucosal injury and rule out complication of AEN such as stricture formation, which occurs in up to 25% of these cases [5].

AEN is a life-threatening cause of patients presenting with bloody emesis. Hence, expeditious workup including endoscopy is recommended in critically ill patients presenting with hematemesis to define the source of bleeding. Although rare, AEN should be considered in the differential diagnosis, particularly in patients with coexisting extensive vascular disease or a history of septic shock. Since the genesis of AEN results from a critical reduction in esophageal blood flow, this entity may be reversible with supportive management that includes prompt attention to the cardiovascular system that optimizes splanchnic blood flow.

References

[1] W. Ullah, A. Mehmood, I. Micaily, and M. S. Khan, "Comprehensive review of acute oesophageal necrosis," *BMJ Case Reports*, vol. 12, no. 2, Article ID e227967, 2019.

[2] S. Beg, "Acute oesophageal necrosis: a case report and review of the literature," *British Journal of Medical Practitioners*, vol. 8, no. 3, 2015.

[3] L. D. Averbukh, M. G. Mavilia, and G. E. Gurvits, "Acute esophageal necrosis: a case series," *Cureus*, vol. 10, no. 3, 2018.

[4] J. Carvão, M. G. Faria, V. M. Pereira et al., "Esophageal and gastroduodenal hemorrhagic necrosis: a unique finding in the setting of septic shock and vasopressor use," *ACG Case Reports Journal*, vol. 5, no. 1, p. e57, 2018.

[5] S. Shafa, N. Sharma, J. Keshishian, and E. S. Dellon, "The black esophagus: a rare but deadly disease," *ACG Case Reports Journal*, vol. 3, no. 2, pp. 88–91, 2016.

2

Small Bowel Obstruction Conservatively Managed in Hospital-at-Home

Margaret R. Paulson[1] **Abdullah S. Eldaly**[2] **Francisco R. Avila**[2] **Ricardo A. Torres-Guzman**[2] **Karla C. Maita**[2] **John P. Garcia**[2] **Luiza Palmieri Serrano**[2] **Omar S. Emam**[2] **Antonio J. Forte**[2] **and Michael J. Maniaci**[3]

[1] *Division of Hospital Internal Medicine, Mayo Clinic Health Systems, Eau Claire, Wisconsin 2321 Stout Road, Menomonie, Wisconsin 54751, USA*
[2] *Division of Plastic Surgery, Mayo Clinic, 4500 San Pablo Road, Jacksonville, Florida 32224, USA*
[3] *Division of Hospital Internal Medicine, Mayo Clinic, 4500 San Pablo Road, Jacksonville, Florida 32224, USA*

Correspondence should be addressed to Michael J. Maniaci; maniaci.michael@mayo.edu

Academic Editor: Daniel C. Damin

In 2020, Mayo Clinic established an Advanced Care at Home (ACH) program. ACH is a virtual hybrid hospital-at-home (HaH) program that combines telemedicine with in-home care services by utilizing a state that is software-driven, vendor-mediate medical supply chain. The program initially focused on acute medical diagnosis but has expanded to oversee surgical and postsurgical patients with continued inpatient needs. Here, we report the first case of a small bowel obstruction (SBO) managed under a HaH program. A 52-year-old lady presented to the emergency department with symptoms suggestive of mechanical SBO. The diagnosis was confirmed with an abdominopelvic computed tomography (CT) scan, and the patient was admitted to the hospital. Based on the patient's presentation and laboratory results, the care team proceeded with conservative treatment including nasogastric tube (NG) placement and suctioning, intravenous (IV) fluid replacement, and daily laboratory studies. She spent the first hospital day in the physical hospital ward so that the surgical team could ensure stability clinically and no urgent need for surgical intervention. On hospital day two, she was transferred home with ACH where the NG suctioning and IV replacement therapy could continue, while the medical team conducted daily virtual visits to ensure continued improvement. Additionally, a paramedic and a nurse performed an in-person, head-to-toe assessment and administered medications to the patient twice daily. She spent 5 days in ACH getting acute care and then was discharged into a postacute phase equivalent to outpatient monitoring called the restorative phase. She was monitored remotely for the duration of the restorative phase for 10 more days, and then she recovered fully. This case highlights that high-acuity patients with SBO can receive invasive treatments like NG tube suction as well as be appropriately monitored for clinical decompensation by a virtual hybrid home hospital program which combines virtual care providers with an in-home vendor-mediated supply chain.

1. Introduction

Hospital-at-home (HaH) programs were first conceptualized by Burton and Regenstreif in 1995 as an alternative for geriatric patients requiring acute medical attention [1]. Four years later, the feasibility of the model was investigated by Leff et al. [2] in a pilot study that recruited 17 adult patients, aged 65 or older, that presented with acute conditions mandating hospitalization. The pilot study concluded that the HaH model was safe, feasible, and cost-effective [2], and the following years witnessed the successful implementation of several HaH programs across the country with satisfactory outcomes [3]. The primary motive of these programs is to reduce the problems the traditional brick-and-mortar hospitals (BAM) frequently face, particularly emergency department (ED) overcrowding and high expenses of inpatient care [3].

In 2020, Mayo Clinic established the Advance Care at Home (ACH) program. ACH combines a virtual provider-staffed command center (CC) with a smart supply chain of healthcare professionals that can deliver care to patients in the comfort of their own homes [4, 5]. The goals of this program are in accordance with Mayo Clinic's intent to provide individualized and adaptable care to the largest number of patients, including those who live in rural and underserved areas.

Since its implementation, ACH has successfully treated hundreds of patients with acute medical conditions, such as decompensated heart failure, pneumonia, and postoperative patients. We report the case of a patient who presented with a small bowel obstruction (SBO) and was successfully managed conservatively under ACH care. To the best of our knowledge, this is the first SBO case treated in a HaH program.

2. Case Presentation

A 52-year-old lady presented to the ED on October 26, 2021, with onset of acute epigastric pain, nausea, and ten accounts of nonbloody emesis a few hours prior to arrival. She described the pain as being sharp in nature and localized to the epigastric region near the xiphoid sternum without radiation. She denied nasal congestion, runny nose, postnasal drip, sore throat, cough, chest pain, shortness of breath, other abdominal pain, back pain, flank pain, pelvic pain, dysuria, hematuria, fever, chills, diarrhea or blood in her stool, or vomiting. She had a past medical history of recurrent small intestinal obstruction treated conservatively in 1999, February 2020, and August 2021. She additionally had a history of migraine headaches, an exploratory laparotomy done in 1986 due to a motor vehicle accident (MVA), and a lumbar spinal fracture at L3-L4 in 2017 caused by an MVA.

Her vital signs at presentation included a blood pressure of 130/72 mmHg, a heart rate of 42 beats per minute, a respiratory rate of 16 breaths per minute, an oral temperature of 36.9°C, and an SpO_2 of 95%. The physical examination was positive for diffuse abdominal tenderness without guarding or rigidity. Abdominopelvic computed tomography (CT) scan showed SBO without evidence of free air, bowel incarceration, or abscess. Laboratory evaluation revealed leukocytosis (WBC 15.6) and an elevated lactate (2.5). The patient was admitted to the hospital where she remained in the ED due to the lack of inpatient ward bed availability. General surgery was consulted, and they advised admission to the hospital to start conservative treatment with gastric decompression, pain control, and intravenous (IV) fluid resuscitation. A nasogastric (NG) tube was placed and connected to low continuous suction. The patient was kept nil per os (NPO) and started on 0.9% normal saline IV at 100 mL/hour. She was admitted to the hospital with the expectation of 5–7 days of acute hospital care, watching for symptom resolution and the return of bowel function.

The following day, the patient reported that her symptoms had improved, and on examination, she had amelioration of abdominal distension and tenderness. The surgical team was encouraged that the conservative treatment was working and surgical intervention was unlikely. Although encouraged by her progress overnight, she did not want to stay an extended period of time in the BAM hospital and inquired if there were any other treatment options. The surgical team requested a consultation by the ACH team to evaluate whether the patient was a potential candidate for continuing treatment at home. The ACH team assessed the patient at bedside to determine her eligibility based on insurance, demographic, social, and clinical criteria for program admission (Figure 1) [4]. She was informed that she would be monitored very closely by a combination of both virtual and in-home personnel, and if any complications that could not be handled arose in the home, she could be rapidly transported back to the BAM hospital. At home, she would be continuously connected to the ACH Command Center (CC), which is staffed by a hospitalist physician, advanced practice providers (APPs), registered nurses (RNs), a pharmacist, and a case manager. This team would constantly assess her clinical situation and, in conjunction with the surgical team, update her medical care plan, and direct the in-home care delivery. In-home services would include APPs for advanced physical examinations, community paramedics, RNs, aides, rehabilitative services, infusion therapy, phlebotomists, and basic radiography technicians. The benefits and risks of the program were discussed in detail with the patient. Benefits included receiving hospital-level care in the comfort of her own home, called the "acute phase," as well as ownership of her postacute care by the same care team as she recovered, called the "restorative phase." The potential risks mentioned included delay in care due to the nature of remote management and service limitations with the use of telemedicine technology, including interruptions, unauthorized access, and technical difficulties. She was also informed that she would not be accrued any additional cost for ACH care, and here, insurance would be billed the same for both BAM and ACH care. Alternatives other than the ACH program were offered to the patient. These comprised remaining at the hospital during the acute phase of illness and seeking care from different postacute service providers after hospitalization, such as skilled nursing facilities or home health agencies. All patient questions were answered. She agreed to participate in the program and was transferred to her home on the same day.

A technological kit that consisted of a tablet for video conferencing, a two-way telephone connected to the CC and encrypted cellular cradle point, and a 72-hour backup power supply. She was also provided a personal emergency response system which consisted of a Bluetooth-connected watch with a panic button that the patient would constantly wear throughout her home hospital stay. No matter where her home location is, if any trouble arose, she would be able to activate the watch panic button which would both instantly connect her to the CC team as well as alert an in-person rapid response team. The equipment was thoroughly checked and tested for functionality. Moreover, the patient and her caregivers verbalized their understanding of how to use the equipment and when and how to contact the CC.

Eligible Patients

Inclusion Criteria	Exclusion Criteria
(i) Clinical stability	(i) Uncontrolled mental illness
(ii) Geography–within 25-30 miles of hospital	(ii) IV pain medication needs
(iii) Social determinants making home unsafe for patients or staff	(iii) Requiring 24/7 assistance with activities of daily living
(iv) Payer coverage	(iv) Unstable arrhythmia
(v) Age (adults only)	(v) Requires telemetry monitoring
(vi) Acute exacerbation requiring inpatient-level care	

Figure 1: Advanced care at home patient eligibility criteria.

On her first day of the ACH acute phase (hospital day #2), the patient was contacted by her virtual bedside registered nurse (RN) to address any concerns and verify the medications and their dosages. The RN reviewed the treatment plan for the remainder of the day. Additionally, a paramedic and a nurse visited the patient twice daily to administer medications and perform complete assessment of the cardiac, gastrointestinal, genitourinary, psychosocial, musculoskeletal, peripheral vascular, and respiratory systems. At that time, the patient was kept NPO and had an NG tube maintained on a home low intermittent suctioning device. The patient received the following medications while at home: acetaminophen suppositories 325 mg, D5W and NaCl 0.45% with KCl 20 mEq/L infusion, enoxaparin injection 40 mg, ketorolac injection 15 mg, lidocaine 5% 1 patch, ondansetron injection 4 mg, ondansetron tablet 4 mg, and pantoprazole injection 40 mg.

On the third hospital day, the general surgery team made their virtual rounds on the patient. The patient reported 2/10 abdominal pain, no nausea, and had started to pass flatus. The surgical team recommended clamping the NG tube for several hours and then conducting a Gastrografin contrast enhanced abdominal radiograph series. As this advanced imaging could not be done in the home, the patient was informed that the ACH standard of care was to transport her back to the BAM hospital in a monitored medical ambulance directly to the radiology department, bypassing the ED or the hospital wards, and have the imaging study completed. Her inpatient status would remain the same, just as a patient in the BAM receiving a radiological study, and there would be no additional cost for this procedure. After completion, she was transported back home and awaited the results. The study revealed passage of contrast from the small bowl to the colon. Later that day, the RN checked the NG tube residual, which was 5 mL after 4 hours of clamping, and the NG tube was then removed.

On hospital day 4, the patient was started on small sips of clear fluids, which she tolerated. No abdominal pain, distension, nausea, or vomiting was reported by the patient to the virtual teams. She was encouraged to start ambulating more in her home to prevent deconditioning. The following day she had her first bowel movement and denied any abdominal pain or discomfort. Her diet was advanced to a full liquid diet per her request. The IV fluids were reduced from 100 mL/hr to 75 mL/hr.

On her fifth day of the ACH acute phase (hospital day #6), no pain, nausea, or vomiting was documented. She reported as feeling quite well, and she was advanced to a low fiber diet. It was decided by the ACH team that she was well enough to be discharged from the hospital and was moved to the postacute care, restorative phase of ACH. The IV fluids were stopped, the IV access was removed, and her medications were changed to oral administration.

During the posthospital restorative phase, the patient received a video call every morning from an RN to perform an assessment, review her vital data, and confirm the medications. Additionally, the patient was requested to call the CC twice daily to report her vitals and any updates related to her condition. She had a virtual visit with a physical therapist who instructed her on exercises she could do at home to improve strength and mobility. Two days after the discharge from the acute hospital phase, the patient returned to work. She was monitored for additional 8 days in the restorative phase, and upon advancing to a regular diet and having an uneventful treatment course, she was discharged from this postacute monitoring phase. The total care time was 16 days, with 1 day in the BAM hospital, 5 days in the hospital-level ACH acute phase, and 10 days in the postacute restorative phase (Figure 2).

3. Discussion

Telemedicine and HaH programs are effective in reducing costs of medical services, in-hospital admission, and readmission rates while improving outcomes and patient satisfaction [6–8]. The potential of these programs has escalated due to the exponential growth of technology in the last decade. Here, we present a patient with a SBO treated with conservative management in our ACH program. The patient was treated in both the acute and postacute phase and was able to avoid a prolonged stay in an inpatient ward. This is important as SBO has traditionally been seen as a condition that was only able to be treated in a BAM hospital setting. By combining virtual telemedicine with in-home, high-acuity care, we were able to accomplish treatment and recovery in an alternative setting.

SBO comprises 4% and 16% of abdominal pain related ED visits and surgical admissions in the US, respectively [9, 10]. These admissions alone result in over 2 billion USD costs annually in the US [10–12]. Postoperative adhesions account for 80% of SBO cases and are associated with higher recurrence rates [10]. Conservative management is the conventional treatment for patients with uncomplicated SBO and is successful in 43–73% of patients. Moreover, most patients show signs of clinical improvement within the first 48 hours [13–15]. IV fluid resuscitation, analgesics, antiemetics, and bowel rest constitute the conservative management of SBO [10]. All these measures can be easily delivered with a HaH program. However, the challenge in managing a patient with SBO at home is the continuous monitoring for signs of clinical deterioration (e.g., fever, leukocytosis, and tachycardia) to permit a timely surgical intervention, if needed, and prevent any compromise to the patient's outcome.

We believe that this challenge can be appropriately addressed by the ACH program as it permits real-time,

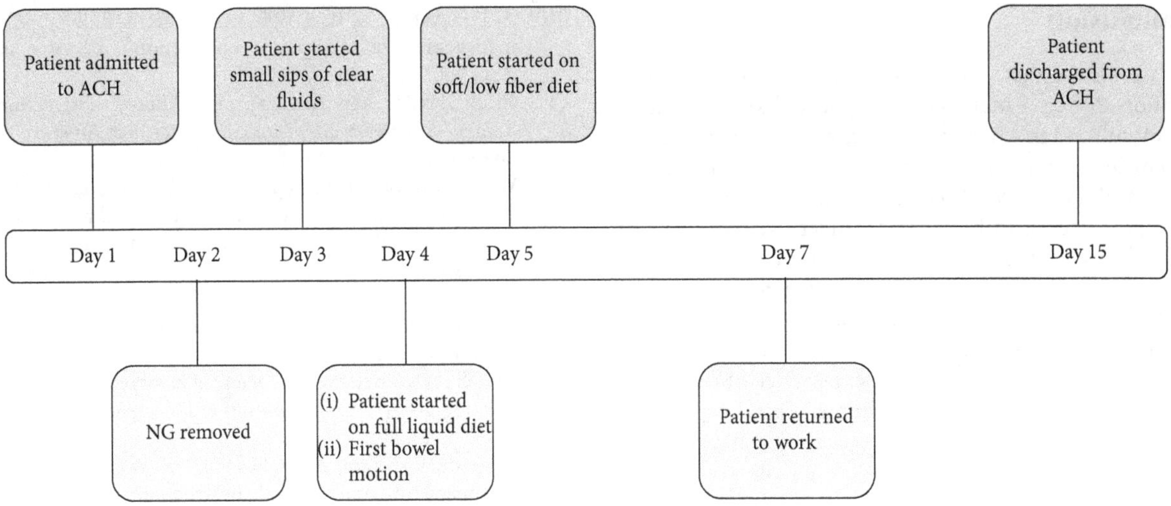

FIGURE 2: Timeline showing 5 days in the acute phase of inpatient-equivalent care and 10 days in the restorative phase of postacute recovery care.

hospital-level monitoring of patients due to synchronous telemedicine with standard HaH services and allows timely interventions when necessary. The patients are observed in their homes using biometric devices that collect the vital data that are normally gathered in the hospital. Furthermore, a two-way telephone permits 24/7 communication between patients, and the medical team and the emergency response system bracelet keeps patients connected to the care team no matter where the location of the home is. This process of synchronous telemonitoring is enabled by the CC where RNs, physician assistants, and advance nurse practitioners collaborate with nonclinical service coordinators to ensure the potency and quality of the service. Additionally, the ACH program is equipped with a highly qualified care team, including nurses, paramedics, phlebotomists, radiology technicians, and oxygen services. This group permits any changes in the management plan to take place smoothly in a time-efficient fashion. Finally, advanced, nontraditional in-home interventions like an NG tube connected to low intermittent suction were able to be performed. The clinical team did not start with such interventions at the onset of ACH in 2020, but as the vendor-mediated supply chain and in-home rapid response system grew and was repeatedly proven to perform at a high level, more advanced treatment options such as the above were added to expand ACH use cases. New interventions require elaborate planning for in-home vendor redundancy in order to meet safety guidelines as well as to provide the opportunity for education on these new treatment modalities for both the in-home vendor and the virtual providers. Often, simulation exercises are performed prior to implementation in real patient care in order to make sure all the components work as expected and the ACH team is satisfied with the quality, safety, and experience.

The second key factor in this case was the lack of inpatient ward bed availability, which resulted in the patient being kept in the ED for 24 hours prior to moving her to ACH. The lack of bed availability likely played a role in the patient's decision to enroll into the ACH program. Many hospital systems suffer from the lack of bed capacity, resulting in patients who should be receiving care in an inpatient ward to instead receive ward-level care in the ED where the patient is boarded [16, 17]. This leads to ED overcrowding, which increases morbidity and mortality for both boarded and ED patients as well as increases the length of stay of the admitted patients leading to decreased patient and staff satisfaction [16]. One solution to this problem is the creation of virtual wards through HaH programs. HaH programs can provide much needed hospital capacity creation and serve as a relief valve for overcrowded facilities. This capacity creation was seen many times during the COVID-19 pandemic in 2020–2022, with many institutions using the HaH model to reduce their BAM admissions [18]. Although ACH was used to manage some postoperative patients who required continuous monitoring, this was the first time an acute SBO was admitted into the program. We did not initially start our ACH program with patients who need complex in-home interventions like NG tube suction and monitoring for bowel perforation and peritonitis. But the growth of our rapid response system and supplier network resulted in our virtual care providers to feel much more comfortable to treat high-acuity surgical patients like SBO in ACH. Once confident in this new mode of care delivery, our ACH team engaged our inpatient surgical colleagues in order to solidify workflows and communication chains so that we could partner in enrolling SBO patients in ACH. Due to this process and partnership, our patient was transferred smoothly from the BAM hospital to ACH, received hospital-level care at her home, and was discharged with a favorable outcome. Furthermore, she returned to work while being monitored by the ACH staff, which is an advantage that could not be achieved under the usual BAM care.

4. Conclusion

This case shows that patients who may need surgical intervention due to a high-acuity diagnosis like SBO can be safely monitored in a hospital-at-home program and receive inpatient-level care including NG suction, laboratory studies, and IV fluids. This case is an example of home building the proper in-home care delivery system overseen by virtual care providers which can offer an alternative care setting in the treatment of SBO. This can have the added benefits of both reducing brick-and-mortar admissions, resulting in improved hospital capacity, and providing the patient with the more comfortable experience of recovering from their illness in their own home. Our hospital will continue to look at ACH as the primary choice in care setting for clinically stable SBO patients. We will continue to conduct studies to discover what other surgical diagnosis can be safely treated inhome hospital.

Disclosure

Figure 1 was created using BioRender.com.

References

[1] M. Anthony, "Hospital-at-home," *Home healthcare now*, vol. 39, no. 3, p. 127, 2021.

[2] B. Leff, L. Burton, S. Guido, W. B. Greenough, D. Steinwachs, and J. R. Burton, "Home hospital program: a pilot study," *Journal of the American Geriatrics Society*, vol. 47, no. 6, pp. 697–702, 1999.

[3] D. M. Levine, K. Ouchi, B. Blanchfield et al., "Hospital-level care at home for acutely ill adults: a randomized controlled trial," *Annals of Internal Medicine*, vol. 172, no. 2, pp. 77–85, 2020.

[4] M. J. Maniaci, R. A. Torres-Guzman, J. P. Garcia et al., "Overall patient experience with a virtual hybrid hospital at home program," *SAGE Open Medicine*, vol. 10, Article ID 205031212210925, 2022.

[5] M. J. Maniaci, K. Maita, R. A. Torres-Guzman et al., "Provider evaluation of a novel virtual hybrid hospital at home model," *International Journal of General Medicine*, vol. 15, pp. 1909–1918, 2022.

[6] A. Qaddoura, P. Yazdan-Ashoori, C. Kabali et al., "Efficacy of hospital at home in patients with heart failure: a systematic review and meta-analysis," *PLoS One*, vol. 10, no. 6, Article ID e0129282, 2015.

[7] A. Vianello, F. Savoia, E. Pipitone et al., "Hospital at home for neuromuscular disease patients with respiratory tract infection: a pilot study," *Respiratory Care*, vol. 58, no. 12, pp. 2061–2068, 2013.

[8] B. Leff, L. Burton, S. L. Mader et al., "Hospital at home: feasibility and outcomes of a program to provide hospital-level care at home for acutely ill older patients," *Annals of Internal Medicine*, vol. 143, no. 11, pp. 798–808, 2005.

[9] B. Long, J. Robertson, and A. Koyfman, "Emergency medicine evaluation and management of small bowel obstruction: evidence-based recommendations," *Journal of Emergency Medicine*, vol. 56, no. 2, pp. 166–176, 2019.

[10] A. J. Hayanga, K. Bass-Wilkins, and G. B. Bulkley, "Current management of small-bowel obstruction," *Advances in Surgery*, vol. 39, pp. 1–33, 2005.

[11] G. E. Hayden and K. L. Sprouse, "Bowel obstruction and hernia," *Emergency Medicine Clinics of North America*, vol. 29, no. 2, pp. 319–345, 2011.

[12] W. Moss and E. M. McFetridge, "Acute intestinal obstruction: a comparative study of 511 cases, with special reference to the lowered mortality achieved by modern methods of therapy," *Annals of Surgery*, vol. 100, no. 1, pp. 158–166, 1934.

[13] S. Di Saverio, F. Coccolini, M. Galati et al., "Bologna guidelines for diagnosis and management of adhesive small bowel obstruction (ASBO): 2013 update of the evidence-based guidelines from the world society of emergency surgery ASBO working group," *World Journal of Emergency Surgery*, vol. 8, no. 1, p. 42, 2013.

[14] D. Seror, E. Feigin, A. Szold et al., "How conservatively can postoperative small bowel obstruction be treated?" *The American Journal of Surgery*, vol. 165, no. 1, pp. 121–126, 1993.

[15] B. T. Fevang, D. Jensen, K. Svanes, and A. Viste, "Early operation or conservative management of patients with small bowel obstruction?" *European Journal of Surgery*, vol. 168, no. 8, pp. 475–481, 2002.

[16] ACEP, "ED crowding," 2021, https://www.acep.org/patient-care/policy-statements/crowding/#sm.000uy2fqlzc4ed610br2m5bif3m23.

[17] P. McKenna, S. M. Heslin, P. Viccellio, W. K. Mallon, C. Hernandez, and E. J. Morley, "Emergency department and hospital crowding: causes, consequences, and cures," *Clinical and Experimental Emergency Medicine*, vol. 6, no. 3, pp. 189–195, 2019.

[18] J. C. Pamplin, B. K. Scott, M. T. Quinn et al., "Technology and disasters: the evolution of the national emergency tele-critical care network," *Critical Care Medicine*, vol. 49, no. 7, pp. 1007–1014, 2021.

3

Ileocaecal Tuberculosis Presenting with Massive Hematochezia: A Rare Clinical Manifestation

Neha Mehta,[1] Man Bahadur Paudyal,[1] Sangam Shah ,[2] Rajan Chamlagain,[1] Moon Shrestha,[1] Ashish Mehta,[3] and Prabin Bhattarai[4]

[1] *Tribhuvan University Teaching Hospital, Maharajgunj 44600, Nepal*
[2] *Maharajgunj Medical Campus, Institute of Medicine, Tribhuvan University, Maharajgunj 44600, Nepal*
[3] *BP Koirala Institute of Health Sciences, Dharan 56700, Nepal*
[4] *Department of Internal Medicine, Maharajgunj Medical Campus, Institute of Medicine, Tribhuvan University, Maharajgunj 44600, Nepal*

Correspondence should be addressed to Sangam Shah; sangam.shah.1997@gmail.com

Academic Editor: Marcel Cerqueira Cesar Machado

Abdominal pain, diarrhea, weight loss, anorexia, and fever are common symptoms of intestinal tuberculosis, while bleeding from the lumen, intestinal obstruction, perforation, and fistula formation are uncommon presentations in ileocaecal tuberculosis. Here, we present a case of a 33-year-old male with intestinal tuberculosis who initially presented with massive bleeding per rectum.

1. Introduction

Tuberculosis is a public health issue in Nepal which is the leading cause of deaths. In Nepal, the incidence of tuberculosis in 2019/20 is 151 per 100,000, with 29% being extrapulmonary [1]. Gastrointestinal tuberculosis is a less-common manifestation of extrapulmonary tuberculosis [2]. Due to overlapping clinical, radiological, and endoscopic characteristics, abdominal tuberculosis is frequently misdiagnosed as Crohn's disease, colonic cancer, and abdominal lymphoma [3]. The signs of abdominal tuberculosis are obscure, creating a delay in diagnosis and treatment, resulting in severe morbidities. The clinical manifestations of abdominal TB differ depending on the site of infection. Abdominal pain, diarrhea, weight loss, anorexia, and fever are common symptoms of intestinal tuberculosis, although bleeding from the lumen, intestinal obstruction, perforation, and fistula formation are uncommon [2, 4]. Here, we present a case of a 38-year-old male with intestinal tuberculosis who initially presented with massive bleeding per rectum.

2. Case Presentation

A 33-year-old male presented to our center with chief complaints of profuse per rectal bleed mixed with stool for three days that was associated with easy fatigability for one week prior to the initial presentation. He also had one episode of black tarry stool. However, he had no complaints of blood in vomit, purpuric rashes, or petechiae. He also had no hematuria, weight loss, night sweats, evening rise of temperature or loss of appetite, cough, chest pain, dyspnea, palpitation, limb edema, loose stools, jaundice, and abdominal distension. Bleeding was absent from other orifices. He had no history of diabetes mellitus, hypertension, cardiac diseases, and pulmonary tuberculosis in the past. He consumed 80 grams of alcohol per day for 15 years, but he did not smoke.

On examination, he was ill looking, conscious, and was well oriented to time place and person. He had pallor and was dehydrated. However, he had no icterus, clubbing, cyanosis, or edema. His pulse rate was 110 beats/minute, blood pressure was 80/60 mm of Hg, body temperature was 98°F (36.6°C), respiratory rate was 19 breaths/minute, and oxygen saturation was 95% in room air. The digital rectal examination showed fresh blood over the examining finger and otherwise normal findings. Abdominal and cardiac examination was normal.

Laboratory investigations showed hemoglobin 10.8 g/dl and hematocrit 31.6%. The total leukocyte count was 11510/ mm^3, neutrophils were 78%, and platelet count was 291000/ mm^3. The prothrombin time was 14 seconds, and the International normalized ratio was 1.08. The albumin level in the blood was 2.4 gm/dl, and total protein was 6.1 gm/dl, total and direct bilirubin were 0.7 and 0.1 mg/dl in the blood. Alanine aminotransferase and aspartate aminotransferase level was 97 U/L and 114 U/L, respectively. HbA_1C level in the blood was 7.2. The level of urea (33 mg/dl), creatinine (1.1 mg/dl), sodium (132 mEq/l), and potassium (3.6 mEq/l) were within normal range. Traces of sugar and albumin (++) were present in the urine examination. The fecal occult blood was found in the stool. *Mycobacterium tuberculosis* was not detected in sputum in the acid-fast bacilli (AFB) stain.

The chest X-ray was normal. Ultrasonography (USG) of the abdomen and pelvis and upper gastrointestinal endoscopy showed normal findings. A Computed Tomography (CT) scan of chest and abdomen showed asymmetric circumferential thickening in the ileocaecal region with lobulated thickened caecum, soft-tissue stranding and necrotic mesenteric lymphadenopathy, and indeterminate lobule in the lung (Figure 1). Colonoscopy showed multiple transverse ulcers with overlying exudates in terminal ileum and ascending and transverse colon. Histopathological examination of the ileum and colon showed patchy ulcers with exudates, granulation tissue, fibrosis, deep lymphoplasmocytic inflammation, and crypt regenerative changes with fibrinoid changes in scattered capillaries and venules and was inconclusive. However, gene XPERT was positive for *Mycobacterium tuberculosis*.

He was diagnosed with ileocaecal tuberculosis. The hemoglobin level dropped to 6.1 g/dl after two days of admission, and he had an episode of weakness associated with profuse sweating and rigor. Fluid resuscitation followed by two pints of whole blood transfusion was performed. After that, his hemoglobin was increased to 10.2 mg/dl. He was managed with four antitubercular drugs and showed significant improvement. Following this, he was discharged on oral antitubercular medications (isoniazid, rifampicin, pyrazinamide, ethambutol, and pyridoxine) after 10 days of admission. On follow-up after two weeks, he was responding well to antitubercular medications with improved symptoms, i.e., no per rectal bleeding, and his liver function test was within the normal range.

3. Discussion

The ileocaecal region is the most usually affected by gastrointestinal TB, accounting for 64%, followed by the jejunum and large intestine. The ileocaecal region is the most involved site in the gastrointestinal tract because it has a prolonged fecal stasis, a high density of lymphoid tissue, a neutral pH environment, and absorptive transport mechanisms that allow ingested mycobacterium to be absorbed [5]. Ileocaecal TB is difficult to diagnose since it resembles other conditions such as Crohn's disease, amebiasis, diverticulitis, or colon neoplasms. Abdominal pain, fever, distention, vomiting, night sweats, weight loss, and diarrhea are all indications of this localization [6]. Intestinal tuberculosis presenting with massive rectal bleeding is a rare manifestation accounting for only 5% of causes of lower gastrointestinal bleed [7]. To our knowledge, this is the first case report from Nepal. The diagnosis becomes more difficult in the absence of active pulmonary tuberculosis. The correct diagnosis is only 50% even in prevalent areas [8]. In undeveloped countries like Nepal, where the loss to follow-up is a big concern, delays in prompt diagnosis and treatment lead to severe morbidity and mortality [9].

The primary site of involvement was the ileocaecal area in our patient, and there were no clinical or radiological signs of pulmonary tuberculosis. The colonoscopy-guided biopsy is the investigation of choice in diagnosing ileocaecal and colonic tuberculosis. The acid-fast staining, culture, and gene XPERT have a sensitivity and specificity of (31%, 100%), (31%, 100%), and (95.7%, 100%) respectively [10]. Histological features of tuberculosis are caseous granulomas with conglomerate epithelioid histiocytes, giant cells with submucosal inflammation of predominantly lymphoplasmacytic type, while the microscopic features are lymphoid aggregates, pyloric metaplasia, dilated submucosal lymphatics, cryptitis, and crypt abscess [11]. However the classic histological features are seen only in 13–33% of patients with colonic tuberculosis [12]. Also, the rest show nonspecific findings. In our patient, histopathological findings did not show classical features of tuberculosis. In addition to caseous necrosis and acid-fast bacilli (which are found in only a small percentage of biopsy specimens from patients with intestinal tuberculosis), the size, number, and confluence of granulomas, the presence of ulcers lined by bands of epithelioid histiocytes, and disproportionate submucosal inflammation may help distinguish intestinal tuberculosis from Crohn's disease [12]. In our patient, there were multiple transverse ulcers suggestive of intestinal tuberculosis. Crohn's disease and intestinal tuberculosis can coexist rarely, and after successful treatment of tuberculosis, reevaluation is mandatory [13].

In a study in China, only 20% of patients were diagnosed with intestinal tuberculosis and the rest 80% were misdiagnosed [14]. Due to mimicking with other diseases such as Crohn's disease, a malignancy [3], misdiagnosis can lead to delay in treatment of other diseases as well as unnecessary drug toxicity from antitubercular therapy. Similarly, therapy with immunosuppressants in intestinal tuberculosis considering Crohn's disease can cause a flare up of tuberculosis and significant morbidity and mortality [8]. A single cost-effective investigation is still not available for intestinal tuberculosis, and the diagnosis reached on the therapeutic basis in 20% of cases [15].

The treatment of gastrointestinal tuberculosis is the same as that of pulmonary tuberculosis constituting a regimen of four drugs isoniazid, rifampicin, pyrazinamide, and ethambutol for initial 2 months followed by isoniazid and rifampicin for 4 months. Surgical treatment is instituted in

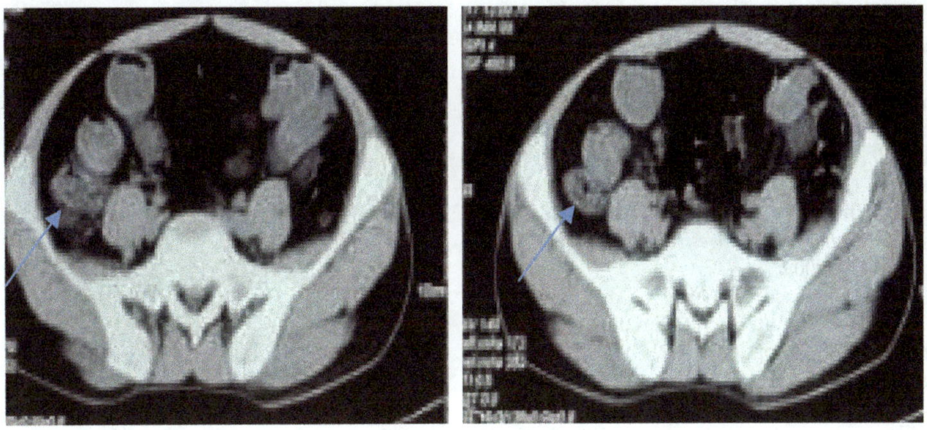

Figure 1: CT of the abdomen showing asymmetric circumferential thickening in the ileocaecal region with lobulated thickened caecum, soft-tissue stranding, and necrotic mesenteric lymphadenopathy.

intestinal obstruction, perforation, and fistulization refractory to ATT. The advancement of colonoscopy and gene XPERT has caused a decline in laparotomies.

Upper and lower gastrointestinal bleeding, fistulas at different sites, obstruction of the gut lumen, stricture formation, intussusception, perforation, anemia, malnutrition, malabsorption, weight loss, deficiency of essential vitamins and minerals, and chronic inflammatory demyelinating polyneuropathy have all been reported in patients with intestinal tuberculosis [13]. Surgical bypassing of concerned intestinal segments, radical excision of implicated segments, or conservative operations such as strictureplasty are used to treat intestinal tuberculosis [13].

Massive hematochezia can lead to rapid fall in the level of hemoglobin level as in our patient which can be managed with the transfusion of whole blood. For complications such as free perforation, substantial bleeding, total obstruction, abscess formation, big fistulas, and unresponsiveness to antimicrobial medications, surgery is the next best option after drug therapy. The most common complication is obstruction; individuals who have multiple and/or lengthy strictures are less likely to respond to medical treatment. Colonoscopic balloon dilation, which has been proved to be a viable option, can be used to treat easily accessible, short, and fibrous tuberculous ileal strictures that are causing subacute obstructive symptoms. Despite the lack of expertise, this approach looks safe and may eliminate the need for surgery. In our case, surgery was not opted for the treatment.

4. Conclusions

Although severe hematochezia is a rare symptom of intestinal tuberculosis, it should be considered a differential diagnosis in patients who come with rectal bleeding in tuberculosis-endemic areas. Physicians should be aware of the misdiagnosis due to the presentation of rectal bleeding that can lead to the potential complications.

Authors' Contributions

NM and MBP wrote the original manuscript and reviewed and edited the manuscript. SS reviewed and edited the original manuscript. NM, MBP, SS, RC, MS, AM, and PB were in charge of the case and reviewed the manuscript.

References

[1] Annual Report: Department of Health Services, Government of Nepal, Ministry of Health and Population, Department of Health Services Kathmandu, 2075.

[2] U. K. Shrestha, D. Shrestha, R. Shrestha, and A. Ghosh, "Clinical profile of 103 patients with abdominal tuberculosis in Nepal," *Journal of Advances in Internal Medicine*, vol. 4, no. 2, pp. 51–56, 2017.

[3] T. Rath, R. Atreya, W. Geißdörfer, R. Lang, A. Nägel, and M. F. Neurath, "A severe case of tuberculosis radiologically and endoscopically mimicking colorectal cancer with peritoneal carcinomatosis," *Case Reports in Gastrointestinal Medicine*, vol. 2017, Article ID 6206951, 4 pages, 2017.

[4] J.-K. Cho, Y. M. Choi, S. S. Lee et al., "Clinical features and outcomes of abdominal tuberculosis in southeastern Korea: 12 years of experience," *BMC Infectious Diseases*, vol. 18, no. 1, pp. 1–8, 2018.

[5] U. Debi, V. Ravisankar, K. K. Prasad, S. K. Sinha, and A. K. Sharma, "Abdominal tuberculosis of the gastrointestinal tract: revisited," *World Journal of Gastroenterology*, vol. 20, no. 40, p. 14831, 2014.

[6] A. Michalopoulos, V. N. Papadopoulos, S. Panidis, T. S. Papavramidis, A. Chiotis, and G. Basdanis, "Cecal obstruction due to primary intestinal tuberculosis: a case series," *Journal of Medical Case Reports*, vol. 5, no. 1, pp. 1–5, 2011.

[7] A. V. B. Kela, V. B. Agrawal, R. Sharma, R. Agarwal, and A. Agarwal, "Ileal tuberculosis presenting as a case of massive rectal bleeding," *Clinical and Experimental Gastroenterology*, vol. 129, p. 129, 2009.

[8] H. Park, T. Kansara, A. M. Victoria, N. Boma, and J. Hong, "Intestinal tuberculosis: a diagnostic challenge," *Cureus*, vol. 13, pp. 2–5, 2021.

[9] V. K. Kapoor and L. K. Sharma, "Abdominal tuberculosis," *British Journal of Surgery*, vol. 75, no. 1, pp. 2-3, 2005.
[10] C. Lowbridge, S. A. M. Fadhil, G. D. Krishnan et al., "How can gastro-intestinal tuberculosis diagnosis be improved? A prospective cohort study," *BMC Infectious Diseases*, vol. 20, no. 1, pp. 1–8, 2020.
[11] P. B. Tripathi and A. D. Amarapurkar, "Morphological spectrum of gastrointestinal tuberculosis," *Tropical Gastroenterology: Official Journal of the Digestive Diseases Foundation*, vol. 30, pp. 35–39, 2009.
[12] R. Kirsch, "Role of colonoscopic biopsy in distinguishing between Crohn's disease and intestinal tuberculosis," *Journal of Clinical Pathology*, vol. 59, pp. 840–844, 2006.
[13] R. C. Chakinala and A. M. Khatri, *Gastrointestinal Tuberculosis*, StatPearls, Treasure Island, FL, USA, 2021.
[14] W. Cheng, S. Zhang, Y. Li, J. Wang, and J. Li, "Intestinal tuberculosis: clinico-pathological profile and the importance of a high degree of suspicion," *Tropical Medicine and International Health*, vol. 24, no. 1, pp. 81–90, 2019.
[15] F. M. Abu-Zidan and M. Sheek-Hussein, "Diagnosis of abdominal tuberculosis: lessons learned over 30 years: pectoral assay," *World Journal of Emergency Surgery*, vol. 14, no. 1, pp. 1–7, 2019.

4

Gastric Siderosis and Ulceration from Intravenous Iron Supplementation Manifesting as Chronic Upper Gastrointestinal Bleeding: A Case Report and Review of the Literature

Donald Ewing,[1] Ava Brozovich,[1] Ethan Burns,[2] Gonzalo Acosta,[2] Courtney Hatcher,[2] Pragnesh Patel,[3] Rose Anton,[4] Bincy Abraham,[1,3] and Leena Samuel[4]

[1] *Texas A&M University College of Medicine, 8447 Bryan Rd., Bryan, TX 77807, USA*
[2] *Houston Methodist Hospital, Department of Medicine, 6550 Fannin St., Houston, TX 77096, USA*
[3] *Houston Methodist Hospital, Department of Gastroenterology, 6550 Fannin St., Houston, TX 77096, USA*
[4] *Houston Methodist Hospital, Department of Pathology and Genomic Medicine, 6550 Fannin St., Houston, TX 77030, USA*

Correspondence should be addressed to Ethan Burns; eaburns312@gmail.com

Academic Editor: Olga I. Giouleme

Iron deficiency is the most common etiology of anemia worldwide and is often managed with varying methods of iron supplementation. Although rare, oral iron supplementation can perpetuate iron deficiency anemia by causing gastric ulceration and upper gastrointestinal bleeding in high-risk populations. However, this complication has not been previously described with intravenous iron supplementation. We present a case of a 63-year-old male with severe iron deficiency anemia on biweekly intravenous iron infusions and weekly packed red blood cell transfusions who presented with melena over several months. Upper endoscopy demonstrated a clean-based gastric body ulcer and nonbleeding gastric varices. Histology of the gastric ulcer was suggestive of iron-induced gastric mucosal injury. This case demonstrates that frequent utilization of intravenous iron and packed red blood cell transfusions may predispose certain patients to the development of iron-induced gastritis and ulceration.

1. Introduction

The prevalence of anemia in the global population is estimated to be 24.8%, with iron deficiency as the most common etiology [1]. Oral iron supplementation is the most conventional treatment modality for iron deficiency anemia (IDA) with intravenous (IV) iron and packed red blood cell (PRBC) transfusions reserved for specific circumstances such as oral iron intolerance, history of gastric surgery, chronic blood loss anemia, malabsorptive syndromes, and severe deficiency/anemia [2]. Adverse effects of oral iron therapy may include a metallic taste, nausea, constipation, diarrhea, and flatulence; nonetheless it is generally well tolerated [2]. Uncommon but potentially serious adverse effects are chronic gastritis, ulceration, and bleeding secondary to oxidative damage to the gastric mucosa [3–5].

Iron-induced gastritis is a rare condition that is scarcely reported in the literature. We present a unique case of iron-induced gastritis due to recurrent PRBC transfusions and IV iron infusions.

2. Presentation of Case

A 69-year-old Caucasian male with history of a precancerous supraglottic mass treated with resection and radiation, compensated alcoholic cirrhosis, and large ascending colon polyp treated with right hemicolectomy 4-years-ago presented with melena for the past 4 months. The patient denied nausea, vomiting, abdominal pain, hematemesis, hematochezia, reflux symptoms, change in bowel habits, or weight loss. He denied use of nonsteroidal anti-inflammatory agents.

The patient had episodes of intermittent melena for the past 3 years requiring blood transfusions, but it had become a daily occurrence in the past 4 months. Prior to presenting for this current admission, the patient had two esophagogastroduodenoscopies (EGD), two colonoscopies,

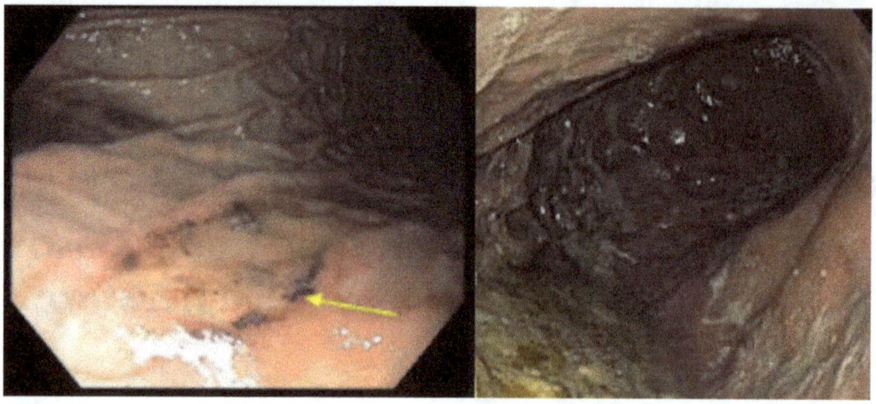

FIGURE 1: (a) EGD at admission. Nonbleeding ulcer located in the gastric body. There is black mucosal discoloration present. Biopsies were taken. (b) Gastric body during repeated EGD 6 months later. Significant residue in the stomach. Ulceration not visualized. EGD: esophagogastroduodenoscopy.

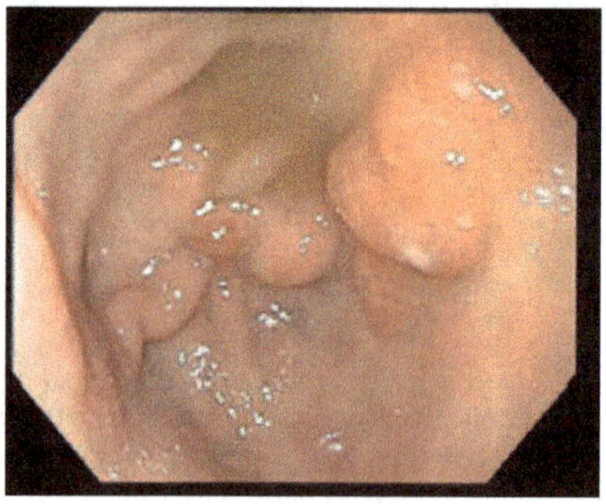

FIGURE 2: Nonbleeding gastric varices.

and one video capsule endoscopy that failed to identify a source of his melena. In the last 2 months, his hemoglobin has ranged between 6.2 g/dL and 7.4 g/dL requiring 2 units of PRBCs weekly as well as biweekly IV iron infusions. He had not used oral iron supplementation in the 6 months prior to admission.

On presentation, the patient was asymptomatic and hemodynamically stable. Rectal exam revealed black, tarry stool in the rectal vault without hemorrhoids or a palpable rectal mass. Blood work was significant for a hemoglobin of 4.4 g/dL and acute kidney injury, for which he received two units of PRBCs. His ferritin was 109 ng/mL, transferrin 194 mg/dL, TIBC 225 ug/dL, iron level 38 ug/dL, and percent iron saturation 16.9%, supporting the diagnosis of IDA. Computed Tomography (CT) of the abdomen and pelvis was notable for cirrhosis. An esophagogastroduodenoscopy (EGD) demonstrated a nonbleeding clean-based ulcer in the gastric body (Figure 1(a)) and nonbleeding gastric varices (Figure 2). Biopsies indicated heavy iron deposition, and immunostaining for *Helicobacter pylori* (H. Pylori) was negative (Figure 3). Iron therapy was discontinued and treatment with a proton pump inhibitor was initiated. The patient's hemoglobin remained stable and he was discharged. On follow-up, the patient's melena had resolved and after 9 months his hemoglobin was stable at 11.2g/dL. Repeated EGD did not locate an ulcer (Figure 1(b)), and histology showed chronic inactive gastritis. Repeated iron staining was not performed.

3. Discussion

According to a population-based study of 3,000 participants in Sweden, the prevalence of peptic ulcer disease (PUD) is approximately 4.1% (gastric=2.0%, duodenal=2.1%) [6, 7], which has decreased over time with treatment of *H. pylori* [7] infections and gastric acid suppression with proton pump inhibitors [8]. In developed countries, the frequent use of aspirin and nonsteroidal anti-inflammatory drugs has become a more common cause of PUD [7]. Iron-induced gastric ulcers are a rare phenomenon and are previously reported in association with oral iron pill therapy [3–5]. To our knowledge, there are no reported cases in the literature demonstrating gastritis or gastric ulceration due to intravenous iron or PRBC transfusions.

Iron deposition in the gastric mucosa is also known as gastric siderosis. Gastric siderosis and mucosal ulceration are diagnosed by EGD and biopsy [9]. Common EGD findings include erosion, orange/black mucosal discoloration, and reactive gastropathy [9]. While gross examination of the gastric ulceration may provide evidence of iron-induced injury, biopsy of the gastric ulcer is required to make a confirmatory diagnosis [10]. Marginean et al. theorized three histological patterns (A, B, and C) regarding the cause of gastric siderosis [10]. Pattern A refers to iron deposition in the macrophages, stromal cells, and focally in the epithelium [10]; this pattern is thought to be associated with gastric inflammation, ulceration, prior mucosal hemorrhage, or possibly oral iron medications [10, 11]. Pattern B, also referred to as "iron-pill gastritis," demonstrates extracellular clumps of crystalline iron deposition with stromal and epithelial deposition and is associated with oral iron medication and mild gastritis [10]. Pattern C has gastric glandular deposition associated with systemic iron overload and hemochromatosis [10]. This patient had mucosal discoloration surrounding the

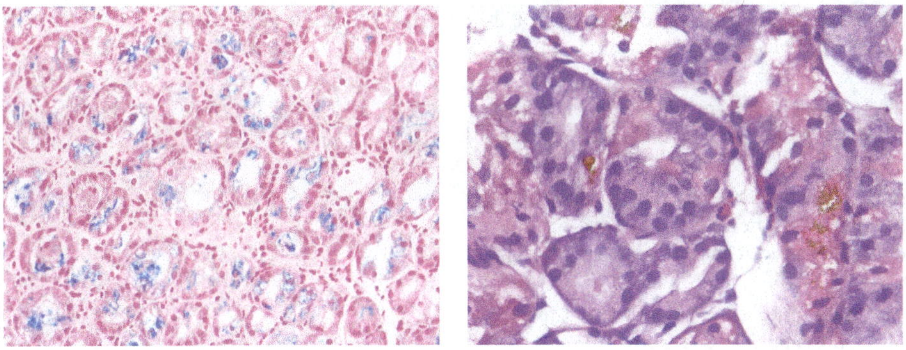

(a) (b)

FIGURE 3: (a) An iron stain with intraepithelial and intraluminal iron (blue stain). Prussian blue, 200x. (b) A high-power view of the stomach shows parietal and chief cells containing intracytoplasmic yellow-orange coarse granules consistent with iron deposition. H&E, 400x.

ulcer consistent with iron-associated injury (Figure 1) and a biopsy most consistent with patterns A and C as iron was found within epithelial cells and within glandular cells, suggesting iron overload (Figure 3) despite labs consistent with iron deficiency.

Iron-associated mucosal injury is a well-recognized process in patients with iron overload and tissue deposition secondary to hemochromatosis, oral iron overdose, and frequent blood transfusions [11]. Although the mechanism is not fully understood, it is thought to involve the Fenton reaction, which describes the iron-mediated generation of reactive oxygen species (ROS) [12]. Superoxide ions convert ferric iron (Fe^{3+}) to ferrous iron (Fe^{2+}) [12]. Ferrous iron reacts with hydrogen peroxide to produce hydroxyl free radicals, which lead to mucosal injury and subsequent inflammation [11, 12]. Additional possibilities include the direct corrosive effect in patients taking oral iron pills but this was not applicable to our patient with no recent oral iron pill therapy [11].

Our patient has a history of compensated cirrhosis secondary to chronic alcohol abuse. Endoscopy also revealed nonbleeding gastric varices which may have also contributed to gastrointestinal bleeding and the patient's need for IV iron and frequent blood transfusions prior to presentation, though no evidence of prior or active bleeding was found. In our patient, his cirrhosis and alcohol abuse, in addition to concomitant IV iron infusions and frequent blood transfusions, may have contributed to gastric siderosis [8, 11, 13]. A study by Hattori reported that 26% of patients with cirrhosis were found to have gastric iron deposition compared to only 4% without cirrhosis [13]. It is possible that cirrhosis can predispose patients to iron-induced gastritis and gastric ulcers if they are receiving additional therapies high in iron concentration, regardless of mode of intake. This case illustrates that patients with underlying risk factors such as alcohol abuse, cirrhosis, and frequent iron intake (regardless of modality) are at increased risk for gastric iron deposition, progression to gastritis and ulceration, and potential upper gastric bleeds. Clinicians should remain vigilant for this possible sequela even if labs do not suggest iron overload. Furthermore, this diagnosis should be on the differential level in patients with treatment-resistant anemia receiving IV iron therapy or frequent transfusions.

4. Conclusion

To our knowledge, this is the first reported case of gastric siderosis, gastritis, and gastric ulceration resulting from IV iron and frequent PRBC transfusions. Iron-induced gastritis is a rare, potentially serious, and paradoxical complication of iron supplementation that may not be recognized as a potential cause of refractory iron deficiency anemia. Clinicians should consider iron-induced gastritis in patients with refractory iron deficiency anemia in the setting of frequent iron supplementation and be aware of additional predisposing risk factors such as cirrhosis.

Abbreviations

WHO:	World Health Organization
IDA:	Iron deficiency anemia
PRBC:	Packed red blood cells
IV:	Intravenous
GI:	Gastrointestinal
CT:	Computed Tomography
EGD:	esophagogastroduodenoscopy
PUD:	Peptic ulcer disease
H. Pylori:	Helicobacter pylori.

References

[1] World Health Organization, "Vitamin and Mineral Nutrition Information System. Worldwide prevalence on anaemia 1993–2005".

[2] S. L. Schrier and M. Auerbach, "Treatment of iron deficiency anemia in adults," *UpToDate*, 2018.

[3] T. Sunkara, M. E. Caughey, S. Nigar, R. Olivo, and V. Gaduputi, "Iron pill gastritis: an under diagnosed condition with potentially serious outcomes," *Gastroenterology Research*, vol. 10, no. 2, pp. 138–140, 2017.

[4] J. G. Hashash, S. Proksell, S. Kuan, and J. Behari, "Iron Pill–induced gastritis," *ACG Case Reports Journal*, vol. 1, no. 1, pp. 13–15, 2013.

[5] L. E. Meliţ, C. O. Mărginean, S. Mocanu, and M. O. Mărginean, "A rare case of iron-pill induced gastritis in a female teenager," *Medicine*, vol. 96, no. 30, p. e7550, 2017.

[6] P. Aro, T. Storskrubb, J. Ronkainen et al., "Peptic ulcer disease in a general adult population: The kalixanda study: A random population-based study," *American Journal of Epidemiology*, vol. 163, no. 11, pp. 1025–1034, 2006.

[7] W. I. Najm, "Peptic ulcer disease," *Primary Care—Clinics in Office Practice*, vol. 38, no. 3, pp. 383–394, 2011.

[8] I. C. Roberts-Thomson, "Rise and fall of peptic ulceration: A disease of civilization?" *Journal of Gastroenterology and Hepatology*, vol. 33, no. 7, pp. 1321–1326, 2018.

[9] G. De Petris, S. Gatius Caldero, L. Chen et al., "Histopathological changes in the gastrointestinal tract due to drugs: An update for the surgical pathologist (part I of II)," *International Journal of Surgical Pathology*, vol. 22, no. 2, pp. 120–128, 2014.

[10] E. C. Marginean, M. Bennick, J. Cyczk, M. E. Robert, and D. Jain, "Gastric siderosis: Patterns and significance," *The American Journal of Surgical Pathology*, vol. 30, no. 4, pp. 514–520, 2006.

[11] J. P. Kothadia, R. Arju, M. Kaminski, A. Mahmud, J. Chow, and S. Giashuddin, "Gastric siderosis: An under-recognized and rare clinical entity," *SAGE Open Medicine*, vol. 4, p. 205031211663210, 2016.

[12] P. Mladěnka, T. Šimůnek, M. Hübl, and R. Hrdina, "The role of reactive oxygen and nitrogen species in cellular iron metabolism," *Free Radical Research*, vol. 40, no. 3, pp. 263–272, 2006.

[13] H. Hattori, "High prevalence of haemosiderin accumulation in the cytoplasm of gastric glands in patients with liver cirrhosis," *Journal of Clinical Pathology*, vol. 57, no. 6, pp. 621–624, 2004.

5

Retroperitoneal Fat Necrosis in Response to an Episode of Acute Pancreatitis

M. B. Gilani,[1] T. Akcan,[1] M. Peterson,[1] and A. Zahid[2]

[1]*Department of Internal Medicine, Marshfield Clinic Health System—Marshfield, Marshfield, WI 54449, USA*
[2]*Department of Hospital Medicine, Marshfield Clinic Health System—Marshfield, Marshfield, WI 54449, USA*

Correspondence should be addressed to M. B. Gilani; gilani.muhammad@marshfieldclinic.org

Academic Editor: Marcel Cerqueira Cesar Machado

Acute pancreatitis can result in fat necrosis, typically occurring in the peripancreatic region within weeks to months, and it generally appears as a low attenuation collection, with minimal heterogeneity. There are no specific imaging features that can diagnose retroperitoneal fat necrosis which may imitate other entities including certain malignancies, which may lead to invasive studies for diagnosis. Herein, we present a case of extensive retroperitoneal fat necrosis beyond the peripancreatic region that developed 10 days after an episode of acute pancreatitis.

1. Introduction

Retroperitoneal fat necrosis can result as a sequela of pancreatitis due to the release of lipolytic enzymes during inflammatory processes, and its presentation varies [1]. On contrast-enhanced computerized tomography (CECT) scan, retroperitoneal fat necrosis generally appears as a low attenuation collection, with minimal heterogeneity which may imitate certain malignancies, such as carcinomatosis and liposarcoma, which may lead to further invasive studies for evaluation [1, 2]. Prior data show the interval between episodes of pancreatitis and the appearance of retroperitoneal fat necrosis varies which is generally from weeks to months rarely in days [3]. We report a case of extensive retroperitoneal fat necrosis that developed within 10 days after an episode of acute pancreatitis.

2. Case Presentation

A 23-year-old man with a past medical history of pilocytic astrocytoma and obstructive hydrocephalus requiring a ventriculoperitoneal (VP) shunt presented with right-sided constant, intense abdominal pain that was ranked as a 10 out of 10 in intensity one day after binge drinking alcohol. The pain was mainly located on the right side of the abdomen that radiated to the back and associated with nausea and 6–8 episodes of vomiting small amounts of yellowish fluid. Initial labs showed an abnormal white blood cell (WBC) count of 18,000 per microliter and an elevated lipase level of 1,260 units per liter; the remaining labs, including comprehensive metabolic panel (CMP) and urinalysis, were in the normal range. A computed tomography (CT) scan of his chest showed retroperitoneal stranding and edema adjacent to the transverse portion of duodenum and posterior to the peripancreatic head (Figure 1). The patient was diagnosed with acute pancreatitis most likely secondary to binge drinking and was not given anything by mouth. His symptoms were managed with intravenous (IV) hydromorphone and fluids. On day three postpresentation, his pain started to improve, and he was transitioned from IV hydromorphone to oral tramadol as needed. On day five, the patient was started on a liquid diet that was slowly advanced as tolerated. The patient was discharged pain-free on day six.

On day nine postpresentation, the patient returned with lower back and groin pain which was 8 out of 10 in intensity. Lab work-up was repeated and showed leukocytosis with white blood cell (WBC) count of 18,500 per microliter and elevated levels of C-reactive protein (CRP) of 22.6 mg/dL and procalcitonin of 2.34 ng/mL. His CMP and lipase activity were within the normal range. A follow-up CT of the

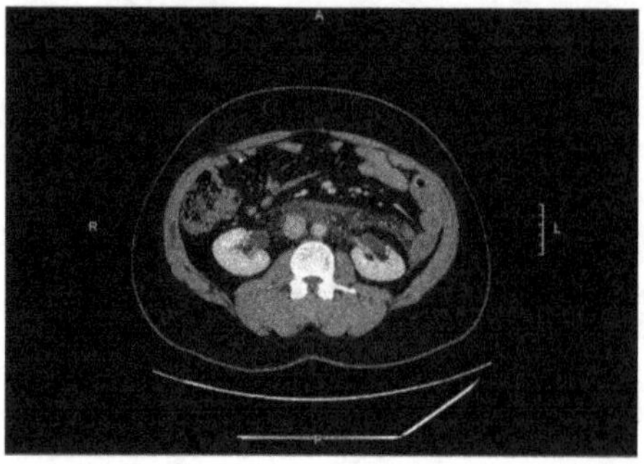

Figure 1: CT imaging of chest shows retroperitoneal stranding and edema adjacent to the transverse portion of duodenum and posterior to the peripancreatic head at day 1.

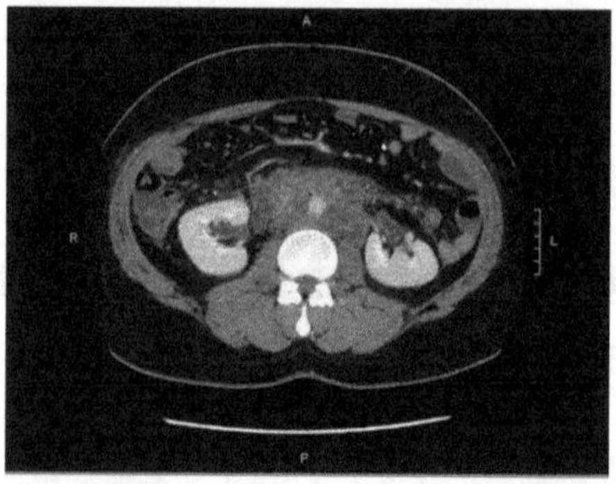

Figure 2: CT imaging of the abdomen and pelvis reveals large retroperitoneal process with dense infiltrative tissue extending along the aorta at day 9.

abdomen and pelvis with contrast was done and revealed a new, large retroperitoneal process with dense infiltrative tissue extending along the aorta starting just below the origin of the superior mesenteric artery (SMA) and extending to the bifurcation measuring about $10.8 \times 9.3 \times 5.2$ cm (Figure 2). Wispy tissue extended up along the pancreas and down the anterior pararenal spaces as well as along the iliac vessels. The retroperitoneal tissue exerted mass effect narrowing the inferior vena cava (IVC) just inferior to left renal vein and uplifted the aorta anteriorly off the spine. The pancreas enhanced normally with no pancreatic duct dilatation. Possible differentials were inflammatory sequelae from recent acute pancreatitis and retroperitoneal fibrosis, but due to the atypical distribution of inflammation, a gastroenterologist was consulted who recommended conservative management including IV hydration and pain control. On day 10, the patient spiked a fever and was empirically started on a piperacillin/tazobactam (Zosyn®) regimen while an infectious disease (ID) specialist was consulted. The ID specialist recommended a tissue biopsy of the retroperitoneal process and further laboratory work-up for infection. A CT-guided aspiration of the retroperitoneal lesion was done and histology testing performed specifically potassium hydroxide preparation (KOH) smear, fungal culture, acid-fast bacillus (AFB) smear and culture, and aerobic and anaerobic cultures with subsequent Gram stain. Other work-up for infections included blastomycosis urinary antigen, interferon gamma release assay, blood cultures, and urinalysis. Results were either inconclusive or negative. Zosyn was continued for a total of seven days and discontinued upon receipt of infectious disease work-up results. The patient was discharged from the hospital and additional CT imaging of the abdomen and pelvis was performed at four (Figure 3) and 12 weeks (Figure 4) that showed significant improvement in retroperitoneal mass appearance.

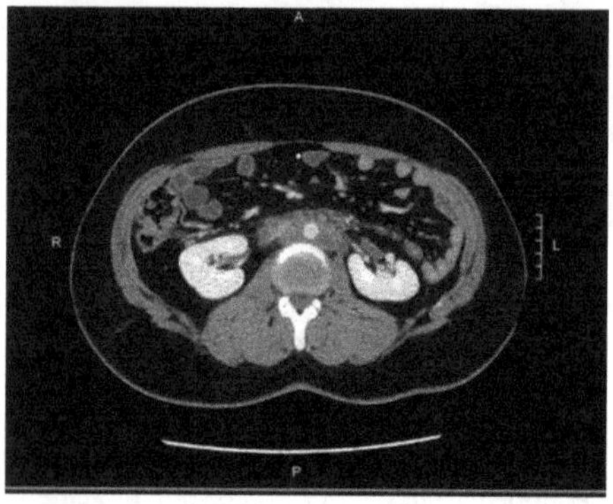

Figure 3: CT imaging of the abdomen and pelvis performed at four weeks shows improvement in retroperitoneal mass appearance.

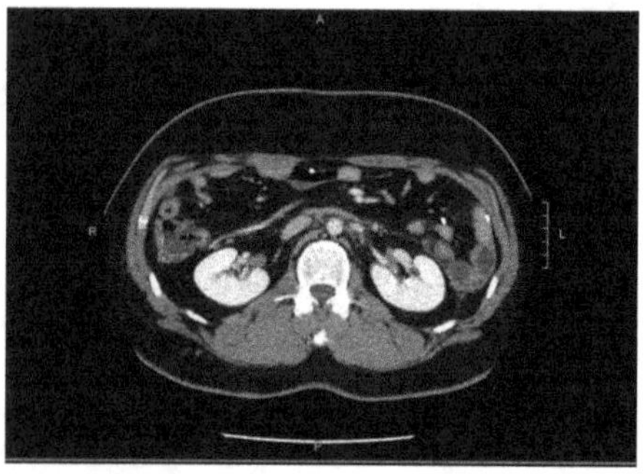

Figure 4: CT imaging of the abdomen and pelvis reveals significant improvement in retroperitoneal mass appearance at 12 weeks.

3. Discussion

Fat necrosis is a known complication of acute pancreatitis [2, 3] that can be detected with contrast-enhanced computerized tomography (CECT) [4]. Conservative management of sterile fat necrosis is an accepted practice and is associated with a low (12%) mortality [5]. According to Smith et al., "The distribution of fat necrosis is typically peripancreatic, with extensions to the origin of the mesentery of the small intestine, the transverse mesocolon, and the omentum" [2].

The initial retroperitoneal stranding seen in our patient was consistent with a typical distribution; however, subsequent CECT findings of extensive fat necrosis have, to our knowledge, not previously been reported in association with pancreatitis. In addition, the development of retroperitoneal fat necrosis occurred within 10 days of acute pancreatitis, which varied from the normal time interval of weeks to several months [3]. The patient in this report showed marked improvement with CECT at 4 and 12 weeks post-pancreatitis, in contrast to a similar case which showed persistence of peritoneal deposits after six months [2].

Consultation with oncology led to a negative work-up for carcinomatosis, based in part of the patient's age and the rapid progression of the mass. Due to the consistent decrease in size of the fat necrosis over time, malignancies were not considered as a potential diagnosis [6]. A literature review found one case of extensive retroperitoneal fat necrosis in a case of renal cell carcinoma [7].

Sterile necrosis has been historically managed conservatively to prevent the introduction of an infectious agent into the body [5]. Retroperitoneal fat necrosis secondary to acute pancreatitis is currently not preventable; this case demonstrates a clinically favorable outcome with conservative management and monitoring with CECT.

Acknowledgments

The authors acknowledge Emily Andreae, PhD, from the Marshfield Clinic Research Institute for manuscript editing assistance.

References

[1] A. Kamaya, M. P. Federle, and T. S. Desser, "Imaging manifestations of abdominal fat necrosis and its mimics," *RadioGraphics*, vol. 31, no. 7, pp. 2021–2034, 2011.

[2] J. P. Smith, J. P. Arnoletti, S. Varadarajulu, and D. E. Morgan, "Post-pancreatitis fat necrosis mimicking carcinomatosis," *Radiology Case Reports*, vol. 3, no. 2, p. 192, 2015.

[3] J. M. Howard, "Studies of acute pancreatitis with retroperitoneal necrosis: "the suet syndrome," improvements in patient survival," *Journal of Hepato-Biliary-Pancreatic Surgery*, vol. 3, no. 3, pp. 195–202, 1996.

[4] E. Villatoro, M. Mulla, and M. Larvin, "Antibiotic therapy for prophylaxis against infection of pancreatic necrosis in acute pancreatitis," *Cochrane Database of Systematic Reviews*, vol. 2010, no. 5, Article ID CD002941, 2010.

[5] E. Zerem, "Treatment of severe acute pancreatitis and its complications," *World Journal of Gastroenterology*, vol. 20, no. 38, pp. 13879–13892, 2014.

[6] H. Devos, L. Goethals, D. Belsack et al., "Fat misbehaving in the abdominal cavity: a pictorial essay," *Polish Journal of Radiology*, vol. 85, pp. e32–e38, 2020.

[7] M. C. Yang and W. J. Lee, "Extensive intra-abdominal-retroperitoneal fat necrosis in a patient with renal cell carcinoma," *Journal of the Formosan Medical Association*, vol. 95, no. 9, pp. 719–721, 1996.

6

Case Report of Rare Type Submucosal Polyp–Angiolipofibroma of Sigmoid Colon

Khin San Aye,[1] **Aung Khine Zan**,[2] **Myo Thet Tin**,[3] **and Than Than Aye**[1]

[1]*Department of Gastroenterology, University of Medicine 2, Yangon, Myanmar*
[2]*Yangon General Hospital, Myanmar*
[3]*Nay Pyi Taw General Hospital (1000-bedded), Myanmar*

Correspondence should be addressed to Khin San Aye; ksaye.08@gmail.com

Academic Editor: Yoshifumi Nakayama

Most of the colonic submucosal mesenchymal polyps are benign tumors. They are formed by more than one type of mesenchymal tissue. The diagnosis of angiolipofibroma depends on the histological findings with the proliferation of vascular, fatty, and fibrous connective tissues. Majority of angiolipofibromas are arising in the kidney and have rare presentation as extra renal region. Here we report a case of 58-year-old female patient with angiolipofibroma of sigmoid colon (8.5 cm x 4 cm size) which was treated successfully with surgical resection. The clinical presentation, operative procedure, pathological features, and medical literature review are presented.

1. Introduction

Most of the colonic polyps are originated in the mucosa and a small subset of them originate from the submucosal mesenchymal. The most common types of submucosal polyp are composed of single type tissue include lipoma, leiomyoma, neurofibroma or mucosal Schwann cell hamartomas, vascular lesion, and gastrointestinal stromal tumor (GISTs) [1]. The mixed mesenchymal lesions are extremely rare. Angiolipofibromas are a form of mesenchymal hamartoma, composed of more than single type tissue including blood vessels, smooth muscle cells, and mature fat cells. Majority of angiolipofibromas arise in the kidney and extrarenal angiolipofibromas have rare presentations [2]. Again, colonic angiolipofibroma is rare benign tumors of the extra renal type with particular histopathologic characteristics.

The aim of this report is to present an unusual case of colonic polyp originating from submucosal with mixed mesenchymal composed of vascular, mature fatty, and fibrous connective tissues.

2. Case Presentation

A 58-year-old female patient presented with one episode of rounded mass protruded from anus during defecation and reduced manually by herself. She was previously healthy person and had normal bowel motion. She had no history of abdominal pain or mass, bleeding per rectum, and weight loss. There was no family history of colonic polyps or colon cancer. On physical examination, there was no significant anemia, no palpable abdominal mass nor tenderness. Stool examination was positive for occult blood. Her hemoglobin was mildly reduced 11.6 gm/dl with hypochromic microcystic type of anemia and a serum carcinoembryonic antigen level (0.32 ng/ml) was normal. Other laboratory tests like blood sugar, renal profiles, and liver profiles were within normal ranges.

A full colonoscopy was performed. A large polyp about 8 cm with rather smooth surface but highly vascular was found at the sigmoid colon, 14 cm from anal verge. The mass was occupied two third circumference of whole colonic lumen (Figure 1). The origin of the polyp or stalk was difficult to

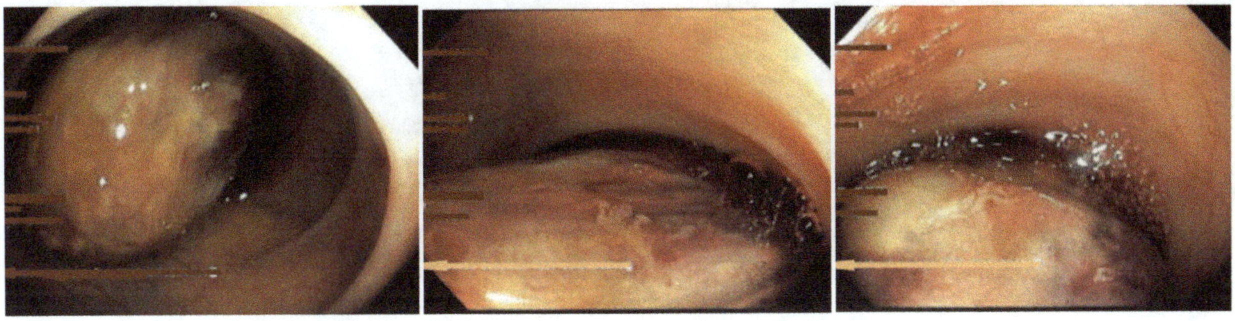

FIGURE 1: Endoscopic finding.

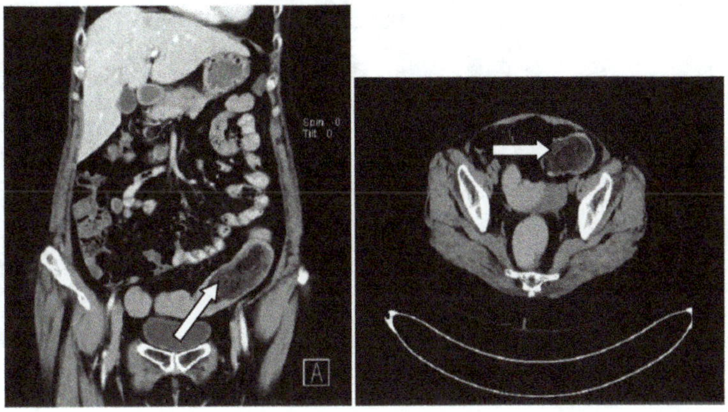

FIGURE 2: CT abdomen.

identify. CT abdomen was done before sent for surgery. The finding was a circumferential well defined arterial contrast enhancing bowel mass measurement of 8.1 cm length arising from the distal part of the descending colon. Entrapped fat attenuations were seen inside the colonic lumen. No mesenteric adenopathy was seen. CT diagnosis was fat containing mesenchymal tumor (GISTS) of descending colon (Figure 2). Patient was planned for surgical resection without biopsy because of risk of hemorrhage.

In laparotomy, a large polypoid lesion about 8 x 3 cm with short stalk was found in sigmoid colon. The serosal surface appeared normal and no adjacent intra-abdominal lymph nodes were enlarged. Affected portion of sigmoid colon was resected and sent for histology examination (Figure 3). No renal mass was seen grossly during operation.

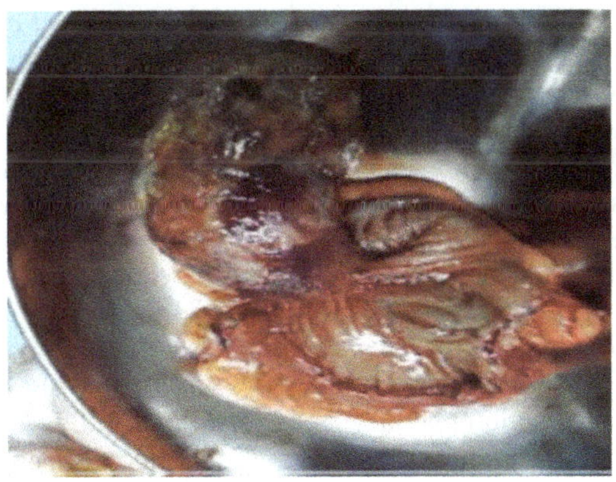

FIGURE 3: Gross surgical section of polyp.

3. Pathologic Report

Macroscopic examination of the excised specimen showed a polypoid growth measured 14 x 9 x 5 cm, of soft consistency, covered by grayish white fleshy mucosa. The luminal surface of polypoidal growth was measured 8.5 x 4 cm. The mucosa surface appeared normal. No hemorrhagic or necrosis was seen (Figure 4).

Histological finding was large pedunculated polyp arising from the wall and composed of mature adipocytes and proliferating large and small vessels of varying nature (capillaries, small veins, venules, arterioles, and small arteries) lined by a thin wall endothelial lining. No vasculitis or thrombosis was noted. There also proliferated smooth muscle spindle cells with eosinophilic cytoplasm embedded in loose myxoid stroma. Histological diagnosis was benign angiolipofibroma polyp, sigmoid colon (Figure 5).

4. Discussion

Colonoscopy is the gold standard procedure for colonic screening of colorectal cancer or polyps [3]. In this case, we

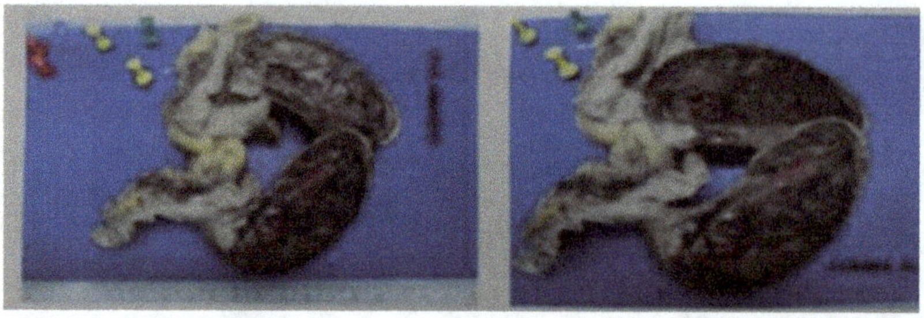

FIGURE 4: Gross pathological section of polyp.

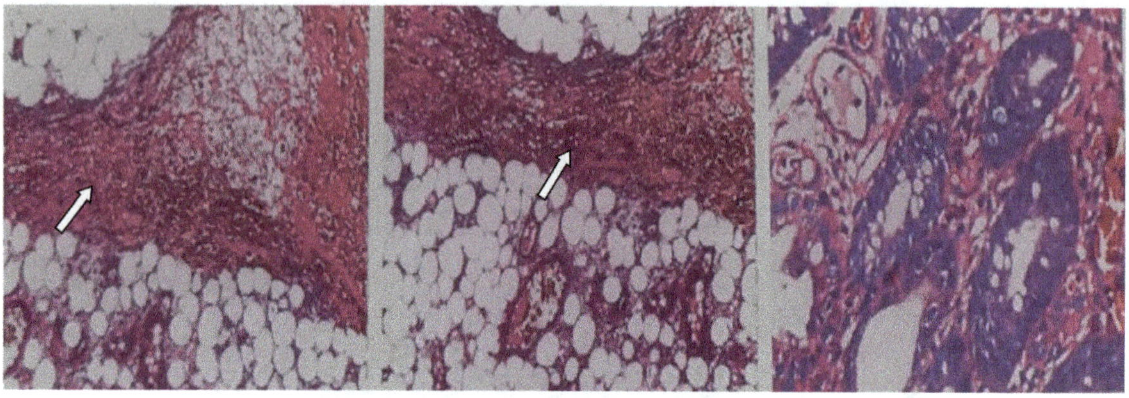

FIGURE 5: Histological finding of polyp.

found submucosal polyp showing a characteristic histological triad of adipose tissue, vessels, and smooth muscle of mixed mesenchymal structures normally present in the submucosa supporting the diagnosis of an angiolipofibroma hamartoma rather than a true neoplasm.

The majority of angiolipofibromas are benign tumors derived from mesenchymal tissue and majorities are arising in the kidney. Extra renal presentations are very rare and reported to be found in the liver, nasal cavity, vagina, spermatic cord, skin, mediastinum, and GI tract. Among GI tract involvement, colonic involvement is rather rare condition [2].

Angiolipofibroma may be a challenging in diagnosis when it arises outside its typical renal location because of its rarity and the histological variation. Typically, angiolipofibroma shows a mixture of adipose tissue, fat, and abnormal vessels, but it may show a wide range of histological appearances. These include tumors where the muscle component is dominant, including epithelioid variants band showing considerable nuclear atypia. Preoperative diagnosis of angiolipofibroma is difficult [4].

Demir et al. described a similar lesion originating in the mesocolon of the sigmoid, composed of vascular proliferation in a fibrofatty tissue background; it was published in the name of "angio lipomatous mesenchymal hamartoma" [5]. Groisman et al. described a cecal submucosal polyp formed by adipose tissue, fibrous tissue, and vascular proliferation and lymph vessels in variable sizes under the name "angiolipofibroma of the cecum" [6]. Another common differential diagnosis is lipomatous neoplasms formed by adipose tissue and commonly found in the right colon [7]. Vascular lesions seen in the gastrointestinal tract formed solely by vascular proliferation include lymphangiomas, hemangiomas, hemangiolymphangiomas, and congenital vascular malformations [8].

Only few cases of colonic angiolipofibroma have been reported in the literature [9–11]. Most of them occurred in middle aged men. The natures of the polyps were polypoid or pedunculated nature and located in the colon mostly on the left sided. Most of the colonic angiolipofibromas are presented as small polyps and can successfully be removed by endoscopically and rarely need surgery, but this case presented as a large lesion and needed surgery.

As the recurrence of colonic polyps, it is known that adenoma recurrence rates are estimated to be around 30-40%, 3 to 4 years after the initial colonoscopy [12, 13]. The risk of recurrent adenomas on the surveillance colonoscopy depends on the findings at the initial diagnosis. The risk is higher in advanced and/or multiple adenomas [14, 15]. Some study mentions the recurrence rate of polyp on left colon and rectum is of higher rate than that on right colon. But there remains controversial whether the location may affect the recurrence of polyps [16]. Although there was no data about recurrent rate of colonic angiolipofibroma after resection, we do follow up this patient as usual postpolypectomy followup. Patient is planning to do recheck colonoscopy and CT abdomen after one year and ultrasound abdomen every six months. Our patient is well and uneventful during followup of 6 months and no renal mass and other pathologies are seen in ultrasound examination.

5. Conclusion

This submucosal mesenchymal, angiolipofibroma polyp case was reported on left side of the colon as the common location but differed from others, which was larger polyp (8.5 x 4 cm) with short or no stalk not favored to be removed endoscopically. Surgical excision is the treatment of choice for large lesion.

References

[1] J. F. Flejou, N. A. Shepherd, B. F. Warren et al., "Non-epithelial tumors of the large intestine," in *Morson and Dawson's Gastrointestinal Pathology*, pp. 739–744, Wiley-Blackwell, Oxford, UK, 5th edition, 2013.

[2] A. I. Sharara and A. Tawil, "Angiomyolipoma of the colon," *Clinical Gastroenterology and Hepatology*, vol. 3, article 35, 2005.

[3] G. C. Harewood and D. A. Lieberman, "Colonoscopy practice patterns since introduction of medicare coverage for average-risk screening," *Clinical Gastroenterology and Hepatology*, vol. 2, no. 1, pp. 72–77, 2004.

[4] J.-S. Chen, L.-J. Kuo, P.-Y. Lin, and C.-R. Changchien, "Angiomyolipoma of the colon: report of a case and review of the literature," *Diseases of the Colon and Rectum*, vol. 46, no. 4, pp. 547–549, 2003.

[5] R. Demir, A. Schmid, W. Hohenberger, and A. Agaimy, "Angiolipomatous mesenchymal hamartoma (angiolipomatosis) of the sigmoid mesocolon," *International Journal of Clinical and Experimental Pathology*, vol. 4, no. 2, pp. 210–214, 2011.

[6] G. M. Groisman, "Angiolipofibroma of the cecum: a rare type of submucosal polyp," *Case Reports in Pathology*, vol. 2013, Article ID 737015, 4 pages, 2013.

[7] O. Tascilar, G. K. Cakmak, B. D. Gün et al., "Clinical evaluation of submucosal colonic lipomas: decision making," *World Journal of Gastroenterology*, vol. 12, no. 31, pp. 5075–5077, 2006.

[8] A. Handra-Luca and E. Montgomery, "Vascular malformations and hemangiolymphangiomas of the gastrointestinal tract: morphological features and clinical impact," *International Journal of Clinical and Experimental Pathology*, vol. 4, no. 5, pp. 430–443, 2011.

[9] J. Pelz, K. Weber, J. Göhl, A. Dimmler, and W. Hohenberger, "Angiomyolipoma of the colon - Case report and review of the literature," *Zeitschrift für Gastroenterologie*, vol. 41, no. 8, pp. 715–718, 2003.

[10] M. Abdulkader, J. Abercrombie, T. A. McCulloch, and P. V. Kaye, "Colonic angiomyolipoma with a monotypic expression and a predominant epithelioid component," *Journal of Clinical Pathology*, vol. 58, no. 10, pp. 1107–1109, 2005.

[11] H. Cheng, M. D. Sitrin, and A. Rani, "Angiomyolipoma in the colon," *Gastrointestinal Endoscopy*, vol. 64, no. 3, pp. 443-444, 2006.

[12] P. F. Pinsky, R. E. Schoen, J. L. Weissfeld et al., "The yield of surveillance colonoscopy by adenoma history and time to examination," *Clinical Gastroenterology and Hepatology*, vol. 7, no. 1, pp. 86–92, 2009.

[13] D. A. Lieberman, D. G. Weiss, W. V. Harford et al., "Five year colon surveillance after screening colonoscopy," *Gastroenterology*, vol. 133, no. 4, pp. 1077–1085, 2007.

[14] M. E. Martínez, R. Sampliner, J. R. Marshall, A. K. Bhattacharyya, M. E. Reid, and D. S. Alberts, "Adenoma characteristics as risk factors for recurrence of advanced adenomas," *Gastroenterology*, vol. 120, no. 5, pp. 1077–1083, 2001.

[15] R. E. Schoen, "Surveillance after positive and negative colonoscopy examinations: Issues, yields, and use," *American Journal of Gastroenterology*, vol. 98, no. 6, pp. 1237–1246, 2003.

[16] Y. Huang, W. Gong, B. Su et al., "Recurrence and surveillance of colorectal adenoma after polypectomy in a southern Chinese population," *Journal of Gastroenterology*, vol. 45, no. 8, pp. 838–845, 2010.

7

Acute Mesenteric Ischemia in a COVID-19 Patient: Delay in Referral and Recommendation for Surgery

Mohammad Hossein Bagheripour[1] **and Mohammad Ali Zakeri**[2,3]

[1]*Department of General Surgery, Faculty of Medicine, Rafsanjan University of Medical Sciences, Rafsanjan, Iran*
[2]*Social Determinants of Health Research Centre, Rafsanjan University of Medical Sciences, Rafsanjan, Iran*
[3]*Non-Communicable Diseases Research Center, Rafsanjan University of Medical Sciences, Rafsanjan, Iran*

Correspondence should be addressed to Mohammad Ali Zakeri; mazakeri@rums.ac.ir

Academic Editor: Yoshihiro Moriwaki

Coronavirus (COVID-19) is more common with symptoms such as fever, dry cough, and shortness of breath. However, it may be associated with COVID-19-induced gastrointestinal (GI) symptoms including acute mesenteric ischemia (AMI). These conditions make the diagnosis of AMI challenging. Timely referral with correct diagnosis and attention to the uncommon symptoms of COVID-19 can play an important role in the management and treatment of AMI in COVID-19 patients. We present a patient with AMI due to thrombotic complications of COVID-19, who referred to the hospital too late and ignored the recommendation for abdominal surgery.

1. Introduction

COVID-19 started rapidly in China and spread around the world quickly. It became a global pandemic, creating a wave of fear, anger, and anxiety among patients and members of the community [1, 2]. Fever, dry cough, and shortness of breath are the most common symptoms of COVID-19. However, studies have reported that the incidence of gastrointestinal (GI) symptoms caused by COVID-19 occurred in up to two-thirds of patients with COVID-19 [3]. Symptoms include anorexia, nausea, vomiting, diarrhea, abdominal pain, and GI bleeding that may occur 1 to 2 days before fever and shortness of breath [4]. Asymptomatic COVID-19 patients and carriers who have no or fewer symptoms during the incubation period make disease diagnosis difficult. There are also a number of GI disorders associated with fever that make it difficult to differentiate between symptoms associated with COVID-19 and other diseases [5].

Acute gastrointestinal problems include AMI, which is characterized by a group of diseases that interrupt blood flow to different parts of the small intestine. AMI leads to ischemia and secondary inflammatory changes and, if left untreated, leads to intestinal necrosis with approximately 50% mortality. Early diagnosis and surgical intervention are the basis of treatment to reduce AMI mortality [6]. This report describes a 78-year-old man with COVID-19, who delayed seeking and undergoing abdominal surgery. The insights gained from this study can help us pay more attention to the gastrointestinal symptoms of COVID-19 patients and correctly identify the clinical features.

2. Case Presentation

A 78-year-old male patient (height: 173 cm, weight: 74 kg, and BMI: 24.7) referred to a public hospital for acute abdominal pain from three days ago after seven days of dyspnea and coughing. He had a history of coronary heart disease and percutaneous coronary intervention 6 years ago. His drug history was metoprolol 25 mg tablets twice per day *(bid)*, Nitrocontin 6.4 mg tablets twice per day *(bid)*, and aspirin 80 mg tablets once daily. The patient reported no history of trauma to his abdomen and no history of substance or alcohol abuse. At presentation, the pulse rate was

105 beats per minute (BPM), the blood pressure (BP) was 80/ 60 mm Hg, the body temperature (BT) was 38.7°C, and the respiratory rate (RR) was 20 breaths/min. The baseline electrocardiography (ECG) showed tachycardia with sinus rhythm and without myocardial infarction (MI) or other arrhythmias. The main symptom was a sudden onset of generalized abdominal pain with periumbilical predominance with 10/10 intensity. He claimed obstipation along with nausea and vomiting in this period. He could not eat during these three days. He suffered from coughing, dyspnea, and tachypnea before onset of the abdominal pain.

He was visited two times in outpatient centers and prescribed with pantoprazole 40 mg once daily, hyoscine 10 mg q8h, and painkillers (Advil) before referring to our hospital. On the last hours of the third day, he was admitted to the COVID-19 emergency department. On the examination of the abdomen, the main findings were abdominal distention with no audible bowel sound and also generalized abdominal tenderness and rebound tenderness. He had an obvious abdominal guarding. Digital rectal examination showed an empty rectal ampulla with no sign of mucosal sloughing. Respiratory sounds were nearly normal.

Main laboratory data were positive specific COVID-19 polymerase chain reaction (PCR) (based on a nasopharyngeal swab). Leuckocytosis (WBC = 11.200) and prerenal azotemia (BUN = 120 mg/dl and CR = 2.5 mg/dl) were seen in the patient. The results of the laboratory are presented in Table 1.

Plane abdominal series radiographies and computed tomography (CT) of the chest were performed. A CT scan of the chest showed no definite findings of COVID 19 and cardiomegaly. There was no pleural effusion (Figures 1 and 2), but ascites and dilated small bowel loops could be seen in the few available axial cuts of the abdomen (Figures 3 and 4).

Supine abdominal X-ray showed prominent dilated small bowel loops and the absence of a completely visible colon. Both findings were in favor of small bowel obstruction (Figure 5). Multiple air fluid levels were visible in the small bowel loops in upright abdominal X-ray, pointing at small bowel obstruction (Figure 6).

After initial resuscitation with 2 liters of lactated ringer's solution and antibiotic therapy with empiric wide-spectrum prophylactic antibiotics (ceftriaxone 2 gr stat and metronidazole 500 mg stat), diagnostic laparotomy was performed. Massive brownish ascites and gangrenous small bowel and colon starting from 15 cm of ligamentum of Treitz to the middle part of the transverse colon were seen. Tissue decay has happened, and the intestine was about to perforate (Figure 7). These findings corresponded to acute mesenteric ischemia due to complete occlusion of the superior mesenteric artery for at least several hours. No therapeutic procedure could be performed, and the abdomen was closed. He died a couple of hours later in the intensive care unit (ICU).

3. Discussion

To the best of our knowledge, death of a patient with COVID-19 who had AMI and required emergency surgery was among the first cases of death due to delayed referral. Studies have shown that the mortality rate related to acute mesenteric arterial occlusion is very high. Necessary measures should be taken for the patient before the progression of ischemia to intestinal gangrene. Patient survival, on the other hand, depends on prompt diagnosis and revascularization [7].

Studies have shown that COVID-19 patients are more likely to develop AMI. Consistent with the present report, Chan et al. described a 73-year-old patient with ischemic colitis and showed that the patient died of cardiac arrest on day 5 of admission due to a hypercoagulable state. All inflammatory markers increased significantly in the patient [8]. Sehhat et al. described a 77-year-old patient and showed that impaired blood flow to the visceral-vascular system could cause life-threatening AMI [9]. Besides, Rashid et al. [10], Faridi et al. [11], Sevella et al. [12], and Shahid et al. [13] also confirmed these findings. Almeida et al. also described three patients with intestinal ischemia and pneumoperitoneum and showed that the pathogenicity of COVID-19 has been increasingly attributed to the systemic inflammatory response leading to intravascular disseminated coagulation [14].

Coagulopathy associated with COVID-19 has recently emerged as a major component of the disease and has led to high mortality [8]. Vartanoglu Aktokmakyan et al. showed the possibility of thrombotic events in patients with COVID-19. This observational study was conducted on 60 patients who underwent emergency surgery and showed that 5 out of 6 COVID-19 patients with acute abdomen (83.3%) underwent surgery due to AMI [15].

The pathogenesis of COVID-19 coagulation has not been fully understood yet. COVID-19 can cause a hypercoagulable state with acute inflammatory changes, which differs from disseminated intravascular coagulation (DIC) in that fibrinogen and D-dimer levels increase [16]. Tang found that disseminated intravascular coagulation and venous thromboembolism were the main causes of death in most COVID-19 patients [17]. However, it is not yet clear whether the coagulation disorders are a secondary response to the systemic inflammatory response or are developed directly by COVID-19. Studies on patients with acute COVID-19 have confirmed the presence of strokes and peripheral ischemia mediated by antiphospholipid antibodies [18].

However, several mechanisms or a combination of them may be responsible for AMI in COVID-19 patients. First, COVID-19 enters the cell through the receptor of the angiotensin-converting enzyme 2 (ACE2) in the alveoli and creates a severe form of infection with a systematic inflammatory response [19]. High levels of proinflammatory cytokines (interleukins 1 and 6 and interferon-g), known as the "cytokine storm," have been reported in these patients [20]. Evidence has shown that inflammation activates coagulation, which in turn increases inflammatory activity, and there is a mutual relationship between inflammation and coagulation [21].

Saving of time is one of the most important challenges in the recovery of AMI patients that should be considered. A retrospective cohort study on 72 patients with AMI showed that a delay in operation (>6 hours after surgical

Table 1: The laboratory findings of the patient.

Variable (hematology test)		Normal reference range
White blood cell count (WBC)	11.200	4000–10000 * 1000/cmm
Red cell count (RBC)	5.20	3.9–5.6 mil/cmm
Hemoglobin (Hb)	16.5	12–16 mmol/L
Hematocrit (HCT)	47.8	36–46%
Platelet count (PLAT)	146	150–450 * 1000/cmm
Sodium (NA)	139	135–145 mEq/l
Potassium (K)	4.9	3.8–5 mEq/l
Blood urea nitrogen (BUN)	120	17–43 mg/dl
Creatinine (CR)	2.5	0.7–1.4 mg/dl
Total bilirubin	1.2	0.1–1.2 mg/dl
Direct bilirubin	0.6	0.1–0.3 mg/dl
C-reactive protein	Positive	Negative/positive
Amylase	593	Up to 110 U/L
Aspartate aminotransferase (AST or SGOT)	106	Up to 31 U/L
Alanine aminotransferase (ALT or SGPT)	76	Up to 31 U/L
Alkaline phosphatase (ALP)	206	64–306 U/L
D-dimer	301	Up to 0.5 mg/L

cmm: cells per cubic millimeter; mil/cmm: million cells/cells per cubic millimeter; mmol/L: millimoles per litre; mEq/L: milliequivalents per litre; mg/dL: milligrams per decilitre; U/L: units per litre; and mg/L: milligrams per litre.

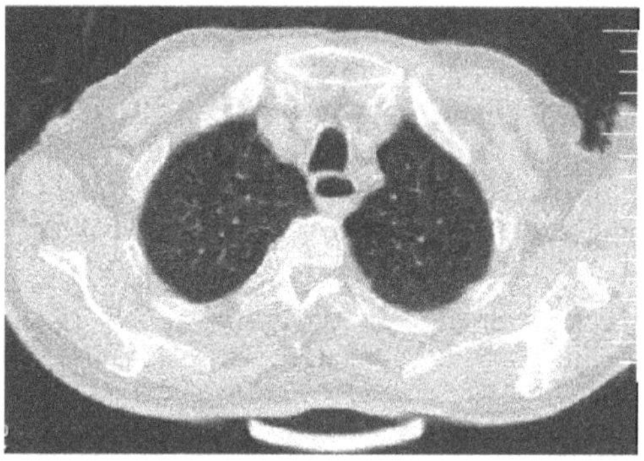

Figure 1: Male patient's chest CT.

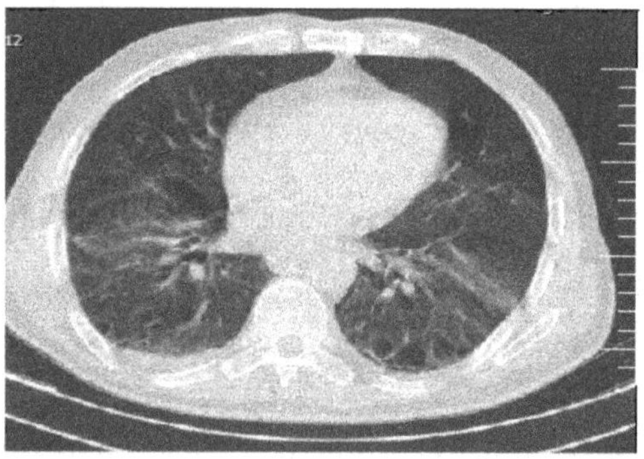

Figure 2: Male patient's chest CT.

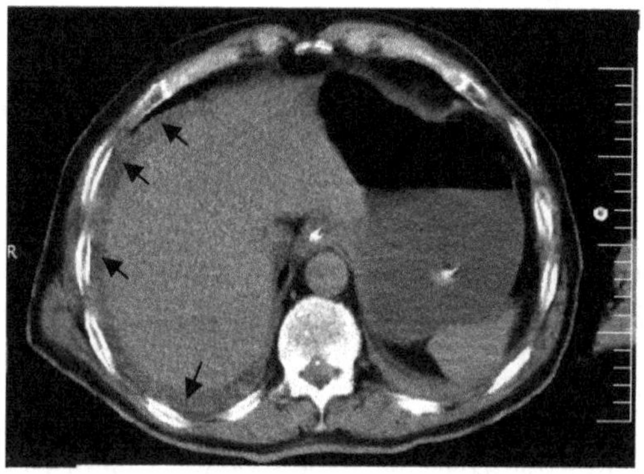

Figure 3: Male patient's abdominal CT (arrows: ascites).

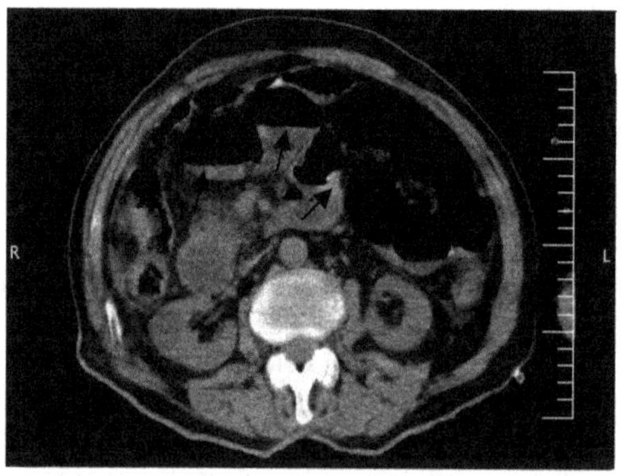

Figure 4: Male patient's abdominal CT (arrows: dilated small bowel loops).

consultation) and delay in surgical consultation (>24 hours after disease onset) were associated with increased mortality [22].

The patient presented in this report experienced acute gastrointestinal symptoms during 3 days, which caused his disease to become acute due to fear of COVID-19 and delayed referral. Fear and anxiety related to referral have been reported in different patients during the prevalence of COVID-19. This has caused acute problems and even death of some patients [23]. Studies have reported a high prevalence of fear and anxiety caused by COVID-19 [24, 25]. Physicians' attention to the mental and psychological condition of patients and involvement of the patients in the

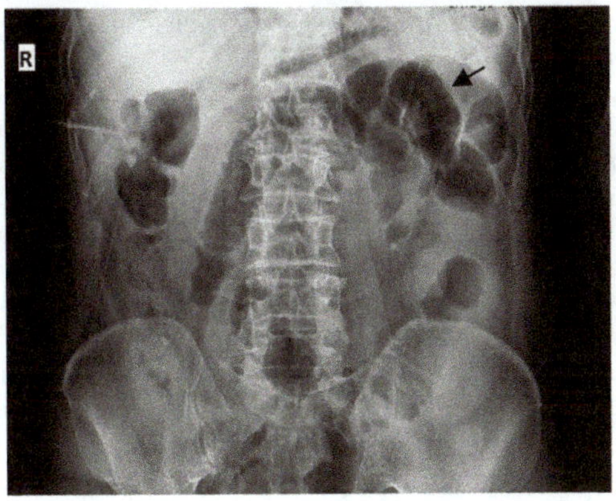

Figure 5: Male patient's supine abdominal X-ray.

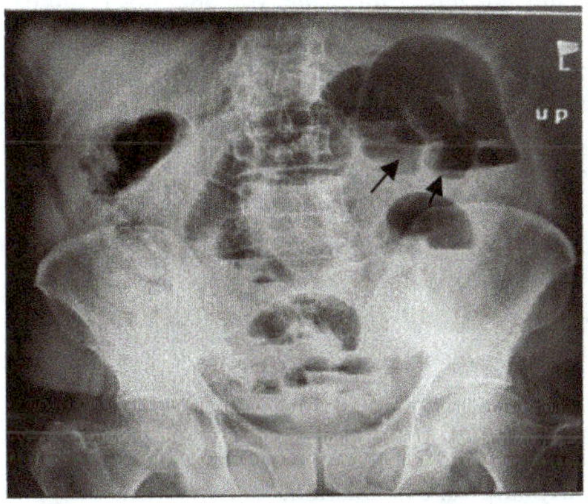

Figure 6: Male patient's upright abdominal X-ray.

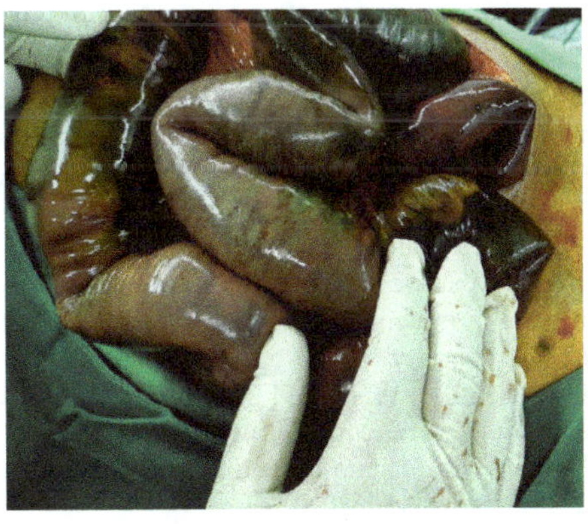

Figure 7: Photo of gangrenous small intestine of the patient.

invasive procedures during the outbreak of COVID-19 are among the most important challenges facing the medical system that can have a direct impact on patient survival. In addition, paying attention to the warning signs and correct diagnostic methods are other issues that should be considered by physicians.

In addition to pulmonary symptoms, gastrointestinal symptoms are increasingly seen in COVID-19. Nausea/vomiting, diarrhea, abdominal pain, abdominal distension, or worsening of systemic conditions (such as sepsis) may be symptoms of patients with severe COVID-19 and AMI [26]. CT can help diagnose AMI. Dilated (>3 cm), thick-walled, and edematous bowel should be considered as signs of AMI. In advanced cases, pneumatosis intestinalis or portal venous gas suggests bowel ischemia. The presence of gas in the intestinal wall should be interpreted with caution because the presence of pneumatosis may be due to mechanical ventilation of the patients with severe COVID-19 [27]. Pirola et al. have described radiologic small bowel alterations including mesenteric ischemia in 50%, small bowel wall thickening in 16%, pneumatosis in 15%, intussusception in 13%, pneumoperitoneum in 3%, and paralytic ileus in 3% in 62 patients with COVID-19 [3].

There are challenges in the management of thromboembolic complications of COVID-19 due to the lack of high quality evidence of the efficacy and safety of various methods of prevention or treatment [28]. One of the suggested methods is thromboprophylaxis with low-molecular-weight (LMW) heparin [10]. Unlike chronic mesenteric ischemia, the treatment of acute arterial mesenteric ischemia requires a thorough bowel evaluation and revascularization by surgical means [7]. AMI can lead to ischemia and secondary inflammatory changes and, if left untreated, intestinal necrosis. Early diagnosis and surgical intervention reduce AMI mortality [6].

For timely intervention, healthcare providers must consider high indicators for recognizing life-threatening complications of COVID-19, such as AMI. On the other hand, information about the warning signs of acute problems of COVID-19 should be provided at the community level to prevent delayed referral of the patients, who should implement the necessary recommendations.

4. Conclusions

According to our information, this is one of the first reports of delayed referral of the patients with COVID-19, which has caused acute and fatal mesenteric ischemia in the patient. AMI should be suspected in the COVID-19 patients with abdominal pain. Early referral and rapid diagnosis among patients with clinical features of COVID-19 as well as attention to the mental state of the patients to participate in treatment are important factors that lead to patient survival. However, further studies are needed to understand the relationship between COVID-19 and the occurrence of AMI and their effects on patients.

Acknowledgments

The authors would like to thank the Social Determinants of Health Research Centre for its support and collaboration (Ethics CODE: IR.RUMS.REC.1399.254) in Ali-Ibn Abi-Talib Hospital, Rafsanjan University of Medical Sciences, Rafsanjan, Iran.

References

[1] M. A. Zakeri, S. M. Hossini Rafsanjanipoor, N. Sedri et al., "Psychosocial status during the prevalence of COVID-19 disease: the comparison between healthcare workers and general population," *Current Psychology*, vol. 40, pp. 1-9, 2021.

[2] M. A. Zakeri, "Iranian psychosocial status during and after COVID-19 outbreak mandatory quarantine: a cross-sectional study," *Journal of Community Psychology*, vol. 49, no. 7, pp. 2506–2516, 2021.

[3] L. Pirola, A. Palermo, G. Mulinacci et al., "Acute mesenteric ischemia and small bowel imaging findings in COVID-19: a comprehensive review of the literature," *World Journal of Gastrointestinal Surgery*, vol. 13, no. 7, pp. 702–716, 2021.

[4] Z. Wu and J. M. McGoogan, "Characteristics of and important lessons from the coronavirus disease 2019 (COVID-19) outbreak in China," *JAMA*, vol. 323, no. 13, pp. 1239–1242, 2020.

[5] J. Ke, N. Lan, T. Wang et al., "Strategies and recommendations for the management of gastrointestinal surgery during the COVID-19 pandemic: experience shared by Chinese surgeons," *Gastroenterology Report*, vol. 8, no. 3, pp. 167–174, 2020.

[6] M. Bala, J. Kashuk, E. E. Moore et al., "Acute mesenteric ischemia: guidelines of the world society of emergency surgery," *World Journal of Emergency Surgery: WJES*, vol. 12, no. 1, pp. 1–11, 2017.

[7] M. C. Wyers, "Acute mesenteric ischemia: diagnostic approach and surgical treatment," in *Seminars in Vascular Surgery*Elsevier, Amsterdam, Netherlands, 2010.

[8] K. H. Chan, S. L. Lim, A. Damati et al., "Coronavirus disease 2019 (COVID-19) and ischemic colitis: an under-recognized complication," *The American Journal of Emergency Medicine*, vol. 38, no. 12, pp. 2758.e1–2758.e4, 2020.

[9] S. Sehhat, H. Talebzadeh, A. Hakamifard et al., "Acute mesenteric ischemia in a patient with COVID-19: a case report," *Archives of Iranian Medicine*, vol. 23, no. 9, pp. 639–643, 2020.

[10] M. Rashid, W. Askar, A. Gaafar, M. Fawzy, and M. Makarem, "Superior mesenteric artery thrombosis as a possible presenting complication of COVID-19," *Medicine Science International Medical Journal*, vol. 9, no. 4, pp. 1–9, 2020.

[11] S. H. Faridi, B. Siddiqui, Y. Afaque, and M. Sohail, "Acute mesenteric ischemia in covid-19 patients: a case series," *Himalayan Journal of Applied Medical Sciences and Research*, vol. 2, no. 4, 2021.

[12] P. Sevella, S. S. H. Rallabhandi, V. Jahagirdar, S. R. Kankanala, A. R. Ginnaram, and K. Rama, "Acute mesenteric ischemia as an early complication of COVID-19," *Cureus*, vol. 13, no. 9, Article ID e18082, 2021.

[13] F. Shahid, S. M. Ali, S. Saleem et al., "Acute mesenteric ischemia due to COVID-19: a case report," *Open Access Journal of Surgery*, vol. 12, no. 2, Article ID 555831, 2020.

[14] A. Almeida, V. V. Azcárate, C. S. Justicia et al., "Severe colon ischemia in patients with severe COVID-2019 infection: a report of three cases," *Revista Espanola de Enfermedades Digestivas*, vol. 112, no. 10, 2020.

[15] T. Vartanoglu Aktokmakyan, M. Tokocin, S. Meric, and F. Celebi, "Is mesenteric ischemia in COVID-19 patients a surprise?" *Surgical Innovation*, vol. 28, no. 2, Article ID 1553350620962892, 2020.

[16] S. Akima, C. McLintock, and B. J. Hunt, "RE: ISTH interim guidance to recognition and management of coagulopathy in COVID-19," *Journal of Thrombosis and Haemostasis*, vol. 18, no. 8, pp. 2057-2058, 2020.

[17] N. Tang, H. Bai, X. Chen, J. Gong, D. Li, and Z. Sun, "Anticoagulant treatment is associated with decreased mortality in severe coronavirus disease 2019 patients with coagulopathy," *Journal of Thrombosis and Haemostasis*, vol. 18, no. 5, pp. 1094–1099, 2020.

[18] Y. Zhang, M. Xiao, S. Zhang et al., "Coagulopathy and antiphospholipid antibodies in patients with Covid-19," *New England Journal of Medicine*, vol. 382, no. 17, p. e38, 2020.

[19] A. Fletcher-Sandersjöö and B.-M. Bellander, "Is COVID-19 associated thrombosis caused by overactivation of the complement cascade? a literature review," *Thrombosis Research*, vol. 194, pp. 36–41, 2020.

[20] M. Levi, T. van der Poll, and H. R. Büller, "Bidirectional relation between inflammation and coagulation," *Circulation*, vol. 109, no. 22, pp. 2698–2704, 2004.

[21] J. H. P. Nascimento, B. F. O. Gomes, P. R. D. Carmo Júnior et al., "COVID-19 and hypercoagulable state: a new therapeutic perspective," *Arquivos Brasileiros de Cardiologia*, vol. 114, no. 5, pp. 829–833, 2020.

[22] I. G. Eltarawy, Y. M. Etman, M. Zenati, R. L. Simmons, and M. R. Rosengart, "Acute mesenteric ischemia: the importance of early surgical consultation," *The American Surgeon*, vol. 75, no. 3, pp. 212–219, 2009.

[23] M. A. Zakeri and M. Dehghan, "The impact of the COVID-19 disease on the referral and admission of the non-COVID-19 patients," *The International Journal of Health Planning and Management*, vol. 36, no. 1, pp. 209–211, 2020.

[24] M. A. Zakeri, M. Dehghan, F. Ghaedi Heidari et al., "Mental health outcomes among health-care workers during the COVID-19 outbreak in Iran," *Mental Health Review Journal*, vol. 26, no. 2, pp. 152–160, 2021.

[25] S. M. Hossini Rafsanjanipoor, M. A. Zakeri, M. Dehghan et al., "Iranian psychosocial status and its determinant factors during the prevalence of COVID-19 disease," *Psychology Health & Medicine*, vol. 26, pp. 1–12, 2021.

[26] A. H. Parry, A. H. Wani, and M. Yaseen, "Acute mesenteric ischemia in severe coronavirus-19 (COVID-19): possible mechanisms and diagnostic pathway," *Academic Radiology*, vol. 27, no. 8, p. 1190, 2020.

[27] L. A. Fitzpatrick, M. D. Rivers-Bowerman, S. Thipphavong, S. E. Clarke, J. A. Rowe, and A. F. Costa, "Pearls, pitfalls, and conditions that mimic mesenteric ischemia at CT," *RadioGraphics*, vol. 40, no. 2, pp. 545–561, 2020.

[28] C. Magro, J. J. Mulvey, D. Berlin et al., "Complement associated microvascular injury and thrombosis in the pathogenesis of severe COVID-19 infection: a report of five cases," *Translational Research*, vol. 220, pp. 1–13, 2020.

8

An Uncommon Presentation of Carcinosarcoma of the Stomach and a Minimally Invasive Approach for Treatment

Anoush Calikyan,[1] Agedi N. Boto,[2] Valeriia Klymenko,[3] and Imran M. Siddiqui[4]

[1]*Frank H. Netter School of Medicine at Quinnipiac University, North Haven, CT, USA*
[2]*St. Vincent's Medical Center, Department of Pathology, Bridgeport, CT, USA*
[3]*St. Vincent's Medical Center, Department of Medical Oncology, Bridgeport, CT, USA*
[4]*St. Vincent's Medical Center, Department of Surgical Oncology, Bridgeport, CT, USA*

Correspondence should be addressed to Anoush Calikyan; anoush.calikyan@quinnipiac.edu

Academic Editor: Naohiko Koide

Carcinosarcoma is a rare malignant neoplasm that is composed of both epithelial and mesenchymal tumor components. Gastric carcinosarcoma is even more rare and is often diagnosed at a late stage. In this report, we investigate a case of early gastric carcinosarcoma with regional lymph node metastasis in a 78 year old woman. The patient underwent partial gastrectomy, lymphadenectomy, and splenectomy. The tumor was confined to the gastric submucosa, and a biopsy specimen led to a histological diagnosis of carcinosarcoma with adenocarcinoma, squamous-cell carcinoma, and undifferentiated pleomorphic sarcoma components. Metastasis was present in one lymph node and displayed osteosarcomatous differentiation. Vigilant monitoring for recurrence and metastatic disease will be required for this patient.

1. Introduction

Carcinosarcoma is an aggressive and malignant neoplasm composed of both epithelial and mesenchymal components. By the time of diagnosis, the cancer has often metastasized to other organs due to its aggressive nature [1]. Diagnosing gastric carcinosarcoma promptly and treating the patient appropriately are critical for better outcomes and reducing recurrence.

We present the case of a 78-year-old woman with a distant history of a duodenal ulcer who was found to have 2 primary synchronous lesions of carcinosarcoma in her stomach. The case is of interest because this type of tumor rarely occurs in the gastric mucosa, particularly as a primary tumor in the stomach. Moreover, the patient was not found to have any distant metastases, highlighting the importance of early detection in the management of this high-grade sarcoma.

2. Case Presentation

A 78-year-old woman presented to the emergency department because of concerns about melena due to gastric bleeding, vague abdominal pain, and fatiguability. She denied hematemesis or hematochezia. She had a remote history of a duodenal ulcer, well-controlled gastroesophageal reflux disease, diverticulosis, hypertension, obesity, and hyperlipidemia. She reported moderate alcohol use.

The physical examination yielded insignificant findings. On initial presentation, the patient was hyponatremic (131 mmol/L), anemic (hemoglobin 7.7 g/dL, hematocrit 24.5%), thrombocytic (769,000 platelets/μL), leukocytic (20,100 white blood cells/μL), and hypoalbuminemic (3.5 g/dL). Endoscopy showed the presence of two gastric masses, and biopsy from endoscopy revealed an undifferentiated pleomorphic sarcoma (UPS). Microscopically, the lesion was found to be an undifferentiated malignant neoplasm with epithelioid, giant cell, and focally spindled cell morphology (Figure 1(a)). Immunohistochemical staining for AE1/AE3, MOC31, CK7, CK20, p40, CDX2, CD3, CD20, PAX 5, HMB-45, S100, SMA, desmin, CD34, CD117, and dog-1 was all negative in tumor cells in the biopsied tissue. CD68 highlighted giant cells, and CD45 was negative in tumor cells (Figures 1(b) and 1(c)). Thus, the immunohistochemical

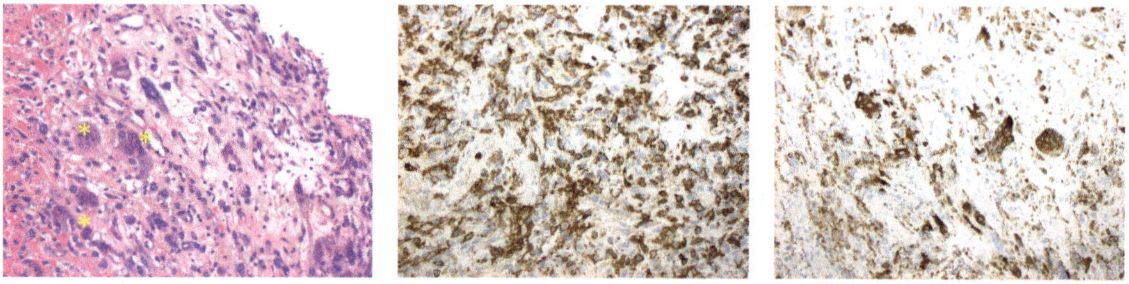

(a) (b) (c)

Figure 1: Initial endoscopic biopsy of tumor at 20x magnification. (a) Microscopic endoscopic biopsy hematoxylin and eosin stain results showed giant cells (*) and interspersed atypical epithelioid and spindle cells. Endoscopic biopsy stained with CD45 (b) and CD68 (c) immunohistochemistry staining in lymphocytes. CD45 was positive in background lymphocytes but negative in atypical cells, and CD68 was positive in giant cells.

profile was not consistent with a carcinoma or lymphoid malignancy. Gene assays indicated the presence of an activating PIK3CA mutation and an inactivating TP53 mutation. Morphology, immunohistochemistry, and gene assays supported a diagnosis of UPS. Endoscopic ultrasound confirmed the presence of a malignant-appearing lesion extending to the second layer (T2) with a malignant-appearing node in the splenic hilum.

Computed tomography (CT) imaging identified the presence of two intraluminal gastric masses arising from the greater curvature of the stomach that measured 3.6 and 2.2 cm in diameter. One large lymph node mass in the splenic hilum was also noted on CT scan. It was positron emission tomography (PET) avid on imaging, raising concern for metastasis to the local lymph nodes. However, on endoscopic ultrasound-guided biopsy, pathology was negative for metastatic nodal disease. Hyponatremia was thought to represent paraneoplastic syndrome of inappropriate antidiuretic hormone (SIADH).

This case was discussed in a multidisciplinary fashion by the tumor board. Owing to the patient's symptoms from anemia as well as the diagnosis of UPS, a plan was made for upfront resection and lymphadenectomy with the likelihood of en bloc splenectomy to achieve complete lymph node clearance.

The patient underwent a robotic longitudinal sleeve-like gastrectomy involving cardia, body, and antrum as well as lymphadenectomy and splenectomy. She had an uneventful postoperative course and was discharged home.

The tumor was located in the body of the stomach and measured 9 cm. Grossly, gastric lesions were found to be ulcerating and fungating, and the gastric mucosa was diffusely covered in fundic gland polyps (Figures 2(a)–2(c)). The gastric lesion was limited to the submucosa. Eleven lymph nodes were dissected, one of which was found to be positive for metastasis and measured 2.0 cm × 1.9 cm × 1.4 cm. This case was thus classified as American Joint Committee on Cancer (AJCC) stage IB. Pathology revealed pT1bN1 carcinosarcoma of the stomach. The biopsy showed not only evidence of UPS with osteoclast-like giant cells and osteosarcoma but also multiple lineages of differentiation including adenocarcinoma and squamous-cell carcinoma (Figures 3(a)–3(d)), which was consistent with a diagnosis of carcinosarcoma. The immunoprofile of the resected tumor showed that the squamous-cell and adenocarcinoma components were both positive for AE1/AE3 and CK7 (Figures 3(e)–3(g)). CDX2 was focally positive in the adenocarcinoma component and predominantly negative in the squamous-cell and sarcomatous components. CK20 was focally positive in the adenocarcinoma component and predominantly negative in the squamous-cell carcinoma component. P40 was positive in the squamous-cell carcinoma component but negative in the adenocarcinoma and sarcomatous components (Figure 3(h)). SATB2 was negative in the sarcomatous component. HMB45, c-kit, and dog-1 were negative. CD138 was focally positive in the UPS, adenocarcinoma, and squamous-cell carcinoma components (Figure 3(i)). Beta-human chorionic gonadotropin (β-hCG) was negative in giant cells, ruling out a choriocarcinoma component (Figure 3(j)). The sarcomatous component (both pleomorphic undifferentiated sarcoma with osteoclast-like giant cells and osteosarcoma components) was positive for vimentin (Figures 3(k) and 3(l)) and negative for AE1/AE3 (Figures 3(e) and 3(g)). Thus, the immunohistochemical profile on the resection supported a diagnosis of carcinosarcoma. Microscopically, lymph node metastasis displayed osteosarcomatous differentiation (Figures 4(a) and 4(b)). Pathology also revealed evidence of lymphovascular invasion (Figure 4(c)).

The patient underwent adjuvant chemotherapy (platinum based) after discussion by the tumor board. The case was discussed with national experts who agreed with the plan of care, given the rarity of the disease.

3. Discussion

Carcinosarcoma is a rare, malignant, and biphasic tumor that has aspects of both carcinoma (a cancer of epithelial tissue) and sarcoma (a cancer of connective tissue). It is often of müllerian origin and arises in the uterus, ovary, and fallopian tube, but it has also been reported to occur in the esophagus, thyroid, lungs, larynx, breasts, and urinary tract [1, 2]. While already rare, carcinosarcoma of the gastric mucosa is much rarer, with a literature review citing fewer than 100 reported cases of gastric carcinosarcoma [3].

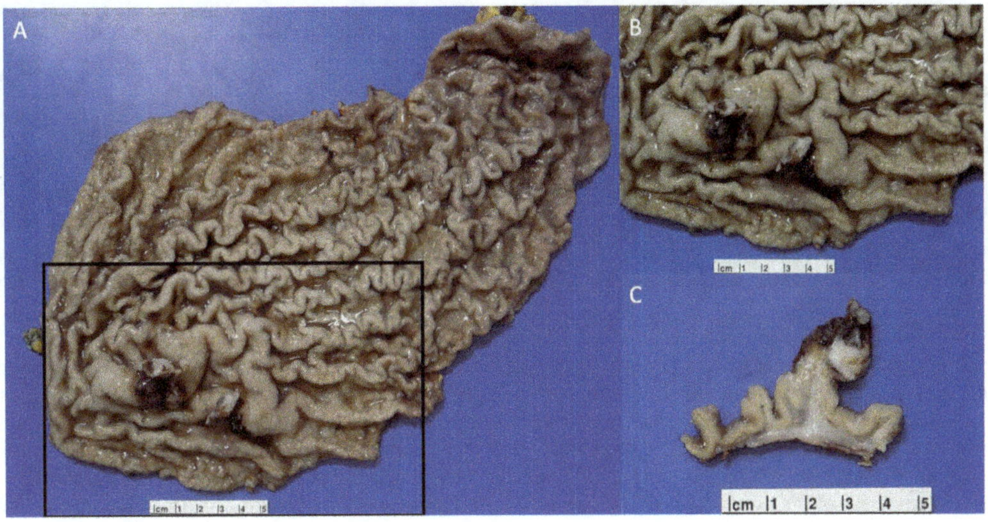

FIGURE 2: Gross lesion. (A) Image shows a fungating mass 3 cm from the margin. (B) Close-up of gross ulcerating and fungating lesion. Also seen is the diffuse granular appearance of the mucosa, which represents fundic gland polyps occurring diffusely throughout the stomach. (C) Internal view of the mass shows that the lesion was ulcerated, fungating, and growing separately from the gastric mucosa.

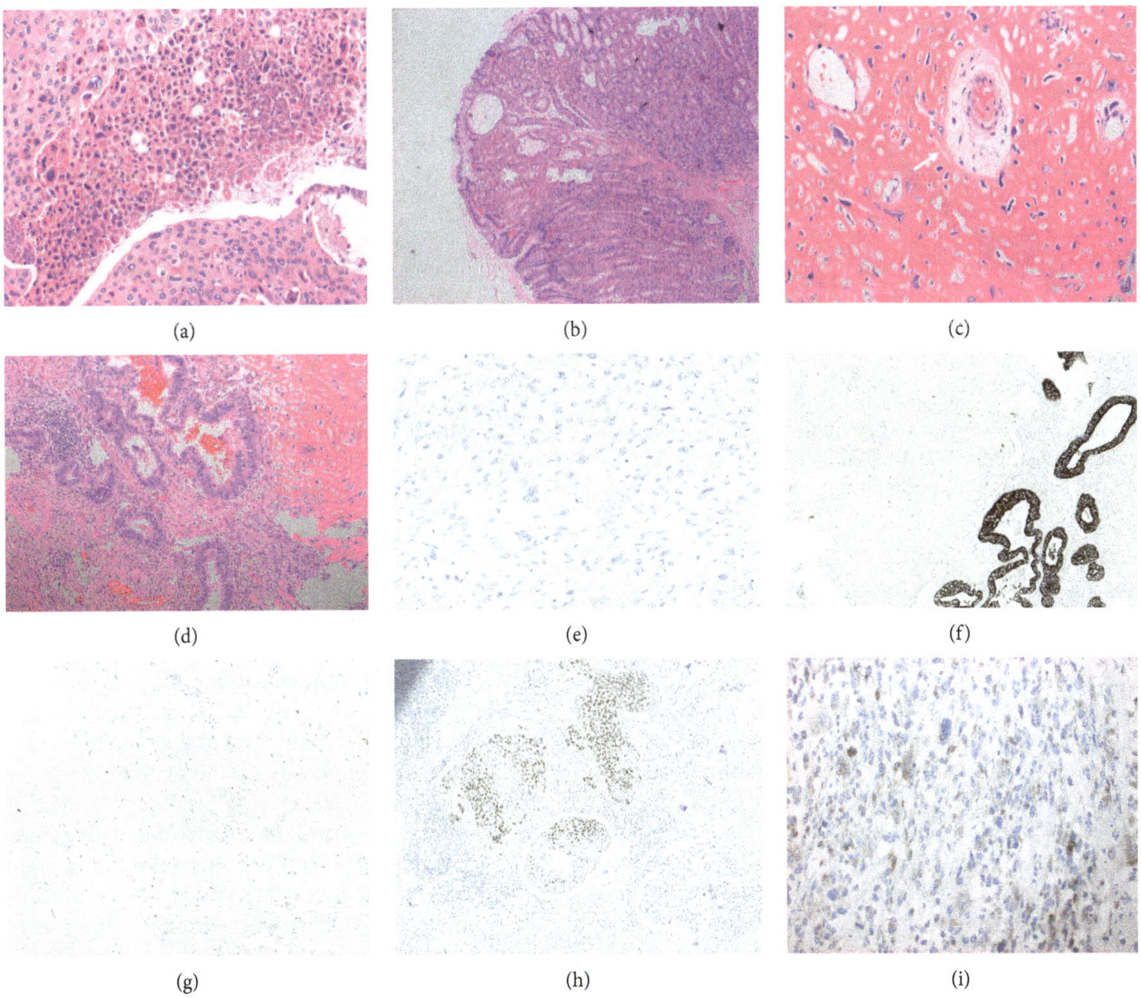

FIGURE 3: Continued.

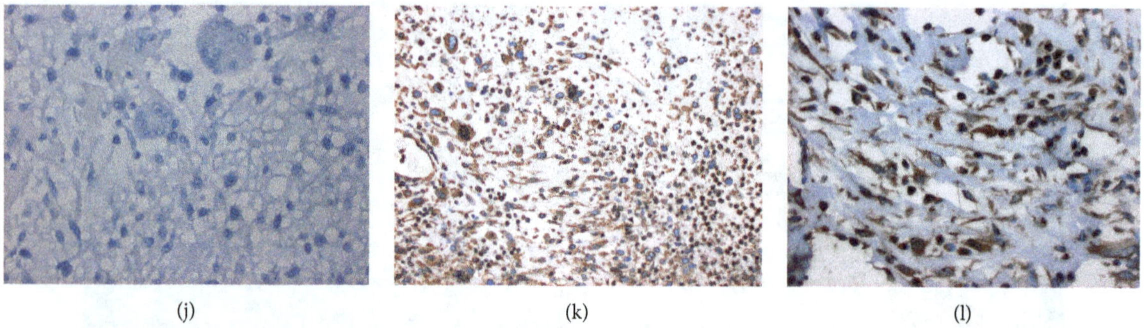

FIGURE 3: Microscopic pathology of the tumor. (a–d) Microscopic images of a fungating polyp. (a) Sheets of squamous cells displayed malignant features including large cell size and keratinization, providing evidence of squamous-cell carcinoma at 10x magnification. (b) The tumor arose in the background of a fundic gland polyp at 4x magnification. (c) Regions of the tumor and the entire lymph node metastasis displayed osteosarcomatous differentiation, evidenced by osteoid (pink) and associated atypical enlarged spindled cells at 20x magnification. (d) Evidence of both adenocarcinoma (left) and osteosarcoma (right) in the same fungating polyp tissue at 10x magnification. (e, f) AE1/AE3 staining. (e) Sarcomatous tissue of the tumor stained negative for AE1/AE3 seen at 20x magnification. (f) Adenocarcinoma component of the main tumor stained positive for AE1/AE3 imaged at 10x magnification. (g) Osteosarcoma component of the main tumor stained negative for AE1/AE3 at 10x magnification. (h) The squamous-cell carcinoma component was positive for P40 seen at 10x magnification. (i) The undifferentiated pleomorphic sarcoma was focally CD138 positive imaged at 20x magnification. (j) Beta-hCG was negative in giant cells, ruling out a choriocarcinoma component, seen at 20x magnification. (k) The undifferentiated pleomorphic sarcoma with osteoclast-like giant cells component was diffusely vimentin positive, seen at 10x magnification. (l) The osteosarcoma component of tumor was vimentin positive, imaged at 10x magnification.

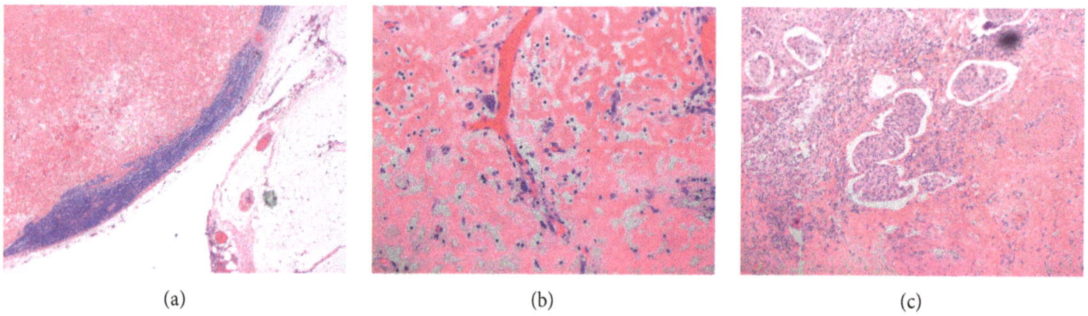

FIGURE 4: Evidence of lymph node metastasis. (a) Osteoid (pink) from osteosarcoma metastasis seen in a lymph node at low power (4x). Note the blue lymphoid cuff on the rim of the lymph node just under the capsule, identifying it as a largely replaced lymph node. (b) Osteoid and atypical spindled cells from osteosarcoma were found in a distant lymph node (higher power of (a) at 20x magnification). (c) Squamous lymphovascular invasion in the main tumor at 10x magnification. Squamous-cell tumor plugs displayed invasion in the lymphatic system.

The pathogenesis of gastric carcinosarcoma is still debated, but there are 2 main theories. The first includes the biclonal origin hypothesis, which suggests that 2 separate tumor cell clones collide. The second theory is the monoclonal origin hypothesis, which indicates that a stem cell is able to differentiate into both epithelial and mesenchymal cells [4]. Sarcomas rarely metastasize to lymph nodes, but they are more likely to do so if they have an epithelioid subtype [5]. In this case, osteosarcoma was found to have metastasized to a lymph node, thus supporting the monoclonal origin theory.

In most patients, the carcinomatous portion of the carcinosarcoma involves adenocarcinoma, but a few reports have described an adenocarcinoma with neuroendocrine differentiation [6] or adenosquamous carcinoma [7], as in our case. The sarcomatous portion of carcinosarcomas is variable, but they can include leiomyosarcoma, rhabdomyosarcoma, and osteosarcoma or can be undifferentiated [8]. The sarcomatous components in the current case included osteosarcoma and UPS with osteoclast-like giant cells. The presence of bone differentiation caused gastric adenocarcinoma with osseous differentiation to be included in the differential diagnosis; however, in that entity, the osseous component is benign, while the osseous component in our case had malignant spindled cells [9]. The presence of osteoclast-like giant cells associated with a carcinoma raised the possibility of primary gastric choriocarcinoma in the differential diagnosis; however, that was not consistent with the observed hCG negativity and cytokeratin negativity in the sarcomatous component, as seen in Figures 3(e)–3(j) [10]. The presence of discohesive individual cells with rare CD138 positivity (Figure 3(i)) raised the possibility of a gastric carcinoma with plasmacytoid morphology [11]; however, the discohesive cells staining weakly for CD138 were cytokeratin negative (Figure 3(e)) and vimentin positive (Figure 3(k)), supporting the diagnosis of carcinosarcoma.

Clinical features of this neoplasm are nonspecific but most commonly include epigastric pain, weight loss, and melena

[3]. The treatment for most patients involves surgical resection by total gastrectomy [1], while some patients undergo chemotherapy [4]. Our case was unique in that the patient was treated with a robotic partial gastrectomy, rather than a total gastrectomy. This approach was used to achieve improved functional outcomes in this elderly patient, while also preserving oncologic principles of wide margins and lymphadenectomy. The unique pathology also made this case very interesting and challenging to treat. Close surveillance will be needed postoperatively to monitor for metastases or recurrence of the gastric tumor. A review of the literature did not reveal a standard postoperative treatment of this disease.

The prognosis for patients with carcinosarcoma remains quite poor, with a mean survival period estimated to be 7–10 months, with 50% of recurrences occurring within the first year postoperatively [12]. To our knowledge, only 6 cases [1, 4, 13–15], including ours, have been diagnosed at an early stage thus far. Interestingly, 4 of the 6 cases showed regional lymph node metastasis, demonstrating the aggressive nature of this tumor. Early identification remains crucial to preventing recurrences and metastasis of this aggressive tumor.

4. Conclusion

Gastric carcinosarcoma is rare and has a poor prognosis. Although surgical resection may improve outcomes, the tumor is aggressive and has often already metastasized before diagnosis. The present study explored the clinical findings, diagnosis, and prognosis of gastric carcinosarcoma. Continued research in this area is required to lessen the burden of this rare disease.

Acknowledgments

The authors thank Dr. Paul Berard, the medical oncologist on this case, for valuable discussion and comments on this case.

References

[1] A. Shioya, N. Kurose, K. Mizutani et al., "Early-stage multi-differentiated gastric carcinosarcoma and post-resection local recurrence: a case report," *Diagnostic Pathology*, vol. 15, no. 1, p. 118, 2020.

[2] O. Gotoh, Y. Sugiyama, Y. Takazawa et al., "Clinically relevant molecular subtypes and genomic alteration-independent differentiation in gynecologic carcinosarcoma," *Nature Communications*, vol. 10, no. 1, Article ID 4965, 2019.

[3] L. Nie, X. Zhou, L. Peng, Y. Fu, Y. Cheng, and Q. Huang, "Histological heterogeneity and distributional difference of gastric carcinosarcoma: report of 4 cases and literature review," *Polish Journal of Pathology*, vol. 69, no. 4, pp. 366–375, 2018.

[4] H. Kuroda, H. Saito, Y. Kono et al., "Carcinosarcoma of stomach confined to the mucosa," *Yonago Acta Medica*, vol. 60, no. 4, pp. 246–250, 2018.

[5] Y. Fong, D. G. Coit, J. M. Woodruff, and M. F. Brennan, "Lymph node metastasis from soft tissue sarcoma in adults analysis of data from a prospective database of 1772 sarcoma patients," *Annals of Surgery*, vol. 217, no. 1, pp. 72–77, 1993.

[6] N. Kuroda, K. Oonishi, S. Iwamura et al., "Gastric carcinosarcoma with neuroendocrine differentiation as the carcinoma component and leiomyosarcomatous and myofibroblastic differentiation as the sarcomatous component. case report," *Apmis*, vol. 114, no. 3, pp. 234-238, 2006.

[7] Y. Sato, T. Shimozono, S. Kawano et al., "Gastric carcinosarcoma, coexistence of adenosquamous carcinoma and rhabdomyosarcoma: a case report," *Histopathology*, vol. 39, no. 5, pp. 543-544, 2001.

[8] R. Cirocchi, S. Trastulli, J. Desiderio et al., "Gastric carcinosarcoma: a case report and review of the literature," *Oncology Letters*, vol. 4, no. 1, pp. 53–57, 2012.

[9] C. D. Olinici, I. Domşa, A. Drăghici, and V. Munteanu, "Heterotopic bone formation in gastric carcinoma. case report and discussion of the literature," *Romanian Journal of Gastroenterology*, vol. 11, no. 4, pp. 331–333, 2002.

[10] S. Gurzu, C. Copotoiu, A. Tugui, C. Kwizera, R. Szodorai, and I. Jung, "Primary gastric choriocarcinoma-a rare and aggressive tumor with multilineage differentiation: a case report," *World Journal of Clinical Cases*, vol. 7, no. 14, pp. 1837–1843, 2019.

[11] Z. Kovacs, S. Gurzu, C. Molnar et al., "Gastrointestinal carcinoma with plasmacytoid morphology: positivity for c-MET, arylsulfatase, and markers of epithelial-mesenchymal transition, as indicators of aggressivity," *Journal of Oncology*, vol. 2019, Article ID 5836821, 11 pages, 2019.

[12] Y. Li, L. Cui, Y. Chen, and F. Wang, "Carcinosarcoma and sarcomatoid carcinoma of the stomach," *Medicine*, vol. 100, no. 12, 2021.

[13] G. Uno, Y. Miyaoka, K. Hukazawa et al., "A case report of gastric carcinosarcoma with abdominal fullness caused by invagination of the tumor into duodenal bulbus," *Gastroenterological Endoscopy*, vol. 53, pp. 3272–3279, 2011.

[14] Y. Yuasa, H. Okitsu, T. Furukawa, A. Kihara, M. Yamashita, and N. Okitsu, "A case of true gastric carcinosarcoma treated using laparoscopy-assisted distal gastrectomy," *Nihon Rinsho Geka Gakkai Zasshi (Journal of Japan Surgical Association)*, vol. 73, no. 5, pp. 1110–1114, 2012.

[15] H. Fujii, K. Iwase, J. Higaki, S. Mikata, M. Imakita, and W. Kamiike, "A case of gastric carcinosarcoma accompaniede by gastric gastrointestinal stromal tumor," *Nihon Rinsho Geka Gakkai Zasshi (Journal of Japan Surgical Association)*, vol. 63, no. 12, pp. 2934–2937, 2002.

9

A Case of Ileocecal IgG4-Related Sclerosing Mesenteritis Diagnosed by Endoscopic Ultrasound-Guided Fine Needle Aspiration using Forward-Viewing Linear Echoendoscope

Yuichi Takano ,[1] Fumitaka Niiya,[1] Takahiro Kobayashi,[1] Eiichi Yamamura ,[1] Naotaka Maruoka,[1] Tomoko Norose,[2] Nobuyuki Ohike,[2] and Masatsugu Nagahama [1]

[1]*Division of Gastroenterology, Department of Internal Medicine, Showa University Fujigaoka Hospital, Yokohama, Kanagawa, Japan*
[2]*Department of Diagnostic Pathology, Showa University Fujigaoka Hospital, Yokohama, Kanagawa, Japan*

Correspondence should be addressed to Yuichi Takano; yuichitakano1028@yahoo.co.jp

Academic Editor: Yucel Ustundag

A 25-year-old woman had undergone removal of a cryptogenic tumor in the left maxillary sinus 1 year prior to presentation. The patient experienced abdominal pain for 4 days with repeated vomiting episodes; therefore, she was transferred to our hospital by an ambulance. Contrast-enhanced computed tomography revealed a 3-cm tumor in the ileocecal region, which caused small bowel obstruction. Contrast imaging of the ileus tube showed extrinsic compression of the ileocecal region. Forward-viewing linear echoendoscope revealed an irregular hypoechoic tumor measuring 3 cm outside the gastrointestinal tract. Using a 25G needle, endoscopic ultrasound-guided fine needle aspiration (EUS–FNA) was performed. Pathological finding was an inflammatory fibrous tissue with diffuse lymphoplasmacytic infiltration, with more than 10 IgG4-positive cells detected in a high-power field. Re-examination of a pathology specimen of the maxillary sinus tumor provided by the previous attending physician revealed that the inflammatory tissue had diffuse lymphoplasmacytic infiltration, which were accompanied by storiform fibrosis and obliterative phlebitis. Immunostaining revealed more than 50 IgG4-positive cells in a high-power field, a finding suggestive of IgG4-related disease. The serum IgG4 level was 21 mg/dl, which was within the normal range. Treatment was initiated with prednisolone at a dose of 50 mg/day, and the dose was later tapered off. CT and MRI performed 2 months later showed complete disappearance of the ileocecal tumor. The final diagnosis was asynchronously occurring IgG4-related maxillary sinusitis and sclerosing mesenteritis.

1. Introduction

IgG4-related disease (IgG4-RD) is an idiopathic inflammatory disorder that affects organs throughout the body [1]. It is characterized by swelling of the affected organs, increase in serum IgG4 level, peculiar histological findings (diffuse lymphoplasmacytic infiltration, storiform fibrosis, obliterative phlebitis, and numerous IgG4-positive cells), and good response to steroid treatment. The most commonly affected organs include the pancreas, parotid glands, lacrimal glands, retroperitoneum (around the aorta), and kidneys, with occurrence in the gastrointestinal tract, spleen, and brain (excluding the pituitary gland) considered rare [2].

Sclerosing mesenteritis is also an inflammatory disease of unknown origin [3]. In recent years, few cases of sclerosing mesenteritis possibly associated with IgG4-RD have been reported [3–12]. These cases were diagnosed by surgical resection or surgical biopsy (laparoscopic biopsy), with no reports available on cases diagnosed by endoscopic ultrasound-guided fine needle aspiration (EUS-FNA). In this study, we report a case of ileocecal IgG4-related sclerosing mesenteritis diagnosed by EUS-FNA using forward-viewing linear echoendoscope. Because the patient showed good response to steroid treatment, surgery could be avoided.

2. Case Presentation

A 25-year-old woman had undergone tumor removal in the left maxillary sinus at the Otolaryngology Department of another hospital 1 year prior to presentation. Pathological diagnosis was inflammatory pseudotumor of unknown origin.

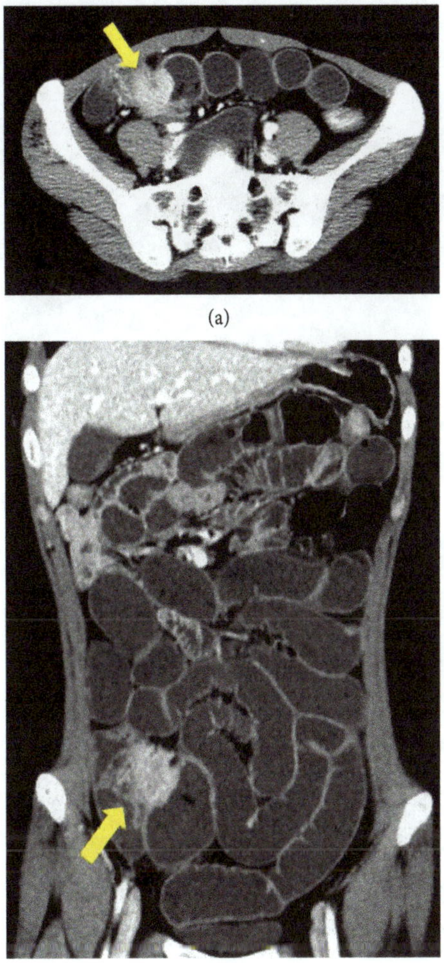

(a)

(b)

Figure 1: (a), (b) CECT showing a 3-cm hypervascular tumor (arrow) in the ileocecal region accompanied by small bowel obstruction.

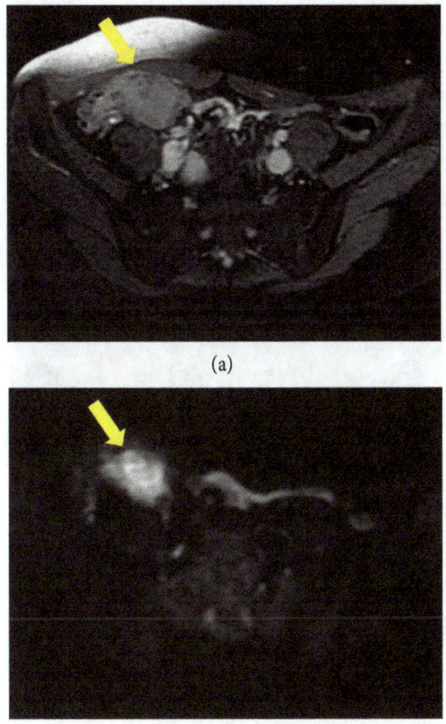

(a)

(b)

Figure 2: (a) MRI T2-weighted images showing mild high intensity lesions in the ileocecal region (arrow). (b) MRI diffusion-weighted images showing decreased diffusion in lesions (arrow).

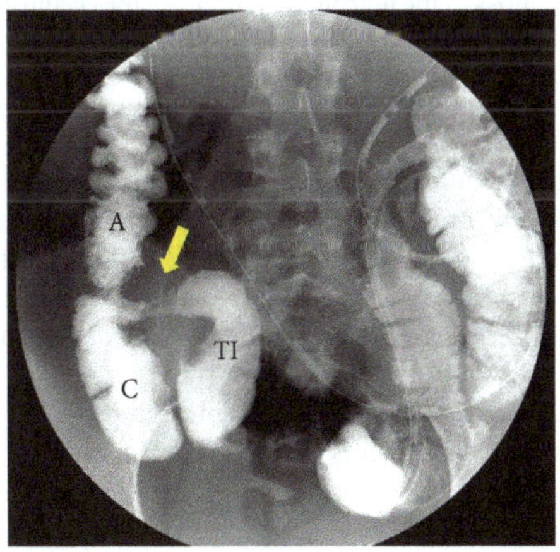

Figure 3: Contrast imaging of the ileus tube showing extrinsic compression of the ileocecal region (arrow). TI: terminal ileum, C: cecum, A: Ascending colon.

The patient had no remarkable family history and did not consume alcohol or smoke. Owing to intermittent abdominal pain for 4 days and frequent vomiting in the morning of the examination day, the patient was transported by ambulance. On arrival, her vital signs were as follows: body temperature, 36.1°C; blood pressure, 115/85 mmHg; and heart rate, 86 beats/min. Physical examination revealed severe tenderness in the right lower abdomen. There were no signs of rebound pain or muscle guarding. Blood test showed WBC count and CRP level of 16740/μl and 10.33 mg/dl, respectively, indicating increased inflammatory response. Further, biochemical measurements were as follows: IgA, 215 mg/dl; IgM, 175 mg/dl; IgE, 246 IU/ml; IgG, 1275 mg/dl; IgG4, 21 mg/dl; ANA, negative; ds-DNA Ab, negative; PR3-ANCA, negative; and MPO-ANCA, negative. No findings were suggestive of an autoimmune disease or vasculitis. The serum IgG4 level was within the normal range. Tumor marker levels were as follows: sIL-2R, 611 U/ml; CA19-9, 9.6 U/ml; and CEA, 2.4 ng/ml; a slight increase in sIL-2R level was observed.

Contrast-enhanced computed tomography (CECT) showed a 3-cm hypervascular tumor in the ileocecal region, revealing small bowel obstruction (Figure 1). The lesion emitted slightly high intensity on simple magnetic resonance imaging (MRI) T2-weighted images and showed decreased diffusion on diffusion-weighted images (DWI) (Figure 2). Accordingly, an ileus tube was rapidly placed after hospitalization. Contrast imaging of the ileus tube showed extrinsic compression of the ileocecal region (Figure 3). While endoscopy of the lower gastrointestinal tract revealed no abnormalities in the mucous membrane of the ileum and cecum, the terminal ileum exhibited extramural compression (Figure 4).

Based on the findings, an extraintestinal tumor of the ileocecal region and small bowel obstruction were diagnosed.

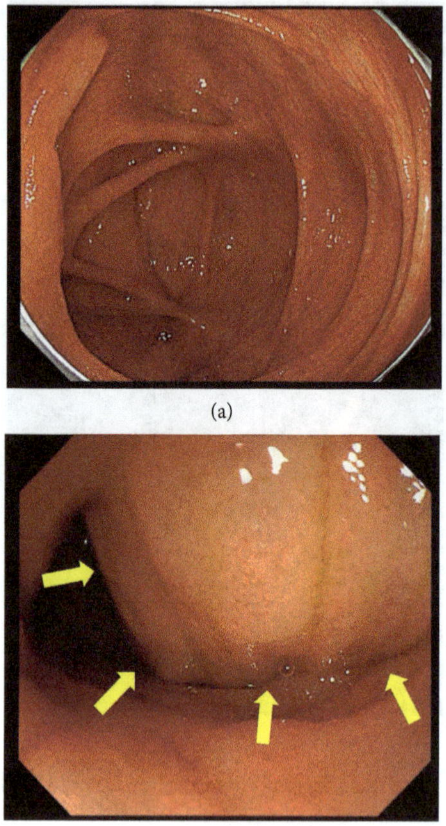

(a)

(b)

FIGURE 4: (a) Endoscopy of the lower gastrointestinal tract showing no abnormalities in the mucous membrane of the cecum and ileum. (b) Extramural compression was detected in the terminal ileum (arrow).

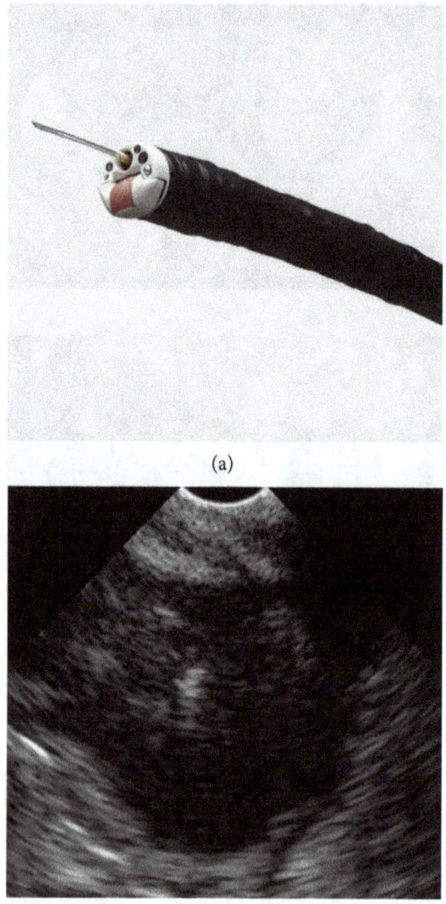

(a)

(b)

FIGURE 5: (a) Forward-viewing linear echoendoscope, TGF-UC180J (Olympus Medical Systems Corp, Tokyo, Japan). (b) EUS revealed an irregular hypoechoic tumor measuring 3 cm outside the gastrointestinal tract.

Differential diagnoses included gastrointestinal stromal tumor (GIST), schwannoma, malignant lymphoma, adenocarcinoma, and inflammatory pseudotumor. Although we considered performing ileocecal resection, we decided to first implement preoperative histological examination after consultation with the surgical department.

A forward-viewing linear echoendoscope (TGF-UC180J, Olympus Medical Systems Corp, Tokyo, Japan) was inserted into the cecum, which revealed a 3-cm hypoechoic tumor with clear boundaries and irregular periphery outside the gastrointestinal tract (Figure 5). Using a 25G needle (Expect™ SlimLine, Boston Scientific Japan, Tokyo, Japan), two sessions of EUS-FNA were performed (Supplementary Video available here). The procedure was completed without any complications. Pathologically, the lesion was found to comprise inflammatory fibrous tissues with lymphoplasmacytic infiltration, and more than 10 IgG4-positive cells were detected in a high-power field (HPF) (Figure 6). While IgG staining was difficult because it involved co-staining, the IgG4/IgG ratio exceeded 40%.

Images and pathological specimens of the maxillary sinus tumor provided by the previous attending doctor were re-evaluated. Contrast-enhanced MRI revealed an irregular tumor showing contrast in the left maxillary sinus (Figure 7). Histologically, the lesion was an inflammatory tissue containing diffuse lymphoplasmacytic infiltration accompanied by storiform fibrosis and obliterative phlebitis. Immunostaining revealed more than 50 IgG4-positive cells in an HPF, which was consistent with IgG4-RD (Figure 7). IgG staining was difficult because it involved co-staining. There were no abnormal findings in other organs throughout the body (lacrimal salivary gland, mediastinal and hilar lymph node, lung, pancreas, bile duct, kidney, artery).

The patient was diagnosed with IgG4-related maxillary sinusitis and sclerosing mesenteritis. The patient weighed 52 kg and prednisolone was started at a dose of 50 mg as 1 mg/kg, which was later tapered off. CT and MRI performed 2 months later showed complete disappearance of the ileocecal tumor (Figure 8). The patient received maintenance therapy with 5 mg/day prednisolone for 1 year thereafter, and IgG4-RD recurrence was not observed.

3. Discussion

In 2001, Hamano et al. reported that serum IgG4 is a marker specific to autoimmune pancreatitis [13]. They later demonstrated IgG4-positive cell infiltration in the pancreatic tissue

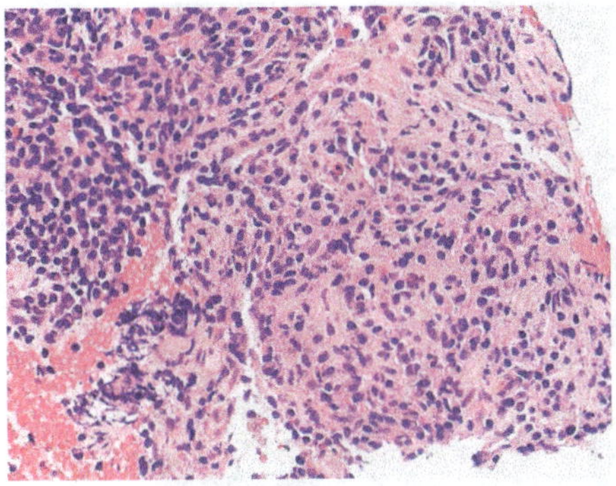

(a)

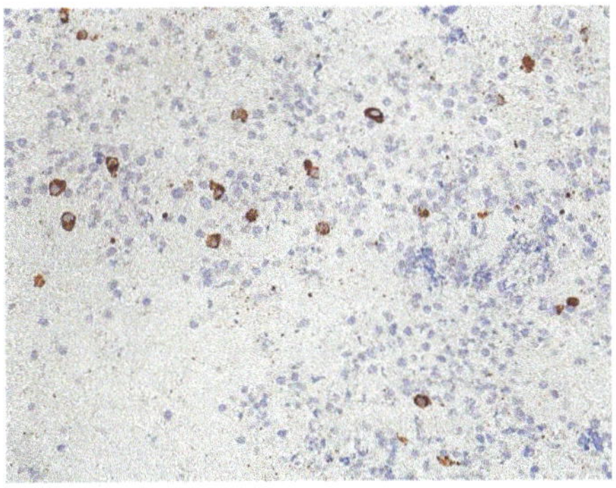

(b)

Figure 6: (a) A specimen obtained by EUS-FNA. Pathologically, the lesion was found to be composed of inflammatory fibrous tissues with lymphoplasmacytic infiltration (Hematoxylin-Eosin Stain, x400). (b) IgG4 staining revealed more than 10 IgG4-positive cells in an HPF (IgG4 Stain x400).

[14]. Another study discovered an inflammatory fibrous disease characterized by increased serum IgG4 level and IgG4-positive cell infiltration in general organs, thereby establishing a novel concept of IgG4-RD [1, 15].

In recent years, few cases of sclerosing mesenteritis possibly associated with IgG4 have been reported. A PubMed search of studies published in 2000–2019 was conducted using the keywords "IgG4" and "sclerosing mesenteritis," and a total of 17 cases (those with ≥10 IgG4-positive cells, excluding reports with fewer or an unspecified number of cells) were found [3–12].

We examined a total of 18 cases including our case (Table 1). The mean age of the patients was 58 years (range: 25–82 years), male: female ratio was 12:6, and mean serum IgG4 level was 95 mg/dl (range: 21–171 mg/dl). Further, the mean IgG4-positive cell count in an HPF was 63 (range: 10–100). Two cases complicated other organ involvements, and the breakdown was retroperitoneal fibrosis and maxillary sinusitis. Regarding diagnostic method, 15 cases underwent surgical resection and 2 underwent laparoscopic biopsy. Only our case was diagnosed with EUS-FNA. None of the cases received steroids except our case. For the 2 cases diagnosed by laparoscopic biopsy, clinical progress was followed up without treatment, and the tumors eventually showed reduction in size [8].

In conclusion, this condition is common among middle-aged men. The serum IgG4 level tends to be within the normal range or slightly increased, and other organ involvements are uncommon. Approximately 90% of the cases were diagnosed by surgical resection, which suggests the difficulty in preoperative diagnosis. Although the first option for the treatment of IgG4-RD is steroid, no cases were treated with steroids other than our case.

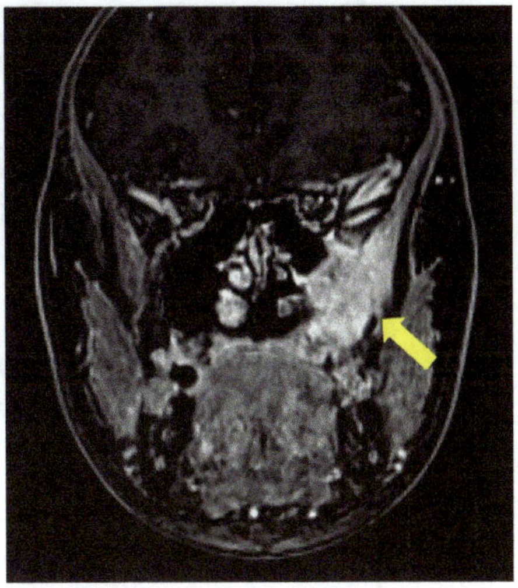

(a)

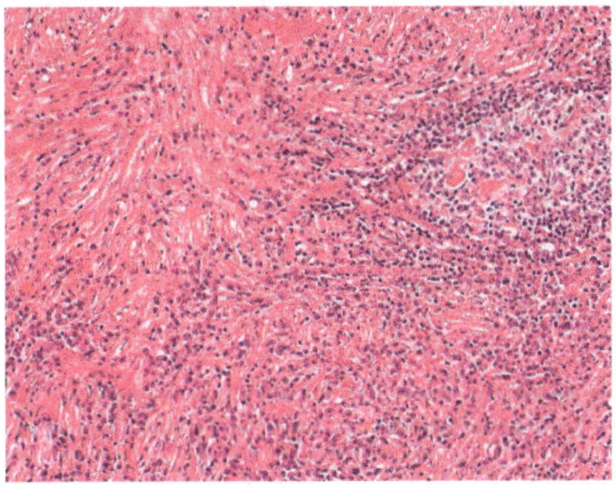

(b)

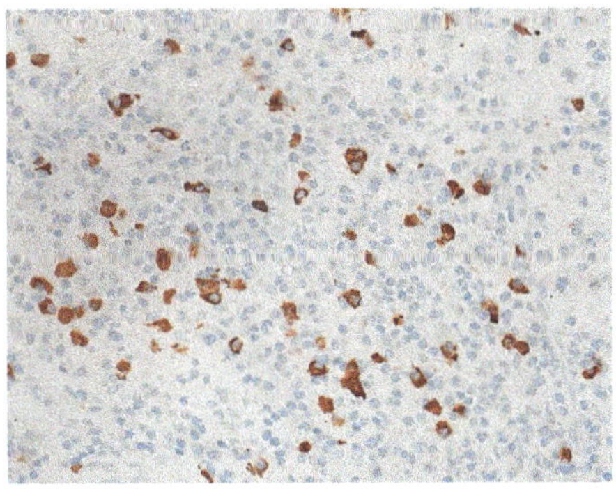

(c)

Figure 7: (a) Contrast-enhanced MRI showing an irregular tumor in the left maxillary sinus (arrow). (b) Pathologically, diffuse lymphoplasmacytic infiltration and storiform fibrosis are observed (Hematoxylin-Eosin Stain, x200). (c) More than 50 IgG4-positive cells are observed in an HPF (IgG4 Stain, x400).

To date, no cases have been diagnosed using EUS-FNA, possibly because lesions tend to be present in deep parts of the gastrointestinal tract, making paracentesis difficult. At present, oblique-viewing linear echoendoscope is usually employed for

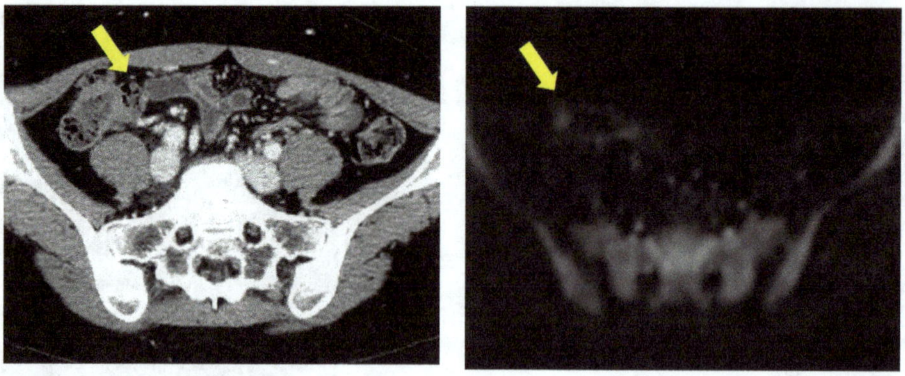

(a) (b)

FIGURE 8: (a) CECT showing complete disappearance of the tumor at 2 months after steroid treatment (arrow). (b) MRI diffusion-weighted images indicate the absence of any lesion (arrow).

TABLE 1: Literature cases.

Case	Age	Sex	Serum IgG4 (mg/dl)	IgG4 positive cells/HPF	Other organ involvement	Diagnosis method	Corticosrereoid	Reference
1	48	F	NA	12	None	Resection	No	[3]
2	74	M	NA	>100	None	Resection	No	[3]
3	46	M	NA	>100	None	Resection	No	[3]
4	52	M	NA	13	None	Resection	No	[3]
5	63	F	NA	16	None	Resection	No	[3]
6	65	M	NA	16	None	Resection	No	[3]
7	82	F	171	130	None	Resection	No	[4]
8	42	M	119	60	None	Resection	No	[5]
9	53	M	127	75	None	Resection	No	[6]
10	64	M	81	38	Retroperitoneal fibrosis	Resection	No	[7]
11	76	M	63.5	56	None	Laparoscopic biopsy	No	[8]
12	77	M	43.2	46	None	Laparoscopic biopsy	No	[8]
13	54	M	105	85	None	Resection	No	[8]
14	77	F	114	253	None	Resection	No	[9]
15	56	F	164	33	None	Resection	No	[10]
16	25	M	90	>50	None	Resection	No	[11]
17	60	M	47	>40	None	Resection	No	[12]
Our case	25	F	21	>10	Maxillary sinusitis	EUS-FNA	Yes	

EUS-FNA. However, in the present case, EUS-FNA was performed from the cecum. Because inserting an oblique-viewing echoendoscope into the cecum involved the risk of intestinal damage and perforation, a forward-viewing echoendoscope was used instead. The puncture was from the lower gastrointestinal tract and there was a risk of perforation and peritonitis. Therefore, EUS-FNA using a thin needle (25G) was performed. The procedure was performed without complications. Even with a 25G needle, enough specimens were obtained, and immunostaining could be performed easily.

In many cases, preoperative diagnoses of malignant diseases, such as GIST, malignant lymphoma, and cancer, are done based on imaging, resulting in surgeries being performed without biopsies. However, in the case of IgG4-RD, steroid is usually effective in shrinking lesions [1]. As such, performing preoperative biopsies is critical. Unnecessary surgery should be avoided as much as possible, particularly in young patients. In the present case, the lesion disappeared after steroid treatment, and small bowel obstruction improved without surgery. Therefore, EUS-FNA proved to be highly beneficial for the patient.

While the serum IgG4 level in our patient was within the normal range, not all patients with IgG4-RD exhibit increased serum IgG4 levels. In fact, an international study revealed that among patients who are histologically diagnosed with type 1 autoimmune pancreatitis (a pancreatic manifestation of

IgG4-RD), 37% had normal serum IgG4 levels [16]. In particular, an increase in the serum IgG4 level tends to be subdued in cases of IgG4-related sclerosing mesenteritis. Histological examination needs to be proactively performed rather than relying solely on serum IgG4 findings.

Recently, cases wherein the serum IgG4 level was normal and IgG4-positive cells were scarcely detected despite showing typical pathological findings of IgG4-RD (storiform fibrosis, obliterative phlebitis, and diffuse lymphoplasmacytic infiltration) have been reported [17–19]. Therefore, further research is warranted because IgG4 may not be a prerequisite for the pathology of the disease.

The elevation of WBC and CRP is not a typical findings in IgG4 related disease. The patient had a bowel obstruction due to the lesion, and it took several days to visit our hospital. Inflammation due to intestinal obstruction may have caused a mild increase in inflammatory response (WBC and CRP).

The diagnosis of IgG4-related sclerosing mesenteritis is still debatable. Avincsal et al. reported that although sclerosing mesenteritis shares histological characteristics with IgG4-RD, given the scarcity of cases with elevated serum IgG4 and other organ involvements, it is possible that many of them are not IgG4-related [8]. They concluded that the possibility of IgG4-RD resulting in lesions in the mesentery is extremely rare.

According to the pathological consensus regarding IgG4-RD published in 2012, a lesion needs to meet the following criteria (at least 3, ideally 4) to be considered an IgG4-RD in a new organ [20]: (1) characteristic pathological findings; (2) increase in serum IgG4 level; (3) good response to steroid treatment; and (4) IgG4-RD in other organs. The present case satisfied criteria 1, 3, and 4, which was considered adequate evidence to warrant the diagnosis of IgG4-related sclerosing mesenteritis.

We treated a case of IgG4-related maxillary sinusitis and sclerosing mesenteritis occurring asynchronously. Although the serum IgG4 level was within the normal range, histological findings and the patient's good response to steroid treatment were consistent with IgG4-RD. Although extremely rare, IgG4-related sclerosing mesenteritis does appear to exist. Biopsies need to be proactively performed to avoid unnecessary surgical interventions. Forward-viewing echoendoscope is useful for conducting biopsy from the deep gastrointestinal tract.

References

[1] J. H. Stone, Y. Zen, and V. Deshpande, "IgG4-related disease," *New England Journal of Medicine*, vol. 366, no. 6, pp. 539–551, 2012.

[2] D. Inoue, K. Yoshida, N. Yoneda et al., "IgG4-related disease: dataset of 235 consecutive patients," *Medicine*, vol. 94, no. 15, p. e680, 2015.

[3] T. S. Chen and E. A. Montgomery, "Are tumefactive lesions classified as sclerosing mesenteritis a subset of IgG4-related sclerosing disorders?" *Journal of Clinical Pathology*, vol. 61, no. 10, pp. 1093–1097, 2008.

[4] Y. Nomura, Y. Naito, N. Eriguchi et al., "A case of IgG4-related sclerosing mesenteritis," *Pathology - Research Practice*, vol. 207, no. 8, pp. 518–521, 2011.

[5] C. Salvarani, R. Valli, L. Boiardi, N. Pipitone, F. Nicoli, and F. Muratore, "IgG4-associated sclerosing mesenteritis," *Clinical and Experimental Rheumatology*, vol. 29, no. 1 Suppl 64, pp. S79–S80, 2011.

[6] H. Minato, J. Shimizu, Y. Arano et al., "IgG4-related sclerosing mesenteritis: a rare mesenteric disease of unknown etiology," *Pathology International*, vol. 62, no. 4, pp. 281–286, 2012.

[7] E. Mori, T. Kamisawa, T. Tabata et al., "A case of IgG4-related mesenteritis," *Clinical Journal of Gastroenterology*, vol. 8, no. 6, pp. 400–405, 2015.

[8] M. O. Avincsal, K. Otani, M. Kanzawa et al., "Sclerosing mesenteritis: A real manifestation or histological mimic of IgG4-related disease?" *Pathology International*, vol. 66, no. 3, pp. 158–163, 2016.

[9] A. Abe, T. Manabe, N. Takizawa et al., "IgG4-related sclerosing mesenteritis causing bowel obstruction: a case report," *Surgical Case Reports*, vol. 2, no. 1, p. 120, 2016.

[10] A. Greenbaum, N. Yadak, S. Perez, and A. Rajput, "Surgical management of isolated mesenteric autoimmune disease: addressing the spectrum of IgG(4)-related disease and sclerosing mesenteritis," *BMJ Case Reports*, vol. 2017, p. bcr- 017-220400, 2017.

[11] M. L. Á. Mejías Manzano, C. Trigo Salado, M. Serrano Jiménez, M. J. Parada Blázquez, and E. Leo Carnerero, "IgG4-related sclerosing mesenteritis, a rare condition that causes abdominal pain," *Revista Española de Enfermedades Digestivas*, vol. 110, pp. 201–203, 2018.

[12] Z. Butt, S. Alam, H. Semeniuk, O. S. Singh, G. S. Chhabra, and I. J. Tan, "A Case of IgG4-related Sclerosing Mesenteritis," *Cureus*, vol. 10, p. e2147, 2018.

[13] H. Hamano, S. Kawa, A. Horiuchi et al., "High serum IgG4 concentrations in patients with sclerosing pancreatitis," *New England Journal of Medicine*, vol. 344, no. 10, pp. 732–738, 2001.

[14] H. Hamano, S. Kawa, Y. Ochi et al., "Hydronephrosis associated with retroperitoneal fibrosis and sclerosing pancreatitis," *The Lancet*, vol. 359, no. 9315, pp. 1403–1404, 2002.

[15] H. Hamano, N. Arakura, T. Muraki, Y. Ozaki, K. Kiyosawa, and S. Kawa, "Prevalence and distribution of extrapancreatic lesions complicating autoimmune pancreatitis," *Journal of Gastroenterology*, vol. 41, no. 12, pp. 1197–1205, 2006.

[16] T. Kamisawa, S. T. Chari, S. A. Giday et al., "Clinical profile of autoimmune pancreatitis and its histological subtypes: an international multicenter survey," *Pancreas*, vol. 40, no. 6, pp. 809–814, 2011.

[17] E. Nakano, A. Kanno, A. Masamune et al., "IgG4-unrelated type 1 autoimmune pancreatitis," *World Journal of Gastroenterology*, vol. 21, no. 33, pp. 9808–9816, 2015.

[18] P. A. Hart, T. C. Smyrk, and S. T. Chari, "Lymphoplasmacytic sclerosing pancreatitis without IgG4 tissue infiltration or serum

IgG4 elevation: IgG4-related disease without IgG4," *Modern Pathology*, vol. 28, no. 2, pp. 238–247, 2015.

[19] Y. Takano, T. Kobayashi, F. Niiya et al., "Serum and histological IgG4-negative type 1 autoimmune pancreatitis," *Clinical Journal of Gastroenterology*, vol. 12, no. 3, pp. 232–238, 2019.

[20] V. Deshpande, Y. Zen, J. K. Chan et al., "Consensus statement on the pathology of IgG4-related disease," *Modern Pathology*, vol. 25, no. 9, pp. 1181–1192, 2012.

10

McKittrick–Wheelock Syndrome: A Rare Case of Secretory Diarrhea

Mohammad Nabil Rayad,[1] Noreen Mirza,[1] Maria Bernardeth Herrera-Gonzalez,[2] Yatinder Bains,[3] and Sarahi Herrera-Gonzalez[3]

[1]*Department of Internal Medicine, St Michael's Medical Center, 111 Central Ave, Newark, NJ 07102, USA*
[2]*Division of Health Sciences, University of Monterrey, Avenida Ignacio Morones Prieto 4500-Pte, San Pedro Garza Garcia, Nuevo Leon 66238, Mexico*
[3]*Department of Gastroenterology, St Michael's Medical Center, 111 Central Ave, Newark, NJ 07102, USA*

Correspondence should be addressed to Sarahi Herrera-Gonzalez; sarahi_h26@hotmail.com

Academic Editor: Daniel C. Damin

McKittrick–Wheelock syndrome commonly presents with a triad of chronic secretory diarrhea, electrolyte disturbances, and renal failure. Secretory diarrhea is due to active ion secretion secondary to secretagogue secretion (cyclic adenosine monophosphate and prostaglandin E2). The mainstay of treatment for these lesions is surgical since it will arrest the loss of electrolytes that may lead to serious clinical consequences. Nonsteroidal anti-inflammatory drugs (NSAIDs) such as indomethacin may be used to decrease electrolyte secretion in patients that desire a nonsurgical approach. Our patient is unique in that this is the first case of a tubular adenoma with high-grade dysplasia leading to MWS and progressing to circulatory collapse with severe electrolyte disturbances. Aggressive replacement of fluids and electrolytes is essential to the survival of these patients.

1. Introduction

Diarrhea is multifactorial in nature and is defined by an increase in stool frequency, volume, or fluidity. Diarrhea is caused by an imbalance in two processes which occur simultaneously including either an increase in the level of section or a decrease in the amount of absorption [1]. There are two main types of diarrheas including secretory or osmotic. Osmotic diarrhea occurs due to production of a gradient by certain nonabsorbable substances [1]. Decreased water absorption and increased secretion due to disrupted epithelial transport of electrolytes cause secretory diarrhea [1]. In secretory diarrhea, stool volume persists regardless of the fasting state and the osmolar gap is usually <50; nonetheless, an osmolar gap of <100 is highly suggestive of secretory diarrhea [2].

McKittrick–Wheelock syndrome is a rare cause of secretory diarrhea and was first reported in 1954 by McKittrick and Wheelock [3]. It is caused by a secretory colorectal tumor that is most frequently a villous adenoma and less commonly adenocarcinoma. These tumors tend to affect various age groups and have a high frequency of malignant conversion [3]. The most common location for these tumors includes the rectum. Furthermore, the complications of these secretory colorectal tumors include severe fluid and electrolyte losses [3]. The mainstay of treatment for these pathological entities includes surgical resection [3]. We present a case of a tubular adenoma with high-grade dysplasia as a cause of secretory diarrhea with hypovolemic shock.

2. Case Presentation

A 74-year-old male with history of hypertension, iron deficiency anemia, schizophrenia, and seizure disorder was brought to the hospital from a nursing home for the evaluation of watery diarrhea for several days followed by hypotension. As per reports from the nursing home, the patient

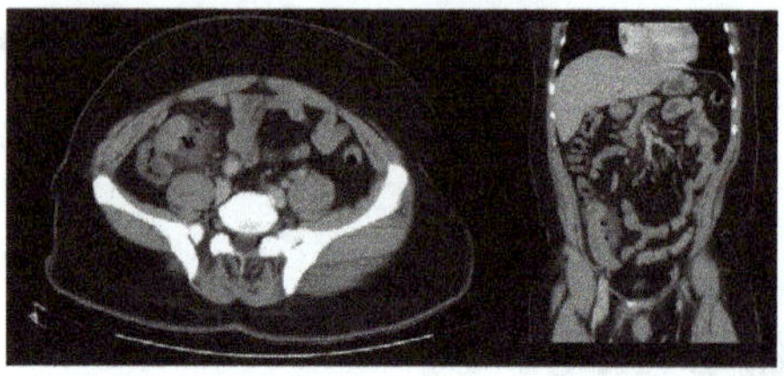

Figure 1: Computed tomography of the abdomen demonstrating mural thickening on the descending and ascending colon with adjacent fatty stranding.

had dementia at baseline oriented only to self and in recent months had become bedridden. On arrival to the hospital, the patient was presumed to be in septic shock with hypotension, tachycardia, and hypothermia. On physical examination, the patient was confused and severely malnourished, with mild diffuse abdominal tenderness and bilateral sacral and buttock pressure wounds. Initial evaluation revealed gross abnormalities with WBC of 106 10*3/μL (4.4–11.00 10*3/μL), Hb of 9.4 g/dL (13.5–17.5 g/dL), MCV of 78 fL (81.2–95.1 fL), platelets of 889 10*3/μL (150–450 10*3/μL), BUN of 59 mg/dL (6–24 mg/dL), Cr of 3.2 mg/dL (0.6–1.2 mg/dL), Na of 138 mmol/L (136–145 mmol/L), K of 4.8 mmol/L (3.5–5.3 mmol/L), Cl of 103 mmol/L (98–110 mmol/L), HCO3 of 12 mmol/L (20–31 mmol/L), and LA of 11.4 mmol/L (0–2 mmol/L). He received resuscitation with intravenous fluids and broad-spectrum antibiotics to which he did not successfully respond and required initiation of intravenous vasopressors. Septic workup was relevant for urinary tract infection. During the first days of hospitalization, a rectal tube was placed due to high volume diarrhea where daily output ranged from 3.2–4.5 liters daily.

Stool studies resulted negative for *Clostridium difficile* on three different occasions, cultures for Salmonella, Shigella, Campylobacter, E. coli O157:H7 were negative, as well as ova, parasite and cryptosporidium, Giardia lamblia antigens. Stool sodium was 89 mEq/L, and K was 21 mEq/L with a stool osmolar gap of 70 mOsm/kg. Fecal lactoferrin was 41.69 (μg/mL).

Computed tomography revealed mural thickening on the descending and ascending colon with adjacent fatty stranding (Figure 1).

Extensive workup for secretory diarrhea was obtained includinggastrin 66 pg/mL (0–115 pg/mL), urine 5HIAA 0.6 mg/24 hrs (0.0–14.9 mg/24 hrs), serotonin <5 ng/mL (21–321 ng/mL), AM cortisol 17.2 μg/dl (7–25 μg/dl), ACTH pg/mL (7.2–63.3 pg/mL), Insulin <1.0 μU/mL (0–17 μU/mL), C-Peptide 3.2 ng/mL (1.1–4.4 ng/mL), glucagon levels were not available at our laboratory. Despite aggressive fluid resuscitation, the patient remained hypotensive on vasopressors. A fasting challenge was done for 48 hrs with no change in diarrhea volume. Octreotide was initiated with three times daily subcutaneous octreotide injections and uptitrated up to 300 mcg without changes on output and hemodynamics. Flexible sigmoidoscopy revealed a fungating, partially obstructing large mass in the distal sigmoid colon about 25 cm from the anal verge (Figure 2).

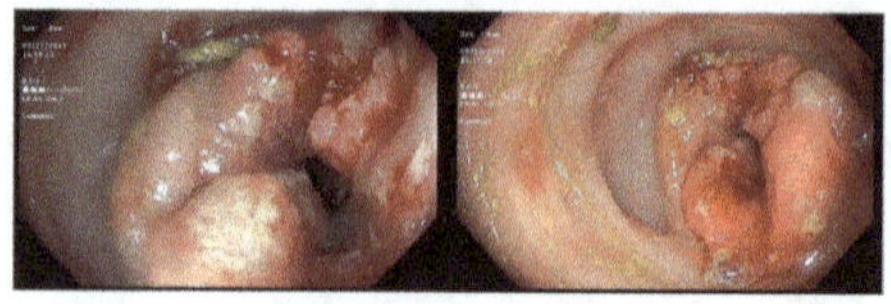

Figure 2: Flexible sigmoidoscopy showing a fungating partially obstructing large mass in the distal sigmoid colon, 25 cm away from anal verge.

Biopsies demonstrated fragments of a tubular adenoma with high-grade dysplasia (intramucosal adenocarcinoma) (Figure 3).

Oncology and surgical consultations were requested; however, the patient was not deemed a surgical or chemotherapy candidate due to functional status and poor overall condition. After discussion with family members, it was decided to withdraw life support and the patient succumbed to his disease.

3. Discussion

Diarrhea is multifactorial in nature and is defined by an increase in stool frequency, volume, or fluidity [1]. It is primarily caused due to the inability of the intestinal lumen to absorb water [1]. However, there are two main processes that can contribute to the development of diarrhea, the first being secretion and the second being absorption. These two mechanisms occur simultaneously; however, absorption tends to take longer. A decrease in the level of absorption or an increase in the level of secretion will lead to the accumulation of water in the lumen and therefore diarrhea will occur [1].

Diarrhea can be further categorized as osmotic or secretory. Osmotic diarrhea occurs when unabsorbed substances draw water from the plasma into the bowel lumen causing the production of an osmotic gradient [1]. On the other hand, decreased water absorption and increased secretion due to disrupted epithelial transport of electrolytes cause secretory diarrhea [1]. To distinguish the two main categories of diarrhea described above, it is imperative to calculate the fecal osmotic gap [1]. The fecal osmotic gap is calculated by the difference of the lumen osmolality, which is approximately equal to the body fluid osmolality (~290 mOsm/kg) and the osmolality of fecal electrolytes (contributed by twice the sum of potassium and sodium) in the lumen [2]. In osmotic diarrhea, the presence of unabsorbed substances (solutes or unmeasured cations) attract water and thus dilute fecal sodium and potassium concentrations. The stool osmolar gap in osmotic diarrhea is therefore >125 mOsm/kg [4]. In secretory diarrhea, the colon is unable to adjust for stool electrolytes, and thus the stool osmolar gap is typically defined as <50 mOsm/kg or <100 mOsm/kg, which varies according to the literature reviewed [4, 5]. The response to the fasting state is also able to differentiate osmotic versus secretory diarrhea. When considering osmotic diarrhea in a fasting state, stool volume decreases, whereas in secretory diarrhea, stool volume persists regardless of the fasting state [1]. The total daily

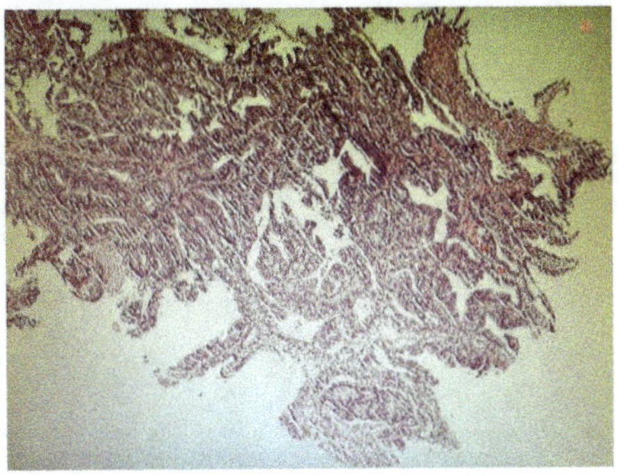

Figure 3: H&E slide: fragments of a tubular adenoma with high-grade dysplasia (intramucosal adenocarcinoma).

volume also differs between the two types of diarrhea with secretory having large volume watery stools of more than 1 liter per day versus osmotic diarrhea having less than 1 liter per day [6]. In our case, the patient's stool osmotic gap was 70 mOsm/kg, without improvement in the fasting state and with a total volume of over 3000 ml/day, supporting the diagnosis of secretory diarrhea.

Secretory diarrhea is typically caused by endocrine disturbances including carcinoid tumors, gastrinomas, VIPomas, and medullary carcinomas of the thyroid [4]. Other common causes include diabetes-related diarrhea, alcohol, and factitious diarrhea (commonly from bisacodyl laxative abuse) [4]. Infections, bile acid malabsorption, inflammatory bowel diseases (Crohn's disease, microscopic colitis, and ulcerative colitis), disordered regulation (post-vagotomy), neoplastic lesions (typically lymphoma, villous adenoma, and colon carcinoma), and idiopathic causes can also give origin to secretory diarrhea [1].

While most colonic polyps are asymptomatic, severe secretory diarrhea has been reported in the past caused due to the presence of colonic adenomas [7, 8]. In general, tubular colon adenomas are known to be precancerous and could undergo malignant transformation. This contrasts with hyperplastic polyps that have no malignant potential. Villous features in a polyp include long "finger-like" protrusions [9]. Tubular adenomas are known to have less than 25% villous features. When a polyp has >75% villous features, it is classified as a villous adenoma. Tubulovillous adenomas are, as the name suggests, adenomas that carry both tubular and villous features [8]. Malignancy risk tends to increase linearly with an increase in the size of the polyp, positive family history of colon cancer, histological type, and degree of dysplasia [10, 11].

McKittrick–Wheelock syndrome is a rare cause of secretory diarrhea and was first reported in 1954 by McKittrick and Wheelock [3]. It is caused by a secretory colorectal tumor that is most frequently a villous adenoma and less commonly adenocarcinoma [11, 12]. Severe secretory diarrhea along with electrolyte disturbances in the form of McKittrick–Wheelock syndrome has also been reported in villous adenomas [8]. Villous adenomas that are ranging from 4 to 18 cm are considered large, and they can cause secretory diarrhea of 500 to 3000 mL/24 hours [4]. The mechanism of action that has been proposed for adenomatous polyps causing large volume secretory diarrhea is due to active ion secretion secondary to secretagogue secretion by adenomas/adenocarcinomas [13]. The secretagogues that are responsible include cyclic adenosine monophosphate and prostaglandin E2 [13]. These lead to the flux of electrolytes and fluids into the lumen [13]. McKittrick–Wheelock syndrome classically presents with a triad consisting of chronic diarrhea, electrolyte disturbances (most commonly hypokalemia), and renal failure [12]. An increase in the number of goblet cells and prostaglandin E2 is responsible for this type of diarrhea [4]. The large surface area of the larger tumors essentially leads to an increase in fluid secretion that triumphs the normal mucosa's ability to reabsorb the presence of extra fluid [14]. Furthermore, the presence of COX-2 expression is known to be higher in tubulovillous adenoma [14].

To work up a patient that presents with chronic diarrhea, it is imperative to conduct a thorough history to identify certain drugs and dietary factors that may be contributing to the patient presentation [13]. Metabolic disorders are routinely diagnosed via blood tests. Infectious causes can typically be ruled out by the examination of stool studies [14]. The most essential step in diagnosis for a patient with chronic diarrhea is colonoscopy to search for the presence of signs of inflammatory bowel disease or the presence of a polyp and colonic neoplasms [14].

The mainstay of treatment for these lesions is surgical. Typical surgical options include transanal resection using an approach, that is, presacral mucosectomy, and abdominal surgery for large tumors [8]. This is the ultimate treatment that will arrest the loss of electrolytes that may lead to serious clinical consequences. In patients that have McKittrick–Wheelock syndrome, nonsteroidal anti-inflammatory drugs such as indomethacin may be used to decrease the electrolyte secretion in patients that desire a conservative nonsurgical approach [8].

4. Conclusion

McKittrick–Wheelock syndrome is a rare syndrome and is most commonly caused by villous adenomas. Our patient is unique in that this is the first ever reported case of a tubular adenoma with high-grade dysplasia leading to a McKittrick–Wheelock presentation and importantly progressing towards circulatory collapse with severe electrolyte disturbances. Aggressive replacement of fluids and electrolytes is essential to the survival of these patients, and it is imperative that clinicians be aware of this rare diagnosis.

References

[1] S. Sweetser, "Evaluating the patient with diarrhea: a case-based approach," *Mayo Clinic Proceedings*, vol. 87, no. 6, pp. 596–602, 2012.

[2] L. R. Schiller, "Secretory diarrhea," *Current Gastroenterology Reports*, vol. 1, no. 5, pp. 389–397, 1999.

[3] L. S. McKittrick and F. C. Wheelock, "Carcinoma of the colon," *Diseases of the Colon & Rectum*, vol. 40, no. 12, pp. 1494–1496, 1997.
[4] C. E. Semrad, "Approach to the patient with diarrhea and malabsorption," *Goldman's Cecil Medicine*, vol. 2012, pp. 895–913, 2012.
[5] W. Karnsakul and C. Lifschitz, "Diarrheal (diarrhoeal) diseases," *Encyclopedia of Food Sciences and Nutrition*, pp. 1804–1813, 2003.
[6] E. Fabian, P. Kump, and G. J. Krejs, "Diarrhea caused by circulating agents," *Gastroenterology Clinics of North America*, vol. 41, no. 3, pp. 603–610, 2012.
[7] J. Louissaint, Y. Schneider, and D. W. Wan, "Case report: tubulovillous adenoma with secretory diarrhea responding to NSAIDs," *American Journal of Gastroenterology*, vol. 110, no. 167, p. S167, 2015.
[8] S. Sanchez Garcia, P. Villarejo Campos, M. D. C. Manzanares Campillo et al., "Hypersecretory villous adenoma as the primary cause of an intestinal intussusception and McKittrick-Wheelock syndrome," *Canadian Journal of Gastroenterology*, vol. 27, no. 11, pp. 621-622, 2013.
[9] M. Taherian, S. Lotfollahzadeh, and P. Daneshpajouhnejad, "Tubular adenoma," in *StatPearls*StatPearls Publishing, Treasure Island (FL), 2021, https://www.ncbi.nlm.nih.gov/books/NBK553180/.
[10] C. O. Mărginean, M. O. Mărginean, I. Simu, A. Horvath, and L. E. Meliţ, "Giant tubular adenoma with malignancy clinical characteristics in a female teenager: case report and a review of the literature," *Medicine (Baltimore)*, vol. 95, no. 40, Article ID e4805, 2016.
[11] A. Popescu, A. M. Orban-Schiopu, G. Becheanu, and M. Diculescu, "McKittrick-Wheelock syndrome - a rare cause of acute renal failure," *Romanian Journal of Gastroenterology*, vol. 14, no. 1, pp. 63–66, 2005.
[12] S. Malik, B. Mallick, K. Makkar, V. Kumar, V. Sharma, and S. S. Rana, "Malignant McKittrick-Wheelock syndrome as a cause of acute kidney injury and hypokalemia: report of a case and review of literature," *Intractable & Rare Diseases Research*, vol. 5, no. 3, pp. 218–221, 2016.
[13] Y. S. Lee, H. J. Lin, and K. T. Chen, "McKittrick-Wheelock syndrome: a rare cause of life-threatening electrolyte disturbances and volume depletion," *Journal of Emergency Medicine*, vol. 43, no. 3, pp. e171–e173, 2012.
[14] M. C. Hsieh, C. J. Chen, and W. S. Huang, "McKittrick-wheelock syndrome," *Clinical Gastroenterology and Hepatology*, vol. 14, no. 4, pp. e41–e42, 2016.

11

Poly (ADP-Ribose) Polymerase 1 Protein Expression in Normal Pancreas and Pancreatic Adenocarcinoma

Roberto Castiglione,[1] Aldo E. Calogero,[1] Enzo Vicari,[1] Giovanna Calabrini,[2] Anna Cosentino,[2] Placido D'Agati,[3] Filippo Fraggetta,[4] and Michele Salemi[5]

[1]*Department of Clinical and Experimental Medicine, University of Catania, Catania, Italy*
[2]*Pathology Unit, Gravina Hospital, Caltagirone, Italy*
[3]*Department "GF Ingrassia" Hygiene and Public Health, University of Catania, Catania, Italy*
[4]*Pathology Unit, Cannizzaro Hospital, Catania, Italy*
[5]*Oasi Research Institute-IRCCS, Troina, EN, Italy*

Correspondence should be addressed to Roberto Castiglione; robertocastiglionen@tiscali.it

Academic Editor: Chia-Tung Shun

Pancreatic cancer is a most frequent cancer in Europe, and the majority of cases of cancer of the pancreas are diagnosed above the age of 65. Radical surgery is the first curative treatment of pancreatic cancer, and alternative or combined therapeutic options, in particular, consist of adjuvant or neoadjuvant chemotherapy, with or without radiotherapy. Many factors, including diet and genetics, have been implicated in the development of cancer of the pancreas. Poly (ADP-ribose) polymerase 1 (PARP-1) protein is required for translocation of the apoptosis-inducing factor (AIF) from the mitochondria to the nucleus. It is involved in programmed cell death processes. Different PARP-1 gene expression proteins have been observed in various tumors such as lung, ovarian, endometrial, skin, and glioblastoma. We evaluated the expression of PARP-1 protein in pancreatic adenocarcinoma and normal pancreas tissues by immunohistochemistry. Protein PARP-1 in the nucleus was found in all samples (normal pancreas and pancreatic adenocarcinoma tissues). No cytoplasmic staining was observed in any sample. PARP-1-positive cells resulted higher in the normal pancreas compared with the pancreas with adenocarcinoma. PARP-1 overexpression in prostate cancer tissue compared with normal prostate suggests a greater activity of PARP-1 in these tumors. These findings suggest that PARP-1 expression in prostate cancer is an attempt to trigger apoptosis in this type of tumor, similarl to that reported in other cancers. This finding suggests that PARP-1-mediated cell death pathways are inhibited in this cancer.

1. Introduction

Gastrointestinal diseases are some of the most common pathologies in the European population. Some of them are characterized by acute symptoms that can lead to serious manifestations such as digestive bleeding and emergency intervention. Other pathologies, however, have a prolonged course over time and tend to become chronic [1, 2], that is, to become permanent, with a heavy impact on the quality of life. In Europe, pancreatic cancer is the sixth most prevalent cancer, accounting for 2.8% of the cancer cases among men and 3.2% among women. With a 5-year survival rate of less than 10%, it is the fifth leading cause of cancer-related deaths [3]. Ninety-four percent of the patients succumb to the disease within the first 5 years of their diagnosis [4]. The majority of the cases of pancreatic cancer are diagnosed after the age of 65, with 60% of the cases at an advanced stage, indicating little improvement in treatment and survival over the past 30 years [3]. Radical surgery offers the only curative treatment of pancreatic cancer, and alternative or combined therapeutic options, in particular, consist of adjuvant or neoadjuvant chemotherapy, with or without radiotherapy [3, 5, 6].

Many factors, including diet, habits, and genetics, have been implicated in the development of pancreatic cancer.

Novel drug combinations have been reported to improve survival, advances in radiation therapy have resulted in less toxicity, and enormous strides have been made in the understanding of the fundamental genetics of pancreatic cancer [5, 6]. These advances not only offer hope but also increase the complexity of medical care. It is clear that multidisciplinary care that provides comprehensive and coordinated evaluation and treatment is the most effective way to manage pancreatic cancer [5, 6].

The poly (ADP-ribose) polymerase 1 (PARP-1) gene, located in the chromosome region 1q42, is 43 kb long and is composed of 23 exons (OMIM 173870). The PARP-1 function may contribute to efficient maintenance of genome integrity [6]. PARP-1 activation is required for the translocation of the apoptosis-inducing factor (AIF) from the mitochondria to the nucleus. The PARP-1 protein is then proteolytically cleaved at the onset of apoptosis by the caspase 3 enzyme [7]. Furthermore, PARP-1 activity and the poly (ADP-ribose) [PAR] polymer mediate PARP-1-induced cell death [7, 8]. *In vivo* pharmacological and genetic studies have revealed that overexpression of PARP-1 is the key mediator of programmed necrotic cell death. In addition, PARP-1 appears to be involved in other programmed cell death processes, such as macroautophagocytic cell death and apoptosis [9]. Microarray analysis of PARP-1 gene expression in more than 8,000 samples has revealed that PARP-1 is highly expressed in several types of tumors compared with the corresponding healthy tissues. Furthermore, PARP-1 mRNA expression in a wide variety of histologically normal tissues is low and uniform [10]. Overall, the most striking differences in PARP-1 expression have been observed in breast, ovarian, endometrial, lung, and skin cancers and in non-Hodgkin's lymphoma [10].

The present study was undertaken to immunohistochemically evaluate and compare the expression of the PARP-1 protein between healthy pancreatic tissue samples and pancreatic adenocarcinoma (PA) tissue samples.

2. Materials and Methods

2.1. Patients and Controls. A comparison was made between seven healthy pancreatic tissue samples obtained during postmortem examination of donors without cancer (four men and three women) and five PA tissues stained with haematoxylin and eosin. At least two operators evaluated the tissue sections. The protocol was approved by the internal Institutional Review Board, and written informed consent was obtained from each PA patient and control donor or, if deceased, from his/her relatives.

2.2. Immunohistochemical Staining. Pancreatic-tissue sections of 4 μm thickness were obtained from all control donors and PA patients. All the sections were formalin-fixed and paraffin-embedded by standard methods. PARP-(F-2), a mouse monoclonal antibody raised against the PARP-1 protein, was used for the immunohistochemical analysis (Santa Cruz Biotechnology, Inc., Heidelberg, Germany; PARP-1 [F-2]: sc-8007). As indicated in the manufacturer's instructions, this antibody, at a dilution of 1 : 300, is known to reliably recognize PARP-1 proteins in PA and healthy tissues in an immunohistochemical analysis. The slides were deparaffinized, rehydrated, subjected to three 5 min cycles in a microwave at 360 W in a citrate buffer, preincubated in citrate buffer with 3% H_2O_2, and thoroughly washed in Tris-buffered saline (TBS) (50 mM Tris-Cl, 150 mM NaCl, pH 7.4) containing 0.05% of Tween 20 (washing buffer). The slides were then preincubated for 30 min in TBS with 3% of bovine serum albumin and, then, with the anti-PARP-1 antibody (1 : 300) in TBS containing 1% of BSA. The slides were then thoroughly washed with a washing buffer, and specific signals were visualized with the LSAB 2 kit (anti-mouse, biotinylated, and peroxidase-labelled streptavidin) and 3,3′-diaminobenzidine-tetrahydrochloride (DAB·4HCl; Dako, Carpinteria CA, USA). After detection, the tissue sections were counterstained with haematoxylin, dehydrated, and mounted in a xylene-based DPX mountant (BDH, Poole, UK) [11].

2.3. Microscopic Evaluation. Slides were examined, and the cells were visually scored at 20X and 40X magnification. To evaluate the percentage of signal-positive tumor cells, microscopic visual fields were chosen such that nontumorous cells were also included. The percentage of PARP-1-positive cells was evaluated independently in a blinded fashion by two co-authors (M.S. and M.A.). No significant difference was found between their observations.

2.4. Statistical Analysis. Results are expressed as mean ± SEM. Data were analyzed by the t-test, and statistical analysis was performed in GraphPad Prism 5 (GraphPad Software, Inc. La Jolla, CA, USA). Statistical significance was assumed at p values lower than 0.05 (Figure 1).

3. Results

Expression of the PARP-1 protein was evaluated in five PA tissue samples. A PARP-1-positive nuclear signal was present in all five samples with a 34% ± 9.5% of nuclei involved (mean ± SEM; Table 1; Figure 2(a)). No cytoplasmic staining was observed in any samples. Healthy pancreatic tissues (seven samples of postmortem tissue) yielded a positive nuclear signal for protein PARP-1 (Table 1; Figure 2(b)) with 81.42% ± 3% of the nuclei involved, whereas no cytoplasmic staining was observed in any of the healthy-tissue samples. The signal was present on the nuclear membrane and in nuclear chromatin in all the samples (healthy and PA tissues). In this study, the percentage of PARP-1-positive cells was lower in tumors of patients with PA than in control tissue samples.

4. Discussion

We found that, in comparison with the controls, the PARP-1 protein was downregulated in PA tissue samples (Table 1). This finding suggests that PARP-1-mediated apoptotic pathways are inhibited in pancreatic cancer. These results

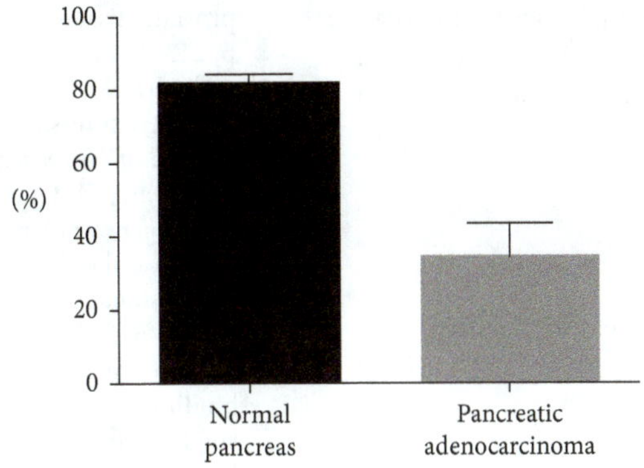

FIGURE 1: T-test data (mean with SEM).

TABLE 1: Characteristics of healthy pancreas tissue donors and of patients with pancreatic adenocarcinoma.

Normal pancreas (autopsy)				Pancreatic adenocarcinoma						
ID	Sex	Age	Positive (cell nuclei %)	ID	Sex	Age	Positive (cell nuclei %)	pT	N	G
1	M	82	75	1	M	90	10	T2	N0	G2
2	F	95	80	2	F	62	55	T2	N0	G2
3	M	94	85	3	M	72	15	T2	N0	G2
4	F	92	85	4	M	61	55	T2	N1	G2
5	M	75	70	5	M	84	35	T2	N0	G2
6	M	78	95							
7	F	84	80							
Mean			81.4				34			
SD			8.0				21.3			
SEM ⊥			3.0				9.5			

ID: identification; pT: tumor stage; N: lymphonodes; G: grading; T-test = 5.4539 ($p < 0.005$); p value = 0.0003(***).

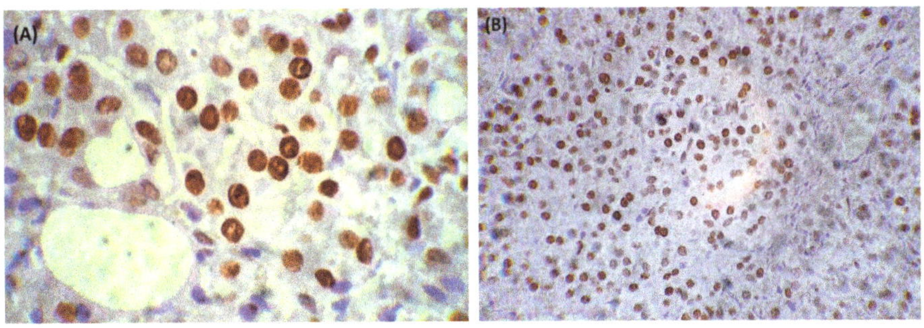

FIGURE 2: (a) Immunohistochemistry of pancreatic adenocarcinoma scored at 40x. Hematoxylin counterstain; (b) immunohistochemistry of normal pancreas scored at 20x. Hematoxylin counterstain.

support the hypothesis that, in some tumors (e.g., melanoma), apoptotic pathways are inhibited at different levels [12].

These results contradict the results of other studies on the expression of the PARP-1 protein in prostate carcinoma [13], glioblastoma [14], squamous cell carcinoma [15], non-Hodgkin's lymphoma, and other cancers such as breast, ovarian, lung, endometrial, and skin malignant tumors [16]. PARP-1 is an abundant, chromatin-associated enzyme present in all eukaryotic cell nuclei, where it plays an important role in the maintenance of genomic integrity and transcriptional control [16,17]. A poly (ADP-ribose) polymerase 1 inhibitor increases an antitumor activity against glioma, intracranial melanoma, lymphoma, and haematological neoplasia [18–21]. Activation of the PARP-1 gene in response to DNA damage is an important mechanism of homeostasis or of triggering apoptosis. Our preliminary data suggest that, in a healthy pancreas, almost 80% of the nuclei express the PARP-1 protein; this level is enough for its proapoptotic activity. In contrast, the PARP-1 protein is expressed to a lesser extent in PA tissues, suggesting that the proapoptotic activity of PARP-1 is lower and that the mechanisms of DNA repair by PARP-1 are less active in PA. These data may partially explain the aggressiveness of PA compared to other cancers. In conclusion, if these results can be reproduced in a larger cohort, then PARP-1 expression can serve as a marker for the differential diagnosis between PA and other pancreatic disorders.

Acknowledgments

The authors thank Dr. Emanuele Gaetano Schilirò, Department of Humanities, University of Catania, Italy, for the accurate linguistic editing.

References

[1] J. P. Gisbert and M. Chaparro, "Acute severe ulcerative colitis: state of the art treatment," *Best Practice & Research Clinical Gastroenterology*, vol. 32-33, pp. 59–69, 2018.

[2] E. Vicari, S. La Vignera, R. Castiglione et al., "Chronic bacterial prostatitis and irritable bowel syndrome: effectiveness of treatment with rifaximin followed by the probiotic VSL#3," *Asian Journal of Andrology*, vol. 16, pp. 735–739, 2014.

[3] M. Bardou and I. Le Ray, "Treatment of pancreatic cancer: a narrative review of cost-effectiveness studies," *Best Practice & Research Clinical Gastroenterology*, vol. 27, no. 6, pp. 881–892, 2013.

[4] D. Xinli, Z. Rihua, X. Yi et al., "Insulin glargine and risk of cancer: a meta-analysis," *International Journal of Biological Makers*, vol. 27, no. 3, pp. 241–246, 2012.

[5] American Cancer Society, *Cancer Facts & Figures 2010*, American Cancer Society, Atlanta, GA, USA, 2010.

[6] C. L. Wolfgang, J. M. Herman, D. A. Laheru et al., "Recent progress in pancreatic cancer," *CA: A Cancer Journal for Clinicians*, vol. 63, no. 5, pp. 318–348, 2013.

[7] S. A. Andrabi, N. S. Kim, S.-W. Yu et al., "Poly(ADP-ribose) (PAR) polymer is a death signal," *Proceedings of the National Academy of Sciences*, vol. 103, no. 48, pp. 18308–18313, 2006.

[8] S.-W. Yu, S. A. Andrabi, H. Wang et al., "Apoptosis-inducing factor mediates poly(ADP-ribose) (PAR) polymer-induced cell death," *Proceedings of the National Academy of Sciences*, vol. 103, no. 48, pp. 18314–18319, 2006.

[9] P. O. Hassa and M. O. Hottiger, "The diverse biological roles of mammalian PARPs, a small but powerful family of poly-ADP-ribose polymerases," *Frontiers in Bioscience*, vol. 13, no. 13, pp. 3046–3082, 2008.

[10] V. Ossovskaya, I. C. Koo, E. P. Kaldjian, C. Alvares, and B. M. Sherman, "Upregulation of poly (ADP-Ribose) polymerase-1 (PARP1) in triple-negative breast cancer and other primary human tumor types," *Genes & Cancer*, vol. 1, no. 8, pp. 812–821, 2010.

[11] M. Salemi, A. E. Calogero, G. Zaccarello et al., "Expression of SPANX proteins in normal prostatic tissue and in prostate cancer," *European Journal of Histochemistry*, vol. 54, p. e41, 2010.

[12] M. Salemi, A. E. Calogero, E. Vicari et al., "A high percentage of skin melanoma cells expresses SPANX proteins," *The American Journal of Dermatopathology*, vol. 31, no. 2, pp. 182–186, 2009.

[13] M. Salemi, A. Galia, F. Fraggetta et al., "Poly (ADP-ribose) polymerase 1 protein expression in normal and neoplastic prostatic tissue," *European Journal of Histochemistry*, vol. 57, p. e13, 2013.

[14] A. Galia, A. E. Calogero, R. E. Condorelli et al., "PARP-1 protein expression in glioblastoma multiforme," *European Journal of Histochemistry*, vol. 56, no. 1, pp. 45–48, 2012.

[15] M. Salemi, D. Giuffrida, M. C. Giuffrida et al., "Three apoptotic genes are upregulated in a patient with Alzheimer's disease and well-differentiated squamous cell carcinoma," *The International Journal of Biological Markers*, vol. 27, no. 1, pp. 60–63, 2012.

[16] S. Eustermann, H. Videler, J.-C. Yang et al., "The DNA-binding domain of human PARP-1 interacts with DNA single-strand breaks as a monomer through its second zinc finger," *Journal of Molecular Biology*, vol. 407, no. 1, pp. 149–170, 2011.

[17] S. Kannan, W. Fang, G. Song et al., "Notch/HES1-mediated PARP1 activation: a cell type-specific mechanism for tumor suppression," *Blood*, vol. 117, no. 10, pp. 2891–2900, 2011.

[18] L. Tentori, C. Leonetti, M. Scarsella et al., "Systemic administration of GPI 15427, a novel poly(ADP-ribose) polymerase-1 inhibitor, increases the antitumor activity of temozolomide against intracranial melanoma, glioma, lymphoma," *Clinical Cancer Research: An Official Journal of the American Association for Cancer Research*, vol. 9, no. 14, pp. 5370–5379, 2003.

[19] A. L. Russo, H.-C. Kwon, W. E. Burgan et al., "In vitro and in vivo radiosensitization of glioblastoma cells by the poly (ADP-ribose) polymerase inhibitor E7016," *Clinical Cancer Research*, vol. 15, no. 2, pp. 607–612, 2009.

[20] B. McEllin, C. V. Camacho, B. Mukherjee et al., "PTEN loss compromises homologous recombination repair in astrocytes: implications for glioblastoma therapy with temozolomide or poly(ADP-ribose) polymerase inhibitors," *Cancer Research*, vol. 70, no. 13, pp. 5457–5464, 2010.

[21] M. Ahmad, A. Torky, F. Glahn, R. J. Scheubel, and H. Foth, "PARP-1 expression and activity in primary human lung cells," *Archives of Toxicology*, vol. 85, no. 6, pp. 669–679, 2011.

12

Colonic Angiosarcoma Arising in Association with Amyloid Deposits

Samar Said, Rondell P. Graham, Tsung-Teh Wu, Saba Yasir, Lizhi Zhang, and Andrew L. Folpe

Department of Laboratory Medicine and Pathology, Mayo Clinic, Rochester, MN, USA

Correspondence should be addressed to Samar Said; said.samar@mayo.edu

Academic Editor: Chia-Tung Shun

Angiosarcoma of the colon is rare, as is colonic amyloidosis. To our knowledge, there have been no reported cases of angiosarcoma arising in association with amyloid deposition. Herein, we described a case of 77-year-old man who presented with hematochezia, and a sigmoid mass was found on colonoscopy. Histologic examination of the resected specimen showed extensive nodular deposition of AL-lambda amyloid material in the colonic wall, as well as high-grade angiosarcoma which was closely intermingled with the amyloid deposits. While the occurrence of both colonic amyloidosis and angiosarcoma in this patient may represent pure coincidence, given the intimate association of the angiosarcoma and the amyloid deposition and the rarity of both of these lesions, we hypothesize that angiosarcoma could be secondary to amyloid deposition.

1. Introduction

Angiosarcoma is a rare malignant vascular neoplasm that involves mainly skin and superficial soft tissue and is extremely rare in the gastrointestinal tract. Most sporadic cutaneous angiosarcomas arise in the setting of significant sun damage and are thought to be related to long-term UV radiation damage [1]. Another important subset of cutaneous angiosarcomas arises following therapeutic radiation or lymphedema, most often in the setting of breast carcinoma [2]. A small number of angiosarcomas have been reported to arise in association with foreign materials, including shrapnel, Dacron vascular grafts, orthopedic prosthetic hardware, and tophaceous gout. Colonic amyloidosis is also rare, and most cases are immunoglobulin light chain-related. It is well known that some types of amyloidosis can be caused by malignancies. For example, calcitonin type amyloid deposits are caused by medullary thyroid carcinoma, and immunoglobulin type amyloidosis can be secondary to plasma cell dyscrasia or lymphoma. The association between sarcoma and amyloidosis was described in only few case reports. However, to our knowledge, there are no reported cases of angiosarcoma arising in association with amyloid deposition. Herein, we report an extremely rare example of colonic angiosarcoma arising in association with nodular amyloid deposits.

2. Case Presentation

A 77-year-old man with history of dementia, chronic kidney disease, gout, malignant melanoma of the skin, osteoarthritis, and gastroesophageal reflux disease presented with hematochezia. A nearly completely obstructing mass lesion in the sigmoid colon was found on colonoscopy. Follow-up staging CT scan of chest, abdomen, and pelvis showed a discrete mass in the distal sigmoid colon measuring approximately 10 cm in length, severe colonic wall thickening involving the distal colon and extending through the rectum, and a 2.5 cm right upper pole renal mass with heterogeneous enhancement worrisome for renal cell carcinoma. The patient underwent open sigmoidectomy. Grossly, there was a $3.4 \times 2.0 \times 0.5$ cm ulcerated mass with raised borders. Sections submitted from the mass demonstrated extensive deposition of amorphous, pale eosinophilic material involving the lamina propria, muscularis mucosa, submucosa, muscularis propria, and subserosa with prominent

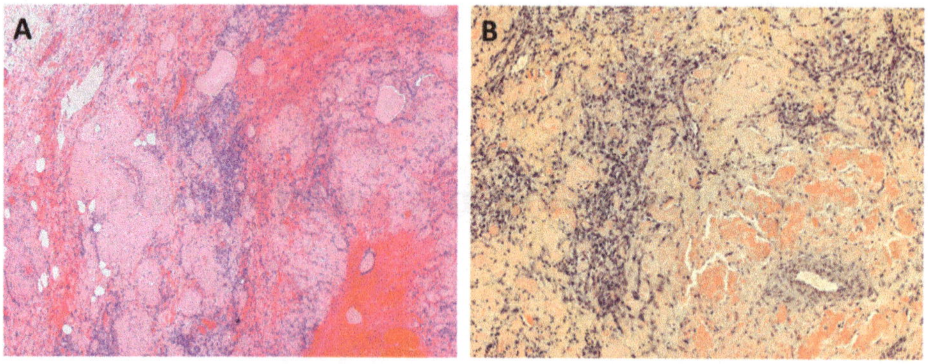

FIGURE 1: (a) Representative low-power image showing sheets of malignant cells and hemorrhage present between areas of extensive amyloid deposition (×40). (b) The amyloid deposits are Congo-Red positive (×100).

involvement of vessels (Figure 1(a)). The material was positive with a Congo red stain (Figure 1(b)) and showed apple-green birefringence under polarized light, characteristic of amyloid. Closely intermingled with and diffusely infiltrating the amyloid deposits, there were sheets of highly atypical, plump spindled cells with amphophilic cytoplasm, oval large nuclei, prominent nucleoli, and frequent mitotic figures (Figures 2(a) and 2(b)). Intracytoplasmic vacuoles containing red blood cells were identified in some of the tumor cells. There were also areas of hemorrhage and blood lakes. The tumor cells were positive for endothelial markers including CD31 (patchy), ERG, and FLI1, confirming the diagnosis of angiosarcoma (Figures 2(c) and 2(d)) and negative for keratins (AE1/AE3), SOX10, S100 protein, and KIT (Figures 3(a)–3(d)). Strong expression of MYC protein by immunohistochemistry was present (Figure 2(e)). Fluorescence in situ hybridization (FISH) showed no evidence of MYC gene amplification.

Amyloid typing by laser microdissection (LMD) followed by high-performance liquid chromatography and tandem mass spectrometry (LC-MS/MS) confirmed the presence of amyloid and was consistent with AL (lambda)-type. No infiltration of plasma cells in the vicinity of amyloid deposits was seen. Due to the patient's advanced dementia, the family decided not to pursue aggressive therapy and opted for palliative care.

3. Discussion

Angiosarcoma is a rare malignant vascular neoplasm that involves mainly skin and superficial soft tissue but may occur in large vessels, deep soft tissue, and parenchymal organs such as the liver, spleen, bone, breast, and heart. It can be primary or secondary. Long-term sun exposure, radiation, chronic lymphedema, and exposure to Thorotrast, polyvinylchloride, and arsenic are known risk factors [1–5]. Angiosarcoma has also reported in association with arteriovenous fistulas in patients with renal failure [6–12], arthroplasty [13, 14], and injection sites [15] and in association with foreign materials that can be introduced to the body during trauma, surgery, and injection or formed in situ. Foreign materials reported to cause angiosarcoma include metals (such as bullets, shrapnel, cardiac defibrillator implants, and orthopedic joint prostheses) [16–20], Dacron graft [18, 21], silicone breast implants [22–24], retained surgical material such as sponge [25–27], and a gouty tophus (where it was hypothesized that the angiosarcoma was induced by the gouty tophus in a mechanism similar to that of foreign body-associated sarcoma) [28]. While development of sarcoma in association with foreign material occurs only rarely in humans, it is a well-documented phenomenon in rodents in which investigators have demonstrated the development of sarcoma after insertion of foreign material [29]. Different types of sarcoma have been reported in this setting including undifferentiated sarcoma, angiosarcoma, osteosarcoma, and chondrosarcoma. There is usually a prolonged latency period between the initial exposure to the foreign material and development of sarcoma [30]. The physical properties of the material seem to play a role in tumorogenesis, as the tumorigenic effect is reduced or lost when the foreign materials are inserted in pulverized or shredded forms, when their surface is rough or when they contain large pores. Formation of thick fibrous capsule around the foreign material is thought to play a role in tumorgenesis as tumorigenic material developed more fibrosis than the nontumorigenic material [30, 31]. MYC amplification, and strong MYC protein expression, initially thought to be limited to secondary angiosarcoma (such as postradiation and lymphedema-associated angiosarcoma) [32], is now known to occur in primary angiosarcoma as well [33].

Colonic angiosarcoma is extremely rare. Wang et al. reported a case of colonic angiosarcoma and summarized the results of 33 previously reported cases [34]. The mean age was 56 years (range 16 to 85 years), and the mean tumor size was 5 cm (range 1.5–12 cm). In more than two thirds of the cases, the tumor was in the left colon (36% in the sigmoid colon and 33% in the anorectal region), whereas 21% were in the cecum, 9% in the ascending colon, and 3% in the transverse and descending colon. Four of the 33 patients had a history of radiation exposure, and in one patient the tumor was associated with retained surgical gauze. An association with renal transplantation, long-term hemodialysis, and chronic colorectal ulcers were also reported (one case each). Clinical symptoms included gastrointestinal bleeding (67%), abdominal/anal pain (46%), intestinal obstruction (24%),

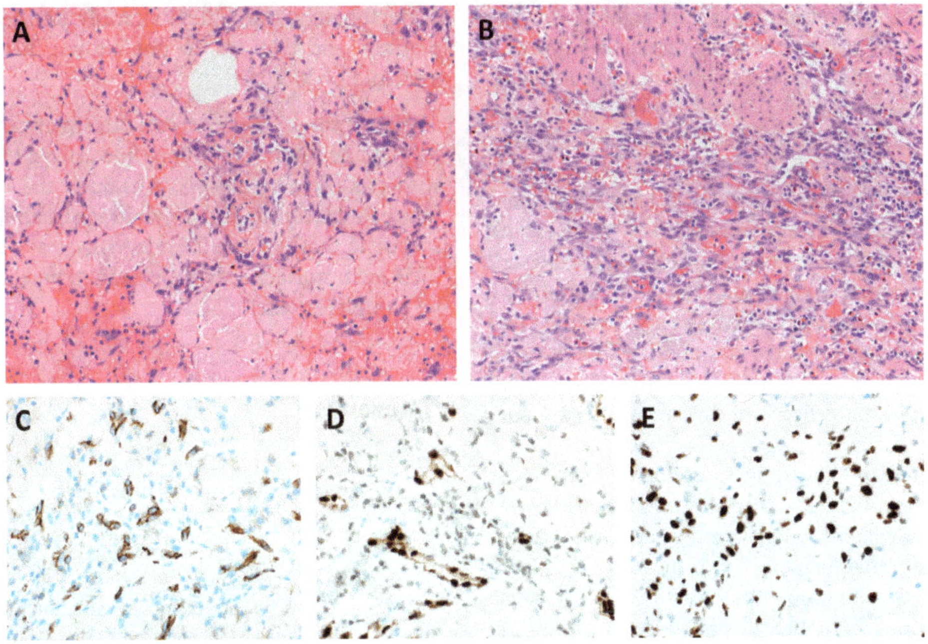

FIGURE 2: (a, b) Diffuse infiltration of amyloid deposits by high-grade angiosarcoma (×200). (c–e) The malignant cells are positive for CD31 (patchy) (c), ERG (d), and MYC (e) (×400).

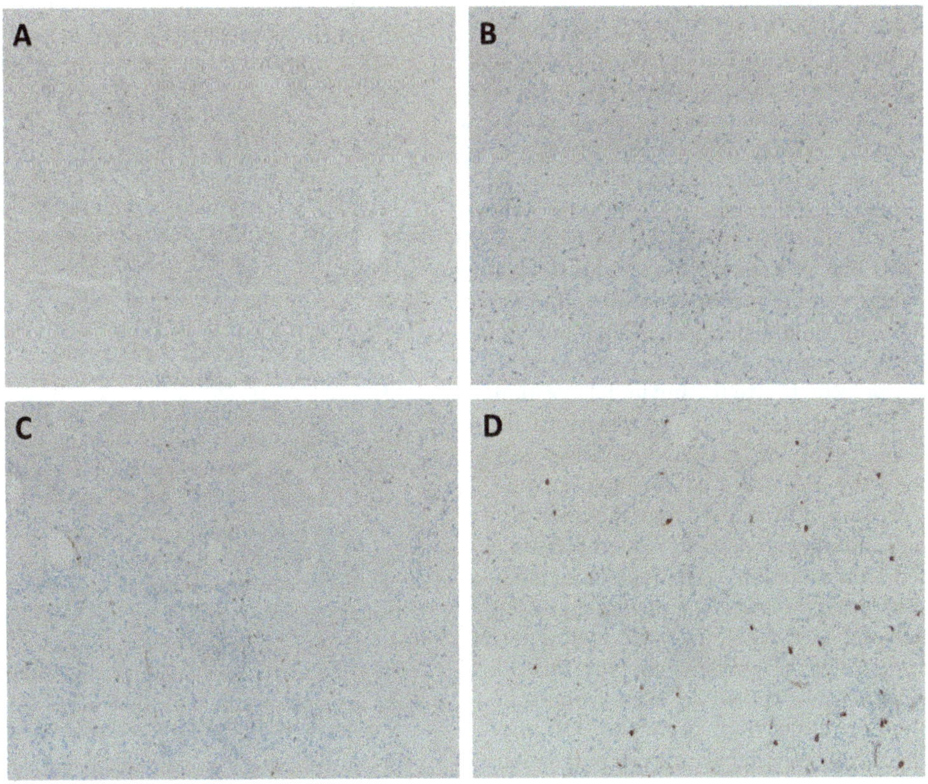

FIGURE 3: (a–d) The tumor cells are negative for keratin AE1/AE3 (a), SOX10 (b), S100 (c), and KIT (d) (×100).

diarrhea (50%), and weight loss (18%). Anemia was present in 42% of patients. Prognosis was poor with a median survival of 4.5 months. Tumor size less than 5 cm and younger age were associated with better prognosis. In general, colonic angiosarcomas are treated surgically, although there may also be a role for adjuvant therapies, including radiation, chemotherapy, and immunotherapy. Gastrointestinal amyloidosis is also rare. Cowan et al. [35] reported 76 patients with gastrointestinal amyloidosis (accounted for 3.2% of patients with amyloidosis), most of which (80%) were due to immunoglobulin light chain. The median age was 61 years (range 34 to 79 years). The stomach was the most affected site involved in 49% of cases followed by the colorectal region (46%), small bowel (42%), and esophagus (8%). Clinical symptoms included weight loss (43%), gastrointestinal bleeding (37%), heartburn (33%), early satiety (33%), diarrhea (29%), and abdominal pain (28%). The amyloidosis was systemic in 79% of cases and localized (i.e., without evidence of an underlying plasma cell dyscrasia or other organ involvement) in 21%. Supportive care was the main treatment for localized gastrointestinal amyloidosis with all patients alive at a median follow-up of 36 months. Patients with systemic AL amyloidosis were treated with anti-plasma cell chemotherapy with 72% survival rate at 4 years.

Amyloid has multiple precursor proteins and can occur in different settings including chronic inflammatory conditions, certain neoplasms, genetic/inherited, and age-related. Hematologic malignancies and medullary thyroid carcinoma are two neoplasms that are known to cause amyloid deposition where medullary thyroid carcinoma causes calcitonin type amyloid and plasma cell dyscrasia and some types of lymphoma can cause immunoglobulin related amyloidosis [36]. Amyloid deposition has also been reported in association with other epithelial neoplasms including urothelial carcinoma, neuroendocrine tumors, pituitary adenoma, gastric carcinoma, nasopharyngeal carcinoma, breast carcinoma, and endometrioid carcinoma and rarely in association with sarcomas including Kaposi's sarcoma, follicular dendritic cell sarcoma, leiomyosarcoma, and pleomorphic sarcoma [37–56]. The relationship between the amyloid and most of the previously mentioned neoplasms, however, is largely unknown. To our knowledge, this is the first case of angiosarcoma arising in association with amyloid deposition. This may represent a purely coincidental occurrence. However, given the intimate association of the angiosarcoma and the amyloid deposition and the rarity of both colonic angiosarcoma and colonic amyloidosis, angiosarcoma could be secondary to the amyloid deposition. It is unlikely that the amyloidosis was secondary to the angiosarcoma, as the area of amyloid deposition was considerably larger than the area involved by angiosarcoma, angiosarcoma was present only within areas of the colon also involved by amyloid, and amyloid deposition has never been previously reported in association with this tumor type. Furthermore, angiosarcomas are rapidly growing, aggressive tumors that usually come quickly to clinical attention. Perhaps most importantly, the amyloidosis type was AL (lambda)-type, which is not known to arise from solid malignancies but rather results from production of amyloidogenic light chains from a clonal plasma cell population. Other factors such as chronic illness or genetic predisposition might have contributed to this exceptional occurrence. AL amyloidosis is the most common type of both systemic and localized amyloidosis. In localized AL amyloidosis, the amyloidogenic light chain is thought to arise from local plasma cell populations, but histologic evidence of monoclonal plasma cell infiltration or lymphoma adjacent to amyloid deposits is not always present [57] (as in this case). Unfortunately, the patient's family decided against further workup, and thus we do not know if his amyloidosis was systemic or localized.

In summary, we report an extremely rare occurrence of a high-grade colonic angiosarcoma arising in close association with colonic amyloidosis. Although the exact relationship between the tumor and amyloid is obscure, it is tempting to speculate that the amyloid deposits may have served as the inciting tumorigenic event, although pure coincident cannot be completely excluded.

References

[1] E. Shustef, V. Kazlouskaya, V. G. Prieto, D. Ivan, and P. P. Aung, "Cutaneous angiosarcoma: a current update," *Journal of Clinical Pathology*, vol. 70, no. 11, pp. 917–925, 2017.

[2] M. Co, A. Lee, and A. Kwong, "Cutaneous angiosarcoma secondary to lymphoedema or radiation therapy - a systematic review," *Clinical Oncology*, vol. 31, no. 4, pp. 225–231, 2019.

[3] G. S. Lipshutz, T. V. Brennan, and R. S. Warren, "Thorotrast-induced liver neoplasia: a collective review," *Journal of the American College of Surgeons*, vol. 195, no. 5, pp. 713–718, 2002.

[4] K. A. Mundt, L. D. Dell, L. Crawford, and A. E. Gallagher, "Quantitative estimated exposure to vinyl chloride and risk of angiosarcoma of the liver and hepatocellular cancer in the US industry-wide vinyl chloride cohort: mortality update through 2013," *Occupational and Environmental Medicine*, vol. 74, no. 10, pp. 709–716, 2017.

[5] M. Salgado, M. Sans, X. Forns et al., "Hepatic angiosarcoma: a report of a case associated with treatment with arsenic salts and a review of the literature," *Gastroenterol Hepatology*, vol. 18, no. 3, pp. 132–135, 1995.

[6] J. D. Kakisis, C. Antonopoulos, K. Moulakakis et al., "Angiosarcoma of a thrombosed arteriovenous fistula in a renal transplant recipient," *Annals of Vascular Surgery*, vol. 56, pp. e1–e4, 2019.

[7] D. Heining, J. Senior, A. Prasad, M. Thomas, A. Bentall, and P. J. Yates, "Multi-system bleeding risk with a cutaneous angiosarcoma at an arteriovenous fistula site," *Oxford Medical Case Reports*, vol. 2018, no. 10, Article ID omy063, 2018.

[8] S. F. Roy, F. M. Ghazawi, A. Alsarheed, K. D. Lach, K. Watters, and E. O'Brien, "Angiosarcoma arising within a nonfunctioning arteriovenous fistula," *International Journal of Dermatology*, vol. 57, no. 12, pp. 1513–1515, 2018.

[9] B. N. L. Costa, C. F. Rivera, M. C. Rodriguez et al., "Angiosarcoma developing in an arteriovenous fistula after kidney transplantation," *Case Reports in Transplantation*, vol. 2017, Article ID 2426859, 3 pages, 2017.

[10] R. A. Aldaabil, A. M. Alkhunaizi, N. A. Al-Dawsari, M. F. Dawamneh, and R. Rabah, "Angiosarcoma at the site of nonfunctioning arteriovenous fistula in a kidney transplant recipient," *Journal of Vascular Surgery Cases and Innovative Techniques*, vol. 2, no. 2, pp. 53–55, 2016.

[11] Y. Oskrochi, K. Razi, J. Stebbing, and J. Crane, "Angiosarcoma and dialysis-related arteriovenous fistulae: a comprehensive review," *European Journal of Vascular and Endovascular Surgery*, vol. 51, no. 1, pp. 127–133, 2016.

[12] A. L. Gale, R. A. W. Marco, S. R. Liberman, D. Zavlin, and A. Echo, "Case report: angiosarcoma in the upper extremity related to a nonfunctioning arteriovenous fistula," *Hand*, vol. 12, no. 5, pp. NP132–NP135, 2017.

[13] S. Terrando, A. Sambri, G. Bianchi et al., "Angiosarcoma around total hip arthroplasty: case series and review of the literature," *Musculoskelet Surgery*, vol. 102, no. 1, pp. 21–27, 2018.

[14] A. Mallick, S. Jain, A. Proctor, and R. Pandey, "Angiosarcoma around a revision total hip arthroplasty and review of literature," *Journal of Arthroplasty*, vol. 24, no. 2, pp. 323–20, 2009.

[15] H. Cheng and P. W. Allen, "Selected case from the Arkadi M. Rywlin International Pathology Slide Seminar," *Advances in Anatomic Pathology*, vol. 18, no. 4, pp. 329–332, 2011.

[16] T. Schneider, J. Renney, and J. Hayman, "Angiosarcoma occurring with chronic osteomyelitis and residual foreign material: case report of a late World War II wound complication," *ANZ Journal of Surgery*, vol. 67, no. 8, pp. 576–578, 1997.

[17] J. Hayman and H. Huygens, "Angiosarcoma developing around a foreign body," *Journal of Clinical Pathology*, vol. 36, no. 5, pp. 515–518, 1983.

[18] A. Agaimy, O. Ben-Izhak, T. Lorey, M. Scharpf, and B. P. Rubin, "Angiosarcoma arising in association with vascular Dacron grafts and orthopedic joint prostheses: clinicopathologic, immunohistochemical, and molecular study," *Annals of Diagnostic Pathology*, vol. 21, pp. 21–28, 2016.

[19] S. C. Smith, K. D. Bernacki, J. W. Haft, and J. B. McHugh, "Internal cardiac defibrillator implant-associated angiosarcoma presenting as suspected implant pouch infection," *Cardiovascular Pathology*, vol. 22, no. 1, pp. 105–108, 2013.

[20] D. J. McDonald, W. F. Enneking, and M. Sundaram, "Metal-associated angiosarcoma of bone: report of two cases and review of the literature," *Clinical Orthopaedics and Related Research*, vol. 396, pp. 206–214, 2002.

[21] O. Ben Izhak, E. Vlodavsky, A. Ofer, A. Engel, S. Nitecky, and A. Hoffman, "Epithelioid angiosarcoma associated with a Dacron vascular graft," *The American Journal of Surgical Pathology*, vol. 23, no. 11, pp. 1418–1422, 1999.

[22] N. R. Smoll, R. D. Farhadieh, R. Ferguson, M. W. Findlay, and D. J. Hunter-Smith, "High-grade angiosarcoma associated with ruptured breast implants," *Plastic and Reconstructive Surgery Global Open*, vol. 1, no. 1, 2013.

[23] M. Takenaka, M. Tanaka, M. Isobe, R. Yamaguchi, M. Kojiro, and K. Shirouzu, "Angiosarcoma of the breast with silicone granuloma: a case report," *The Kurume Medical Journal*, vol. 56, no. 1-2, pp. 33–37, 2009.

[24] N. D. Saunders, J. S. Marshall, and R. C. Anderson, "A case of chest wall angiosarcoma associated with breast implants," *The Journal of Thoracic and Cardiovascular Surgery*, vol. 134, no. 4, pp. 1076-1077, 2007.

[25] K. Cokelaere, J. Vanvuchelen, P. Michielsen, and R. Sciot, "Epithelioid angiosarcoma of the splenic capsule," *Virchows Archiv*, vol. 438, no. 4, pp. 398–403, 2001.

[26] O. Ben-Izhak, H. Kerner, B. Brenner, and C. Lichtig, "Angiosarcoma of the colon developing in a capsule of a foreign body: report of a case with associated hemorrhagic diathesis," *American Journal of Clinical Pathology*, vol. 97, no. 3, pp. 416–420, 1992.

[27] Y.-T. Joo, C.-Y. Jeong, E.-J. Jung et al., "Intra-abdominal angiosarcoma developing in a capsule of a foreign body: report of a case with associated hemorrhagic diathesis," *World Journal of Surgical Oncology*, vol. 3, no. 1, p. 60, 2005.

[28] A. L. Folpe, C. A. Johnston, and S. W. Weiss, "Cutaneous angiosarcoma arising in a gouty tophus," *The American Journal of Dermatopathology*, vol. 22, no. 5, pp. 418–421, 2000.

[29] K. G. Brand, K. H. Johnson, L. C. Buoen, and L. Golberg, "Foreign body tumorigenesis," *CRC Critical Reviews in Toxicology*, vol. 4, no. 4, pp. 353–394, 1976.

[30] T. A. Jennings, L. Peterson, C. A. Axiotis, G. E. Friedlaender, R. A. Cooke, and J. Rosai, "Angiosarcoma associated with foreign body material: a report of three cases," *Cancer*, vol. 62, no. 11, pp. 2436–2444, 1988.

[31] F. Bischoff and G. Bryson, "Carcinogenesis through solid state surfaces," *Progress in Experimental Tumor Research*, vol. 5, no. 5, pp. 85–133, 1964.

[32] J. Manner, B. Radlwimmer, P. Hohenberger et al., "MYC high level gene amplification is a distinctive feature of angiosarcomas after irradiation or chronic lymphedema," *The American Journal of Pathology*, vol. 176, no. 1, pp. 34–39, 2010.

[33] W. Shon, W. R. Sukov, S. M. Jenkins, and A. L. Folpe, "MYC amplification and overexpression in primary cutaneous angiosarcoma: a fluorescence in-situ hybridization and immunohistochemical study," *Modern Pathology*, vol. 27, no. 4, pp. 509–515, 2014.

[34] Q. Wang, T. Zhao, B.-T. Mi et al., "Primary colonic angiosarcoma seen in a patient on calcium channel blocker: a case report with summary analysis of 32 other cases from the literature," *American Journal of Case Reports*, vol. 19, pp. 254–261, 2018.

[35] A. J. Cowan, M. Skinner, D. C. Seldin et al., "Amyloidosis of the gastrointestinal tract: a 13-year, single-center, referral experience," *Haematologica*, vol. 98, no. 1, pp. 141–146, 2013.

[36] E. D. Williams, C. L. Brown, and I. Doniach, "Pathological and clinical findings in a series of 67 cases of medullary carcinoma of the thyroid," *Journal of Clinical Pathology*, vol. 19, no. 2, pp. 103–113, 1966.

[37] D. Sirohi, J. Gandhi, M. B. Amin, and D. J. Luthringer, "Amyloidosis of the bladder and association with urothelial carcinoma: report of 29 cases," *Human Pathology*, vol. 93, pp. 48–53, 2019.

[38] R. R. Vanga, S. Dhingra, and K. Patel, "Insulin expressing pancreatic neuroendocrine tumor associated with intratumor amyloidosis," *Clinical Gastroenterology and Hepatology*, vol. 15, no. 10, pp. A35–A36, 2017.

[39] S. O. Brannan, N. G. Lessan, P. Hiscott, and B. Damato, "A choroidal amyloid-rich neuroendocrine tumor," *Archives of Ophthalmology*, vol. 117, no. 8, pp. 1081–1083, 1999.

[40] N. Al-Kaisi, F. W. Abdul-Karim, G. Mendelsohn, and G. Jacobs, "Bronchial carcinoid tumor with amyloid stroma," *Archives of Pathology & Laboratory Medicine*, vol. 112, no. 2, pp. 211–214, 1988.

[41] S. Faruqi, K. Gumparthy, and Z. Wahbi, "Elevated CA 19-9 levels observed in association with a pulmonary neuroendocrine tumour and amyloid," *Internal Medicine*, vol. 52, no. 1, pp. 105–109, 2013.

[42] A. Samad, R. Attam, J. Jessurun, and S. E. Pambuccian, "Psammoma bodies and abundant stromal amyloid in an endoscopic ultrasound guided fine needle aspirate (EUS-FNA) of a pancreatic neuroendocrine tumor: a potential pitfall," *Diagnostic Cytopathology*, vol. 42, no. 9, pp. 766–771, 2014.

[43] M. Shintaku, H. Tado, K. Inayama, T. Murakami, and T. Suzuki, "Ductulo-insular pancreatic endocrine tumor with amyloid deposition: report of a case," *Pathology International*, vol. 65, no. 4, pp. 197–201, 2015.

[44] S. N. Levine, S. Ishaq, A. Nanda, J. D. Wilson, and E. Gonzalez-Toledo, "Occurrence of extensive spherical amyloid deposits in a prolactin-secreting pituitary macroadenoma: a radiologic-pathologic correlation," *Annals of Diagnostic Pathology*, vol. 17, no. 4, pp. 361–366, 2013.
[45] C. O. Sung, Y.-L. Suh, and D. K. Lee, "Extensive spherical amyloid deposition of pituitary adenoma presenting as pituitary apoplexy," *Clinical Neurology and Neurosurgery*, vol. 110, no. 4, pp. 424-425, 2008.
[46] T. Iwase, S. Nishizawa, S. Baba et al., "Intrasellar neuronal choristoma associated with growth hormone-producing pituitary adenoma containing amyloid deposits," *Human Pathology*, vol. 26, no. 8, pp. 925–928, 1995.
[47] K. Aoyagi, K. Koufuji, S. Yano et al., "Early gastric carcinoma associated with amyloidosis: a case report," *The Kurume Medical Journal*, vol. 49, no. 3, pp. 153–156, 2002.
[48] M. Munichor, H. Cohen, H. Kerner, S. Szvalb, and T. C. Iancu, "Localized amyloidosis in nasopharyngeal carcinoma diagnosed by fine needle aspiration and electron microscopy," *Acta Cytologica*, vol. 44, no. 4, pp. 673–678, 2000.
[49] J. M. Sabate, M. Clotet, S. Torrubia et al., "Localized amyloidosis of the breast associated with invasive lobular carcinoma," *The British Journal of Radiology*, vol. 81, no. 970, pp. e252–e254, 2008.
[50] M. Kotru, H. Chandra, N. Singh, and A. Bhatia, "Localized amyloidosis in endometrioid carcinoma of the uterus: a rare association," *Archives of Gynecology and Obstetrics*, vol. 276, no. 4, pp. 383-384, 2007.
[51] I. Agha, R. Mahoney, M. Beardslee, H. Liapis, R. G. Cowart, and I. Juknevicius, "Systemic amyloidosis associated with pleomorphic sarcoma of the spleen and remission of nephrotic syndrome after removal of the tumor," *American Journal of Kidney Diseases*, vol. 40, no. 2, pp. 411–415, 2002.
[52] M. F. Chiaramonte, D. Lee, L. V. Abruzzo, M. Heyman, and B. L. Bass, "Retroperitoneal follicular dendritic cell sarcoma presenting as secondary amyloidosis," *Surgery*, vol. 130, no. 1, pp. 109–111, 2001.
[53] S. Onishi, N. Hojo, I. Sakai et al., "Secondary amyloidosis and eosinophilia in a patient with uterine leiomyosarcoma," *Japanese Journal of Clinical Oncology*, vol. 35, no. 10, pp. 617–621, 2005.
[54] M. I. Kudrina, E. A. Markina, V. V. Sura, and A. A. Vorob'eva, "Secondary amyloidosis in patient with Kaposi's sarcoma," *Ter Arkh*, vol. 71, no. 12, pp. 53–56, 1999.
[55] D. S. Shimm, G. L. Logue, M. B. Rohlfing, and J. T. Gaede, "Primary amyloidosis, pure red cell aplasia, and Kaposi's sarcoma in a single patient," *Cancer*, vol. 44, no. 4, pp. 1501–1503, 1979.
[56] J. Favreau, L. P. Legresley, and C. Beaudry, "Kaposi's sarcoma associated with primary amylosis, with chronic renal insufficiency," *Canadian Medical Association*, vol. 103, no. 8, pp. 1683–1687, 1973.
[57] S. M. Said, C. Reynolds, R. E. Jimenez et al., "Amyloidosis of the breast: predominantly AL type and over half have concurrent breast hematologic disorders," *Modern Pathology*, vol. 26, no. 2, pp. 232–238, 2013.

13

Serious Complications of EUS-Guided Hepaticoesophagostomy due to Transmural Stent Migration

Mateusz Jagielski, Michał Zieliński, Jacek Piątkowski, and Marek Jackowski

Department of General, Gastroenterological and Oncological Surgery, Collegium Medicum Nicolaus Copernicus University, Toruń, Poland

Correspondence should be addressed to Mateusz Jagielski; matjagiel@gmail.com

Academic Editor: Chia-Tung Shun

Thoracic complications, such as biliopleural fistula and bile leaking into the right pleural cavity, are serious adverse events of transmural endoscopic ultrasound- (EUS-) guided biliary drainage involving EUS-guided hepaticoesophagostomy (EUS-HES). In this article, the authors present endoscopic treatment of biliopleural fistula as a serious thoracic complication of EUS-HES. The authors highlight key components of EUS-guided transmural biliary drainage and their experience with particular emphasis on endoscopic treatment of thoracic complications.

1. Introduction

Transpapillary drainage of bile ducts during endoscopic retrograde cholangiopancreatography (ERCP) is a common and effective treatment for symptomatic patients with mechanical jaundice in the course of biliary obstruction [1–3]. When the drainage through duodenal papilla during ERCP fails, percutaneous transhepatic biliary drainage becomes the treatment of choice [1–6]. Therapeutic endoscopic ultrasound (EUS) techniques were developing intensively in the recent decades. If ERCP is unsuccessful or cannot be performed due to anatomical changes caused by the presence of neoplastic lesions or previous surgeries, EUS-guided transmural drainage of the biliary duct by establishing extra-anatomic anastomoses in the intrahepatic (hepaticoesophagostomy or hepaticogastrostomy) or extrahepatic (choledochoduodenostomy or cholecystoduodenostomy) biliary ducts provides an alternative method of treatment [1–6].

EUS-guided hepaticoesophagostomy is one of the least common methods of extra-anatomical biliary drainage [7]. In this paper, rare and serious complication of EUS-guided hepaticoesophagostomy was presented.

2. Case Presentation

A 57-year-old male patient with malignant biliary obstruction caused by unresectable pancreatic head tumor (adenocarcinoma) was admitted to our medical center due to symptoms of obstructive jaundice. The patient was qualified for symptomatic endoscopic treatment. During ERCP, malignant infiltration of the duodenal wall in the peripapillary region preventing localization of the major duodenal papilla was stated. During the endoscopic examination, with no possibility of transpapillary palliative biliary drainage, the patient underwent transmural drainage of the biliary duct by establishing extra-anatomic anastomoses (Figures 1(a)-1(c)). A linear array echoendoscope was introduced into the stomach, but due to left hepatic lobe hypertrophy in the endosonographic imaging, the echoendoscope was withdrawn into the esophagus. The dilated intrahepatic biliary ducts in the left lobe hepatic segments III were visible through the esophagus wall. Color Doppler ultrasound was used prior to performing an EUS-guided puncture through the esophagus wall to confirm the absence of vascular structures in the potential puncture line. The dilated biliary ducts in the left hepatic lobe were punctured

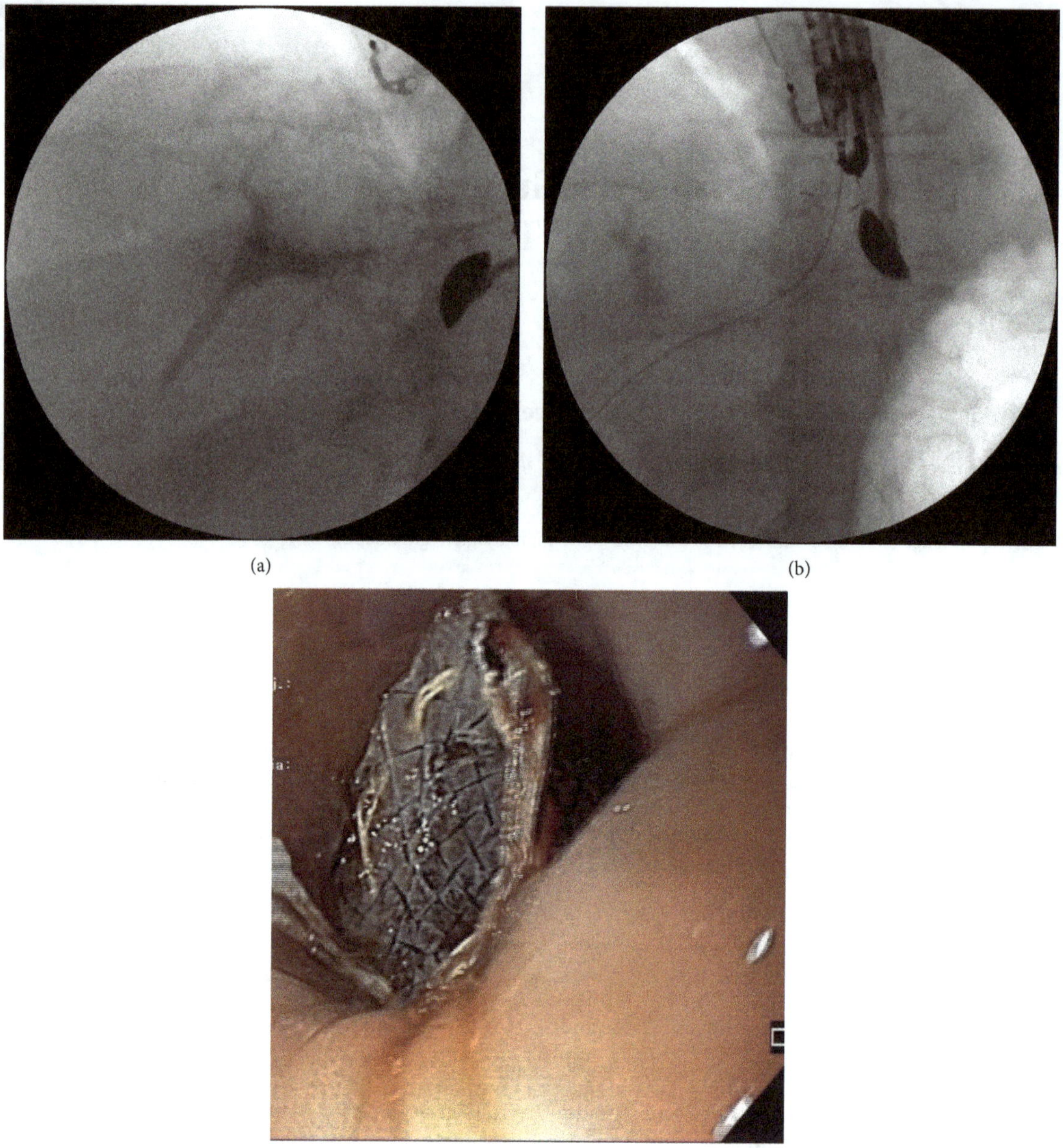

(a)

(b)

(c)

Figure 1: (a–c) EUS-guided hepaticoesophagostomy in a 57-year-old patient with an irresectable tumor of the pancreatic head and left hepatic lobe hypertrophy.

using a 19G needle (EchoTip Ultra 19, Cook Medical, Bloomington, Indiana, USA) under endosonographic control. Following stylet removal, bile content aspiration was performed to confirm an intraductal needle tip location. Next, the contrast agent was administered via the intraductal needle under fluoroscopic control to obtain an antegrade cholangiogram (Figure 1(a)). After flushing the needle with saline solution, a rigid 0.035-inch guidewire (Dreamwire; Boston Scientific Corp., Marlborough, Massachusetts, USA) was introduced through the needle lumen into the bile duct. The guidewire was introduced into the left bile duct and then directed towards the common bile duct with the intention of gaining access to the duodenal lumen so as to continue the procedure using the rendezvous approach or to perform antegrade deployment of the transpapillary stent. Following several unsuccessful attempts to access the duodenum due to malignant stricture of the main bile duct or duodenum, the needle was withdrawn, while the position of the guidewire was maintained and fistula was established using a 10 Fr cystostome (Cook Endoscopy, Ireland). Half-coated self-expanding endoprosthesis (GIOBOR, diameter of 10 mm, length of 10 cm; Taewoong Medical, Gyeonggi-do, Korea) was introduced through the newly formed fistula under endosonographic and fluoroscopic guidance (Figures 1(b) and 1(c)). The catheter was then introduced through the endoprosthesis into the bile duct, and a contrast agent was administered for a follow-up cholangiographic examination to confirm correct positioning of the transmural

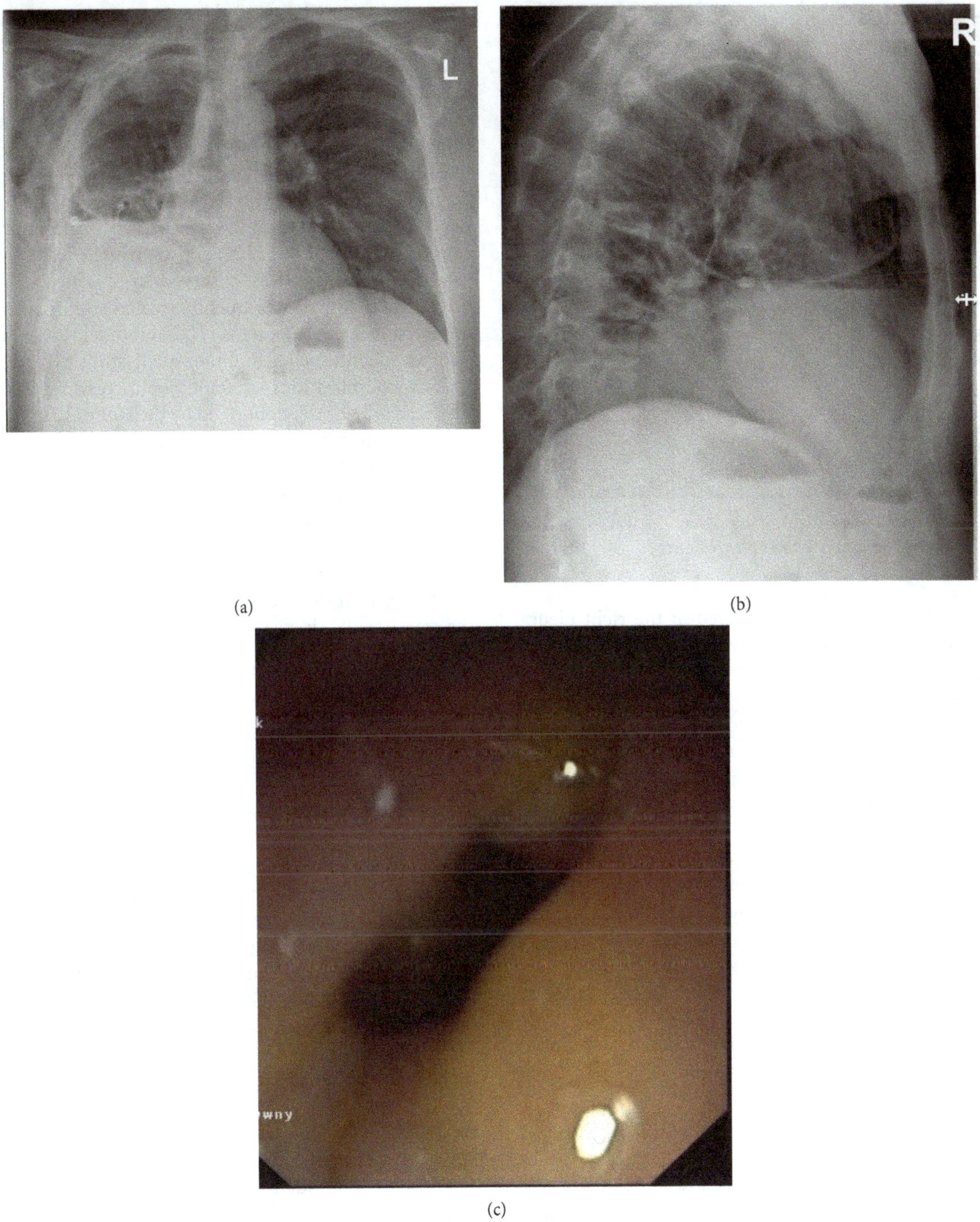

Figure 2: (a–c) Late complication of endoscopic treatment in the form of biliopleural fistula. Right pleural cavity drainage.

endoprosthesis, correct biliary drainage, and the absence of any leaks from the biliary tract. Decrease of cholestasis parameters in blood tests was observed after the endoscopic procedure. The patient was discharged home in good general condition after three days.

Twenty four days after the endoscopic procedure, the patient was admitted again to our department due to symptoms related to fluid in the right pleural cavity (Figures 2(a) and 2(b)). The clinical condition was dominated by dyspnoea. No signs of pleuritis were stated. In the physical examination, lowering of murmur over the right lung was stated. Basing on the clinical image and results of imaging examinations, the late complication of EUS-HES—transmural stent migration resulting in biliopleural fistula and bile leaking into the right pleural cavity—was diagnosed (Figures 2(a)–2(c)). The patient required drainage of the right pleural cavity (Figures 2(a) and 2(b)). This complication was successfully managed endoscopically (Figure 3). The distal end of the dislocated endoprosthesis was located in the biliary duct of the left hepatic lobe, but the

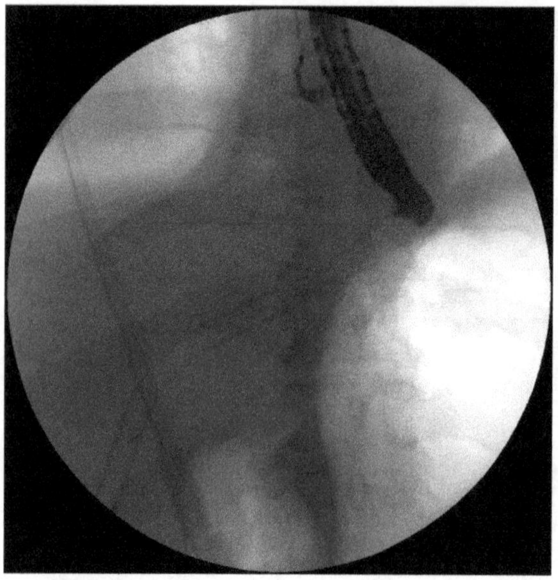

FIGURE 3: Endoscopic treatment of biliopleural fistula as a complication of endoscopic hepaticoesophagostomy

proximal end of this stent was located in the right pleural cavity. During the endoscopic procedure, access through esophageal fistula to the dislocated stent was achieved under the control of the fluoroscopic image. Through the lumen of dislocated endoprosthesis, a rigid 0.035-inch guidewire (Dreamwire; Boston Scientific Corp., Marlborough, Massachusetts, USA) was introduced into biliary ducts. By the use of guidewire, across the dislocated transmural stent, another biliary self-expanding metal stent (using "nstent-in-stent" technique) with a diameter of 10 mm and length of 8 cm (Evolution® Biliary Controlled-Release Stent-Partially Covered, Cook Endoscopy, Ireland) was introduced and esophagobiliary anastomosis was splinted via the right pleural cavity (Figure 3). Seven days after the procedure, the patient was discharged home in good general condition without any symptoms to continue the oncological treatment. During the six-month follow-up, no complications were observed.

3. Discussion

EUS-guided extra-anatomical anastomoses of bile ducts to the gastrointestinal tract have been reported as an effective alternative to percutaneous biliary drainage, when ERCP is ineffective [1–9]. However, in some patients, transgastric or transduodenal approach to biliary ducts is not possible [7–9]. In these cases, EUS-guided hepaticoesophagostomy remains treatment of choice [7–9]. Nevertheless, EUS-guided hepaticoesophagostomy is the least known method of endoscopic extra-anatomical biliary anastomoses [7–9]. Only this year, the first case series of efficacy and safety of EUS-guided hepaticoesophagostomy was published [7]. Earlier on, the EUS-guided hepaticoesophagostomy procedure was being described as case reports [8, 9].

Rugivarodom et al. presented a retrospective study of the first case series of patients with malignant biliary obstruction who underwent EUS-guided hepaticoesophagostomy (EUS-HES) [7]. Technical success was achieved in 100%, and clinical success was achieved in 90.9% of the patients [7]. Treatment-related complications were reported in 27.27% of the patients (with no major procedure-related complications) [7]. Rugivarodom et al. described EUS-HES as a technically feasible and safe procedure for biliary drainage, especially in patients who have undergone left hepatic lobe hypertrophy [7]. The authors observed treatment complications in 3 out of 11 (27.27%) patients: bile leakage leading to mild peritonitis was observed in 1 patient and stent migration that was subsequently treated endoscopically was observed in 2 other patients [7]. No thoracic complications, such as pneumomediastinum or mediastinitis [7], which are serious complications of endoscopic treatment involving EUS-HES [8, 9], were observed by the authors in their study.

In case of lack of access to the extrahepatic biliary ducts, which is more preferred access in extra-anatomical endoscopic biliary duct anastomoses to the gastrointestinal tract, the intrahepatic access is performed (EUS-HES or EUS-HGS) [1–9]. In case when access to the intrahepatic ducts is possible, the gold standard is transgastric access in the form of EUS-HGS [1–9]. However, in some cases, when access to the intrahepatic ducts is not possible, especially in cases of advanced tumors with hypertrophy of left hepatic lobe, endoscopic anastomosis of intrahepatic ducts with esophagus (EUS-HES) may be a treatment of choice [7–9]. Both in EUS-HES and EUS-HGS, a special half-coated self-expanding endoprosthesis is located transmurally [7–9]. Uncoated half of the transmural stent is located intrahepatically, while the remaining part of the stent stays in the transmural anastomosis [7–9]. In our opinion, the EUS-HGS is a safer and more effective procedure than EUS-HES. Firstly, for EUS-HGS, dedicated half-coated self-expanding endoprosthesis is produced to reduce adverse events, for example, in the form of stent's migration, which is described here. There are no dedicated transmural stents for EUS-HES and stents for EUS-HGS are used during the EUS-HES procedure, which increases risk of complications. Secondly, EUS-HES is technically more demanding procedure than EUS-HGS, which is an additional adverse event's factor. Undoubtedly, EUS-HES requires higher technical skills of the endoscopist in the special experienced interventional endoscopic centers. Thirdly, during EUS-HES, distance between the bile ducts and gastrointestinal tract is usually bigger than during EUS-HGS, which is a result of anatomical conditions and severely increases the risk of stent migrations.

As it was stated above, complication of EUS-HES can be prevented by the use of specially designed transmural stents, which is the matter of the future. Additionally, EUS-HES procedures should be performed in the special experienced interventional endoscopic centers by an advanced endoscopist, which will increase the safety of the procedure. In our opinion, these are the only factors that may at the moment prevent described complication due to transmural stent migration.

Due to small amount of data concerning this procedure in current literature, complications and their management are very rarely available. For this reason, this publication is of substantive value because it shows endoscopic treatment of biliopleural fistula and bile leaking into the right pleural cavity as a rare complication of EUS-guided hepaticoesophagostomy.

Disclosure

The funders had no role in the design of the study; in the collection, analyses, or interpretation of data; in the writing of the manuscript; or in the decision to publish the results.

References

[1] M. Jagielski, M. Zieliński, J. Piątkowski, and M. Jackowski, "Outcomes and limitations of endoscopic ultrasound-guided hepaticogastrostomy in malignant biliary obstruction," *BMC Gastroenterology*, vol. 21, no. 1, p. 202, 2021.

[2] J.-M. Dumonceau, A. Tringali, I. Papanikolaou et al., "Endoscopic biliary stenting: indications, choice of stents, and results: European society of gastrointestinal endoscopy (ESGE) clinical guideline - updated october 2017," *Endoscopy*, vol. 50, no. 9, pp. 910–930, 2018.

[3] A. C. Moss, E. Morris, and M. Mathuna, "Palliative biliary stents for obstructing pancreatic carcinoma," *Cochrane Database of Systematic Reviews*, vol. 2, 2006.

[4] R. Z. Sharaiha, M. A. Khan, F. Kamal, and A. Tyberg, "Efficacy and safety of EUS-guided biliary drainage in comparison with percutaneous biliary drainage when ERCP fails: a systematic review and meta-analysis," *Gastrointestinal Endoscopy*, vol. 85, no. 5, pp. 904–914, 2017.

[5] D. Jain, M. Shah, U. Patel, A. Sharma, and S. Singhal, "Endoscopic ultrasound guided choledocho-enterostomy by using lumen apposing metal stent in patients with failed endoscopic retrograde cholangiopancreatography: a literature review," *Digestion*, vol. 98, no. 1, pp. 1–10, 2018.

[6] J. K. Park, Y. S. Woo, D. H. Noh et al., "Efficacy of EUS-guided and ERCP-guided biliary drainage for malignant biliary obstruction: prospective randomized controlled study," *Gastrointestinal Endoscopy*, vol. 88, no. 2, pp. 277–282, 2018.

[7] M. Rugivarodom, P. Aswakul, K. Techathuvanan, A. Chang, and V. Prachayakul, "Efficacy and safety of EUS-guided hepaticoesophagostomy (EUS-HES) for malignant biliary obstruction: the first case series," *Surgical Endoscopy*, 2021, In press.

[8] R. Z. Sharaiha, A. N. Kalloo, and M. A. Khashab, "EUS-guided hepatoesophagostomy for transesophageal biliary drainage (with video)," *Gastrointestinal Endoscopy*, vol. 76, no. 1, pp. 227-228, 2012.

[9] N. Okuno, K. Hara, N. Mizuno et al., "Risks of transesophageal endoscopic ultrasonography-guided biliary drainage," *Gastrointestinal Intervention*, vol. 6, no. 1, pp. 82–84, 2017.

14

Severe Hyperbilirubinemia: A Rare Complication of Lyme Disease

Maarij Baig,[1] Lin Zheng ,[2] and Alka Farmer[2]

[1]*Internal Medicine Residency Program, Inspira Medical Center in Vineland, Vineland, NJ 08360, USA*
[2]*Division of Hospital Medicine, Department of Medicine, Cooper Medical School of Rowan University, Camden, NJ 08103, USA*

Correspondence should be addressed to Lin Zheng; zheng-lin@cooperhealth.edu

Academic Editor: Engin Altintas

Gastrointestinal signs and symptoms are common in the early stages of Lyme disease. However, hyperbilirubinemia from Lyme disease is extremely uncommon. There are only two case reports in literature attributing Lyme disease to hyperbilirubinemia. Here we report a case of severe hyperbilirubinemia as the presenting symptom of Lyme disease. Other plausible etiologies have been ruled out after extensive workups, including liver biopsy. His hyperbilirubinemia gradually resolved after being started on doxycycline. With high incidence of Lyme disease, it should be considered for patients who present with hyperbilirubinemia in endemic areas with possible tick exposure.

1. Introduction

Lyme disease is a multisystemic infection caused by the tick-borne spirochete, Borrelia burgdorferi. Gastrointestinal involvement, such as acute hepatitis, could present in the early stages of Lyme disease [1]. However, hyperbilirubinemia secondary to Lyme disease is extremely uncommon. There are only two case reports in literature attributing Lyme disease to hyperbilirubinemia; one of which was in a pediatric patient [2, 3]. Here we present a rare case of hyperbilirubinemia secondary to Lyme disease.

2. Case Presentation

A 23-year-old male presented to our hospital with jaundice, fever, and arthralgia in early September. He had been in his usual state of health until approximately six days prior to his presentation. He had experienced diffuse arthralgia and a temperature of 38.9°C. He was also told he had yellowing of his eyes and skin, which prompted his visit to the Emergency Department. The patient had a past history of splenectomy five years prior to presentation resulting from a motor vehicle accident. Most recently, the patient states he had discontinued his intravenous heroin and moved from a tent in a rural town into a group home and restarted Suboxone.

On the day of presentation, initial vitals showed a temperature of 36.7°C, blood pressure of 102/56 mmHg, heart rate of 105 beats per minute, respiratory rate of 20 breaths per minute, and oxygen saturation of 98% on room air. On physical exam, the patient was severely jaundiced with scleral icterus. Examination of the abdomen, joints, skin, and lymph nodes was unremarkable and there were no stigmata of chronic liver disease. His initial laboratory tests showed WBC $25.6 \times 10^3/\mu L$, creatinine of 4.5 mg/dL, total bilirubin 11.4 mg/dL (direct 9.8 mg/dL, indirect 1.6 mg/dL) (Figures 1 and 2), Alanine aminotransferase (ALT) of 46 U/L (Unit/Liter), aspartate aminotransferase (AST) of 59 U/L, and Alkaline Phosphatase (ALK) of 127 U/L (Figure 3).

Abdominal ultrasound was negative, while CT of the thorax, abdomen, and pelvis showed diffuse pulmonary infiltrates, extensive parenchymal changes bilaterally in the lung bases with mediastinal lymph nodes and mesenteric portal hepatic adenopathy. He was started on intravenous piperacillin-tazobactam for possible pulmonary infection.

Extensive workup for conjugated hyperbilirubinemia included viral hepatitis screen, α antitrypsin antibody (A1AT), ceruloplasmin, CMV, HIV, antinuclear antibody (ANA), and antismooth muscle antibody, all of which were negative. His LDH was 439 U/L (normal).

There was the concern for tick-borne disease because the patient lived in a tent in the Mid-Atlantic region. Peripheral blood smears were negative for any parasite. Serum screening tests for Lyme disease, Babesiosis, and Ehrlichiosis were ordered. He was started on empirical doxycycline on the third hospital day.

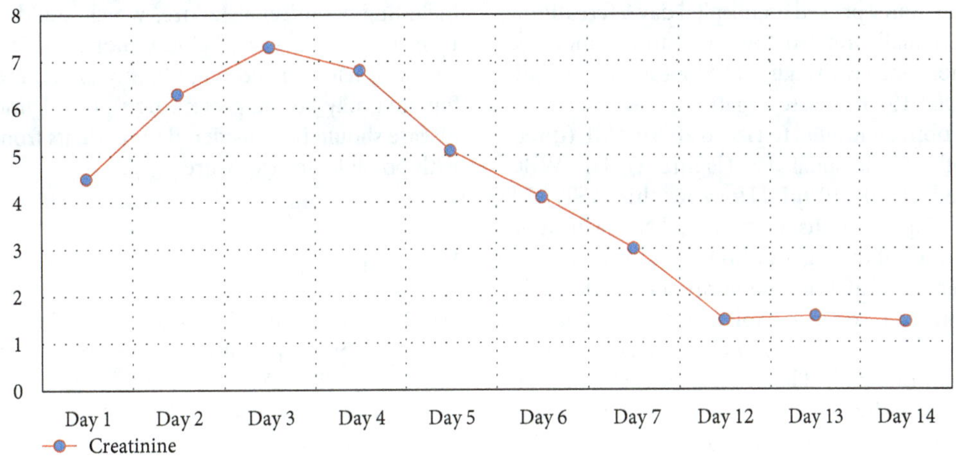

FIGURE 1: Serum creatine level (in mg/dL) by the hospital day.

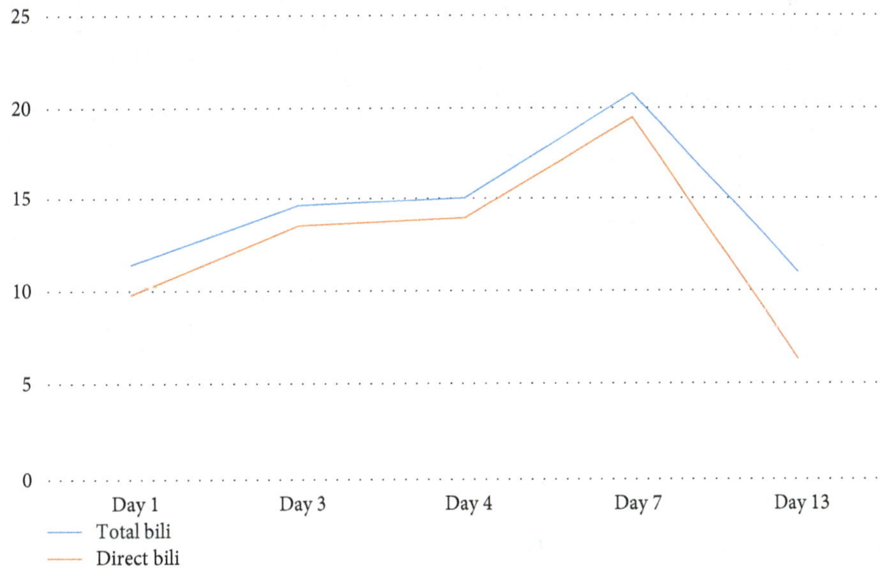

FIGURE 2: Total and direct bilirubin level (mg/dL) by the hospital day.

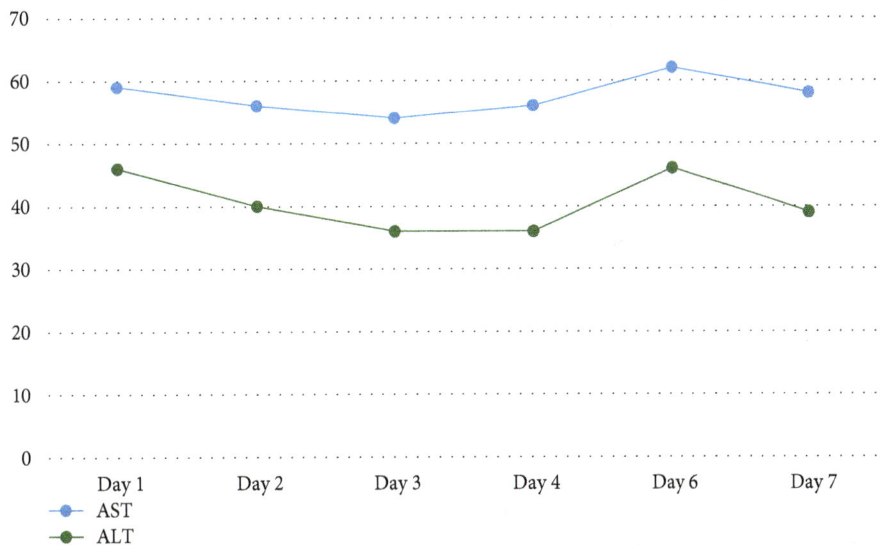

FIGURE 3: Alanine aminotransferase (ALT, in U/L) and aspartate aminotransferase (AST, in U/L) by the hospital day.

His acute renal injury peaked on hospital day 3 (creatinine 7.3 mg/dL) then gradually trended down. Creatinine improved to 3.0 mg/dL on hospital day 7 (Figure 1). Stool studies, including *Escherichia coli* 0157:H7, were negative.

His total bilirubin continued to rise to 20.6 mg/dL (direct 19.3 mg/dL) on the 7th hospital day (Figure 2), His WBC remained elevated at $20 \times 10^3/\mu L$. However, his AST/ALT remained normal (Figure 3). His International Normalization Ratio (INR) was normal throughout his hospitalization.

The patient remained afebrile and normotensive throughout his stay. Magnetic resonance cholangiopancreatography (MRCP) was subsequently performed and showed no evidence of obstruction or intrahepatic dilatation. Repeat US was performed due to worsening of the laboratory findings and showed heterogeneous echotexture of liver suggesting fatty/fibrotic change. The gallbladder was contracted but no stones were present. Hepatic vessels were patent with appropriate direction of flow. He eventually underwent liver biopsy, which was otherwise negative.

Serum screening tests were predominantly negative except for a positive ELISA screen for Lyme disease, which was subsequently confirmed by Western blot. He was continued on doxycycline. His bilirubin steadily declined. He was discharged home with outpatient follow-up. The patient remained asymptomatic throughout the course of his stay, without abdominal pain or pulmonary symptoms.

3. Discussion

Gastrointestinal signs and symptoms are common in the early stages of Lyme disease. One study showed 40% of patients with possible Lyme disease could have abnormal Liver Function Tests (LFTs) [4]. G-glutamyl transpeptidase (GGT) (28%) and alanine transaminase (ALT) (27%) were the most frequently elevated liver function tests among Lyme disease patients [4]. However, hyperbilirubinemia is highly uncommon. Abnormal bilirubin was only seen in 3 out of 115 cases in this study [4]. Similarly, no single case of hyperbilirubinemia was reported in another study, in which a total 314 patients with Lyme disease were included [5]. To the best of our knowledge, this is the first case of hyperbilirubinemia (20 mg/dL) of this extreme attributed to Lyme disease.

Although highly uncommon, Lyme disease should be considered in the differential diagnosis of hyperbilirubinemia, particularly in patients who are at risk of severe infection and end organ damage and are living in an endemic area or have recently travelled to an endemic area, regardless of the presence of rash. Our patient lived in a tent in a wooded area in the Mid-Atlantic region. He presented to the hospital with fever in September. These risk factors should prompt the workup for tick-borne disease.

The combination of ELISA to detect IgM and IgG anti-B. Burgdorferi antibodies and Western blot provides the greatest sensitivity and specificity for the laboratory diagnosis of Lyme disease. Our patient confirmed for *Borrelia burgdorferi* infection. He responded to doxycycline treatment. Extensive workups for other causes of jaundice, including liver biopsy, were negative. He also had multiple end organ damage, including acute renal failure, which could be attributed to Lyme disease associated glomerulonephritis [6].

In conclusion, although highly uncommon, hyperbilirubinemia may be the presenting sign of Lyme disease. Lyme disease should be considered for patients from endemic areas with possible tick exposure.

References

[1] S. A. Zaidi and C. Singer, "Gastrointestinal and hepatic manifestations of tickborne diseases in the United States," *Clinical Infectious Diseases*, vol. 34, no. 9, pp. 1206–1212, 2002.

[2] I. Dadamessi, F. Brazier, A. Smaïl, R. Delcenserie, J. L. Dupas, and J. P. Capron, "Hepatic disorders related to Lyme disease. Study of two cases and a review of the literature," *Gastroentérologie Clinique et Biologique*, vol. 25, no. 2, pp. 193–196, 2001.

[3] K. S. Edwards, S. Kanengiser, K. I. Li, and M. Glassman, "Lyme disease presenting as hepatitis and jaundice in a child," *The Pediatric Infectious Disease Journal*, vol. 9, no. 8, pp. 592–593, 1990.

[4] H. W. Horowitz, B. Dworkin, G. Forseter et al., "Liver function in early Lyme disease," *Hepatology*, vol. 23, no. 6, pp. 1412–1417, 1996.

[5] A. C. Steere, N. H. Bartenhagen, J. E. Craft et al., "The early clinical manifestations of Lyme disease," *Annals of Internal Medicine*, vol. 99, no. 1, pp. 76–82, 1983.

[6] F. R. Mc Causland, S. Niedermaier, V. Bijol, H. G. Rennke, M. E. Choi, and J. P. Forman, "Lyme disease-associated glomerulonephritis," *Nephrology Dialysis Transplantation*, vol. 26, no. 9, pp. 3054–3056, 2011.

15

Concurrent Tumors Revealed by an Autopsy-A Case Report and Literature Review

Miruna Cristian,[1,2] Mădălina Boşoteanu,[1,3] Mariana Aşchie,[1,2,4] Angelica Potamian,[5] Cătălin Adrian Boşoteanu,[1] and Gabriela Izabela Bălţătescu[1,2]

[1]*Department of Clinical Pathology, "St. Apostle Andrew" Emergency County Hospital, Constanta, Romania*
[2]*Center for Research and Development of the Morphological and Genetic Studies of Malignant Pathology-CEDMOG, "Ovidius" University of Constanta, Constanţa, Romania*
[3]*Faculty of Medicine, "Ovidius" University of Constanta, Constanţa, Romania*
[4]*Academy of Medical Sciences, Bucharest, Romania*
[5]*Department of Radiology, Clinical Pneumophthisiology Hospital, Constanta, Romania*

Correspondence should be addressed to Miruna Cristian; miruna.cristian@yahoo.com

Academic Editor: Daniel C. Damin

Introduction. Multiple primary malignant neoplasms are an uncommon phenomenon, given the very low incidence of two or more different tumors, while neoplasm may be limited to a single organ or may involve multiple separate anatomical organs. The main purpose of this study is to highlight the importance of morphological and immunohistochemical tests to distinguish the origin of the primary tumor. *Case Presentation.* We report the case of a 65-year-old deceased male, presenting multiple tumors in the lung, stomach, kidneys, and adrenal organs. The main symptoms presented by the patient were dyspnea with a range of 77% with oxygen saturation, fatigability, and productive cough. Histopathological examination revealed a solid and papillary lung adenocarcinoma, concurrent with tubular gastric adenocarcinoma. Immunohistochemical testing was mandatory by using a panel of seven monoclonal mouse antibodies (TTF-1, Napsin A, CK7, CK20, p40, synaptophysin, and chromogranin A). The pulmonary tumoral immunophenotype (positive for TTF-1, Napsin A, CK7; negative for CK20, p40, synaptophysin, and chromogranin A) confirms the diagnosis of primary lung ADC and invalidates the hypothesis of a metastasis arisen from a gastric adenocarcinoma or other forms of lung cancer. *Conclusion.* The importance of the ancillary test is to distinguish a primary tumor from a metastatic one.

1. Introduction

Multiple primary malignant neoplasms (MPMN) are an uncommon phenomenon as their incidence scarcely reaches 0.99% for two or more different tumors [1]. The criteria for multiple malignant tumors, defined in 1932 by Warren and Gates [2], is that each tumor must present a form of malignancy which clearly differentiates from the other tumors, while the possibility of one of them being a metastasis from the other must be excluded [3]. Neoplasms may either be limited to a single organ or involve multiple separate anatomical organs.

The North American Association of Central Cancer Registries (NAACCR) classifies MPMN into two categories: (1) synchronous, in which cancers occur at the same time (the Surveillance Epidemiology and End Results Programme (SEER) definition is within two months) [4] and (2) metachronous, in which the cancers follow in sequence, more than six months apart [4]. Synchronous MPMN, with lung and gastric cancer, is a rare event. In a retrospective study of Kurishima et al. (2009), 3.2% of 1391 patients with lung cancer (LC) had previous or simultaneous gastric cancer (GC) and smoking had been proven to be a risk factor, as the proportion of smokers was higher among lung cancer patients with GC than those without [5].

LC is one of the deadliest diseases worldwide with a 5-year survival rate of approximately 15% [6]. Globally, the overall lifetime risk of LC is about 1/13 for men and 1/16 for women [7]. There are two main forms of primary LC, classified by the type of cells in which the cancer starts to grow: non-small-cell lung cancer (NSCLC) and small-cell lung cancer (SCLC). NSCLC is the major subtype of LC, which can be further divided into ten subtypes, adenocarcinoma (ADC) is the most prevalent one, with the most common predominant type—acinar pattern [8]. Small cell lung cancer (SCLC) is distinguished from NSCLC by its rapid doubling time, high growth fraction, and the early development of widespread metastases [9]. Lungs are also a frequent target for metastases of extrapulmonary cancers with or without known primary tumors. Metastases of extrapulmonary tumors are found in 20 to 50% of cases and 4% of them are represented by metastatic carcinoma of unknown primary localization [10]. GC is the fourth most common malignancy and is still the second cause of death by malignancy worldwide [11]. The disease becomes symptomatic in an advanced stage [12]. It usually occurs sporadically and mainly affects people over the age of 45, highlighting the fact that males are two times more often affected than females [13]. From the morphological point of view, according to the World Health Organization guidelines, the most frequent subtype is the tubular adenocarcinoma, followed by the papillary and mucinous types [14]. Based on the Lauren classification, most studies showed the intestinal subtype to be the most common, followed by the diffuse and then the indeterminate type [15, 16]. Hematogenous metastases to the stomach are rare, despite its rich blood supply, with a postmortem incidence of 0.2–9% [17]. Metastatic lung cancer to the gastrointestinal (GI) tract is uncommon and very rare, ranging from 0.5 to 14% of cases [17]. They are commonly asymptomatic, and the diagnosis is usually proved during autopsy.

A differential diagnosis between primary lung adenocarcinoma and pulmonary metastasis from another primary site is essential for setting up of a proper treatment. Ancillary tests are extremely helpful, especially when the biopsy results are histologically ambiguous, the most useful biomarkers being Napsin A and thyroid transcription factor-1 (TTF-1) [18, 19].

The main purpose of this study is to highlight the importance of morphological and immunohistochemical tests to distinguish the origin of the primary tumor, in the case of a 65-year-old deceased male, presenting multiple tumors within the lung, stomach, kidneys and adrenal organs.

2. Case Presentation

2.1. Clinical Findings. We report a case of multiple tumors found in the pulmonary, gastric, renal, and adrenal territories, in a 65-year-old overweight and chronic smoking male patient. His medical history revealed a right pulmonary tumor with adrenal metastases, assessed at the Clinical Pneumophtisiology Hospital of Constanta, Romania, in November 2019. In December 2019, he presented to the Emergency Department of "St. Andrew" County Hospital, Constanta, Romania, complaining of dyspnea with a range of 77% in oxygen saturation, fatigability, and productive cough. The computed tomography (CT) scan of the chest showed minimal right pleural effusion with an ipsilateral pulmonary mass, lymphadenopathy of the mediastinal and retrocrural spaces, and bilateral adrenal masses (Figures 1(a) and 1(b)). The laboratory tests showed neutrophilic leukocytosis, a nonspecific inflammatory syndrome, severe azotic retention with low levels of creatinine clearance, and an estimated glomerular filtration rate suggestive of chronic renal failure. During the hospitalization, the patient was treated with antibiotics, diuretics, systemic corticosteroids, and expectorants, followed by amelioration of the respiratory symptoms. Unfortunately, the patient's condition quickly deteriorated, he passed away, and an autopsy was performed.

2.2. Autopsy Findings. The autopsy revealed a male patient weighing 72 kg and measuring 167.0 cm in length (body mass index: 25.82). Macroscopically, a 4×3 cm poorly defined lesion was found in the middle lobe of the right lung, with multiple bilateral necrotic nodules, varying in size from 0.5 cm to 1.5 cm in diameter (Figure 2(a)). The gastric examination diagnosed an ulcerative and infiltrative lesion, measuring 1 cm in the greatest dimension (Figure 2(c)). Moreover, multiple poorly defined lesions were found in both kidneys and the adrenal glands (Figures 2(b) and 2(d)). The specimens obtained from the autopsy were sent to the Clinical Service of Pathology for morphological evaluation.

2.2.1. Microscopical Features. The selected autopsy specimens were fixed in 10% formalin and paraffin-embedded, and then stained with hematoxylin and eosin (H&E). The histopathological examination of the standard pulmonary samples revealed a malignant polygonal epithelial proliferation, with pleomorphic nuclei, frequent atypical mitoses, with a clear nucleoli, and moderately eosinophilic cytoplasm. Malignant cells were predominantly arranged in a solid growth pattern, focally presenting papillary features (Figure 3(a)). Lymphovascular invasion and tumoral necrosis were also noted. The presumptive morphological diagnosis was primary lung adenocarcinoma.

Renal and adrenal lesions were characterized by malignant epithelial proliferation with cytological and architectural modifications like those found in the lungs, presenting with a massive alveolar growth pattern, extensive foci of necrosis, and neoplastic cell emboli in the lymphovascular spaces (Figures 3(c) and 3(d)).

Morphological evaluation of the lesion found in the stomach also revealed a malignant epithelial proliferation of the gastric mucosa with glandular differentiation, which extended to the muscular layer, accompanied by lymphovascular invasion (Figure 3(b)). The cytological and architectural features were consistent with the diagnosis of a moderately differentiated primary gastric adenocarcinoma. These findings raised the question whether the lung tumor

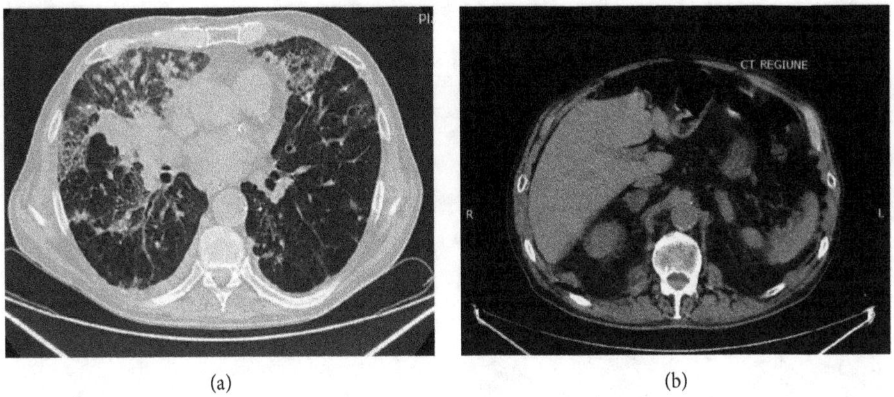

FIGURE 1: Thoracic CT at the initial diagnosis, without intravenous administration of contract material (increased creatinine levels): (a) dense mediastinal pulmonary mass localized in the medium lobe of the right lung, which meets the pulmonary hilum, and cannot be separated from the mediastinal structures, mediastinal, and retrocrural lymphadenopathies; (b) adrenal glands with diffuse increased sizes and spontaneous tissue density.

was a primary mass, or a metastasis from the malignant tumor of the stomach.

The slides were evaluated by a Nikon Eclipse E600 microscope and representative photos were taken from digital whole slide images, obtained with a HuronTISSUEScope™ 4000XT scanner [20].

2.3. Immunohistochemistry Evaluation. Immunohistochemical evaluation was performed on four-μm thick sections of a representative formalin-fixed, paraffin embedded tissue block from the lung tumor. After epitope retrieval, tissue sections were incubated with a panel of seven monoclonal mouse antibodies, ready to use, from BIOCARE Medical (Table 1). A positive reaction for the TTF-1 biomarker was seen considering that at least 1% of the tumor cells were positive [21] and for Napsin A, when a cytoplasmic staining of more than 10% of the tumor cells was found [22]. In the present study, a positive immunoprofile for TTF-1 (Figure 4(a)), a cytoplasmic immunostaining for Napsin A (Figure 4(b)) and a diffuse and intense membranous staining reaction for the cytokeratin 7 (CK7) biomarker (Figure 4(c)) were remarked. Negative results were noticed for cytokeratin 20 (CK20), p40, synaptophysin, and chromogranin A biomarkers (Figure 4(d)).

3. Discussion

MPMNS are very rare tumors which pose difficulties in setting up a correct diagnosis, in conjunction with planning a prompt therapeutic protocol. According to Warren and Gates criteria, the diagnosis of MPMN requires the following mandatory criteria: (a) each tumor should present a definite picture of malignancy, (b) each tumor should be histologically distinct, and (c) the possibility that one is the metastasis of the other must be excluded [2]. Clinically, MPMN is often confused with the metastasis or recurrence of primary malignant tumors since both are characterized by new lesions [23]. Metastatic tumors derive from primary lesions, with the same pathological characteristics and similar developmental processes and prognosis [24]. Conversely, MPMN refers to the development of a *de novo* malignant lesion, with morphological features completely different from those of the original tumor, consequently involving a different prognosis [24, 25].

Globally, earlier studies showed that the combination of gastric and lung cancers is very rare, with a maximum 0.4% incidence [26, 27]. In the study of Duchateau et al., only three patients from 860 NSCLC patients had synchronous or metachronous GC [27]. In the present report, we add new insights to this simultaneous occurrence of two different tumors and highlight the role of ancillary tests in their confirmation.

According to a retrospective study of Kurishima et al., the proportion of men was higher among patients with lung cancer and GC than those without, while the proportion of smokers was higher among lung cancer patients with GC than those without [5]. About twenty-seven of the 45 patients had smoking-related cell types of lung cancer (squamous cell carcinoma and small-cell lung cancer) and the proportion of these morphological subtypes was elevated in patients with lung cancer and GC than those who did not present both lung cancer and GC [5]. In the present report, we noticed that the patient was a smoker for more than 20 years, considered a major risk factor for LC associated with GC.

GC is the second most common cancer worldwide and stands for 8% of all cancers, causing more deaths than lung cancer [28]. Despite the decreasing worldwide incidence, GC accounts for 3% to 10% of all cancer-related deaths [29]. Gastric metastasis from lung adenocarcinoma is extremely rare and this process is not yet completely explained. One hypothesis suggests that certain cytokines may affect the organ specificity in hematogenous metastases, which are usually submucosal and sometimes ulcerated [17]. These lesions are found more commonly in the upper and middle thirds of the stomach, radiographically mirroring a bull's eye sign and endoscopically resembling a volcano or presenting an umbilicated tip [17]. Most of gastric metastases are submucosal; thus, they generally remain asymptomatic [17].

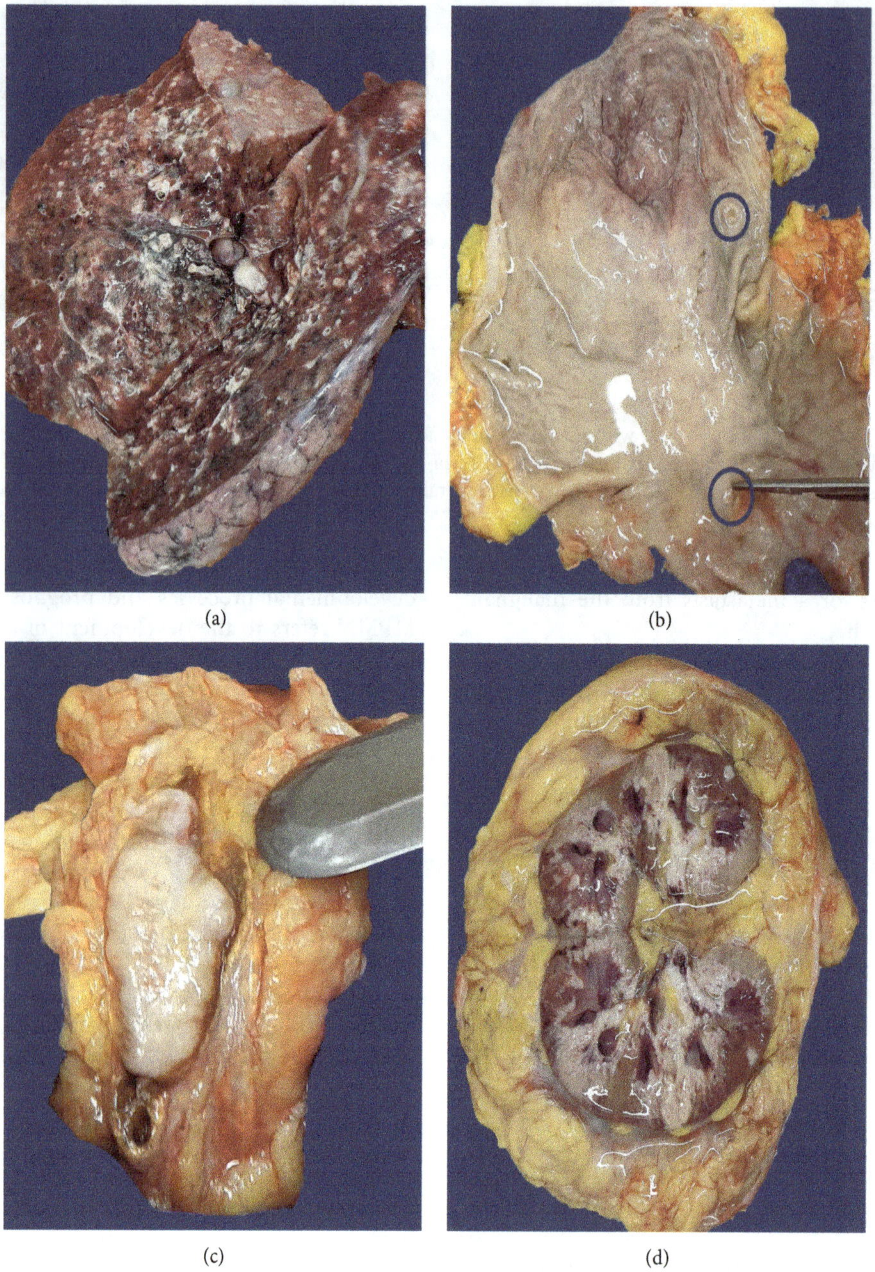

FIGURE 2: Gross findings of the autopsy specimens: (a) 4 × 3 cm poorly defined lesion in contact with the pulmonary hilum, and multiple foci of necrotic nodules, localized in the right lung. (b) Gross view of the gastric mucosa with one ulcerative, infiltrative lesion. (c) Whitish-yellow, poorly defined lesion in the right adrenal gland. (d) Left kidney showing a surface of cut section with multiple poorly defined lesions with diffuse disposition.

On the other hand, lung cancer is primarily known to be associated with upper aerodigestive cancer [30–33] and lung cancer seems to be one of the most common second primary cancers in patients with GC [30, 31].

In this current case, the morphological features of the tumors found in the lung suggest the diagnosis of solid and papillary adenocarcinoma with secondary metastases in the kidney and adrenal glands. Aiming for a correct diagnosis and excluding differential diagnoses, ancillary tests were applied. Adenocarcinoma (ADC) is the most frequent cell type of lung cancer, accounting for over 50% of cancers [34]. Solid predominant ADC was significantly correlated with male gender and smoking history [35]. It was significantly associated with aggressive tumor characteristics including larger tumor size, higher prevalence of lymphovascular invasion, and lymph node metastasis [35]. In the present case, extensive areas of solid pattern malignant proliferation associated with necrosis, lymphovascular invasion, and lymph node metastasis explained its aggressive behavior.

Immunohistochemical techniques are mandatory for a proper diagnosis. The TTF-1 biomarker is a member of the homeobox protein NKX2 (which in humans is encoded by the NKX2-1 gene) family of homeodomain transcription factors which is found in epithelial cells of the thyroid gland

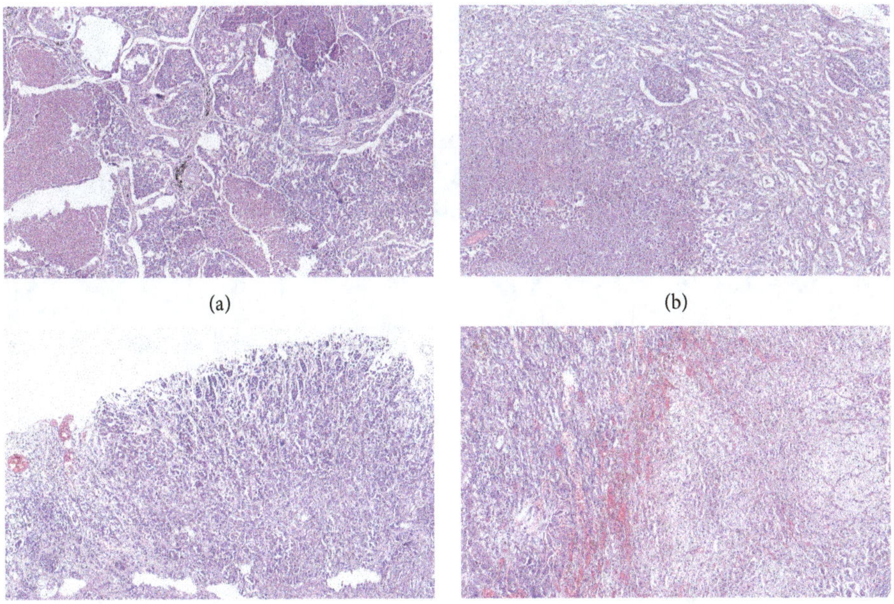

(a) (b) (c) (d)

Figure 3: Microscopical features of (a) lung tumor composed of malignant cells, predominantly arranged in an alveolar growth pattern, defined by solid sheets and tumor nests (H&E, 40X); (c) gastric mucosal lesion-malignant epithelial proliferation with adenocarcinoma morphology (H&E, 100X); (b) renal lesion; and (d) adrenal lesion-malignant epithelial proliferation with cytological and architectural modifications like that found in the lungs, presenting with massive alveolar growth pattern and extensive foci of necrosis (H&E, 40X).

Table 1: Antibodies used for immunohistochemical evaluation.

Antibody	Isotype	Clone	Antigen retrieval	Dilution	External control
Thyroid transcription factor-1 (TTF-1)	IgG1	8G7G3/1	TTF-1	1:100	Lung adenocarcinoma
Napsin A	IgG1	TMU-Ad 02	Synthetic peptide of a part of the N-terminus of human Napsin A	1:100	Lung adenocarcinoma
CK7	IgG1	OV-TL 12/30	CK7	1:100	Ovarian or breast cancer
CK20	IgG2a	Ks20.8	CK20	1:100	Colon carcinoma
p40(M)	IgG1	BC28	Amino acids 5–17 of p40	1:100	Lung squamous cell carcinoma
Synaptophysin	IgG1	27G12	Synaptophysin	1:150	Small cell lung carcinoma
Chromogranin A	IgG1 + IgG1	LK2H10 + PHE5	Chromogranin A	1:100	Pancreas or adrenal gland

and lung, being expressed in pulmonary ADCs and thyroid carcinomas. It is not found in ADCs arising from other sites and, accordingly, are now routinely used to distinguish primary lung cancer from lung metastasis [36]. TTF-1 staining might be also useful in localizing the tumor origin of ADCs encountered outside of the lung [36]. This biomarker has been shown to stain approximately 65–70% of lung ADC cases and rarely provokes a positive reaction in lung squamous cell carcinomas (SCC) [37–39]. Napsin A is an aspartic proteinase expressed in type II pneumocytes, highly sensitive, specific marker for lung ADC, as 85–90% of patients have a positive immunostain, while a negative reaction has been seen in nearly all cases of lung SCC [37–39]. The antibody cocktail of TTF-1 + Napsin A has proved a sensitivity of 91% and 95% specificity for lung ADC versus lung SCC [37]. In cases where TTF-1 and Napsin A are both positive, the specificity of lung ADC versus lung SCC has been shown to be 100% [37]. Considering the present case of MPMN, the positive antibody cocktail of TTF-1 + Napsin A confirms earlier studies of high sensitivity and specificity for lung ADC.

Metastatic carcinoma of unknown primary origin is a perplexing but common problem, accounting for up to 10% to 15% of all solid tumors at presentation [36]. TTF-1 is expressed in lung ADCs and thyroid carcinomas but not in ADCs arising from other sites [36], which confirms the results in this case of primary lung ADC.

The immunohistochemical expression patterns of CK7 and CK20 biomarkers constitute a useful tool to distinguish the site of origin of metastatic carcinomas when a malignant gastrointestinal tumor is simultaneously found. According to the survey conducted by Chu et al. on 435 cases of epithelial

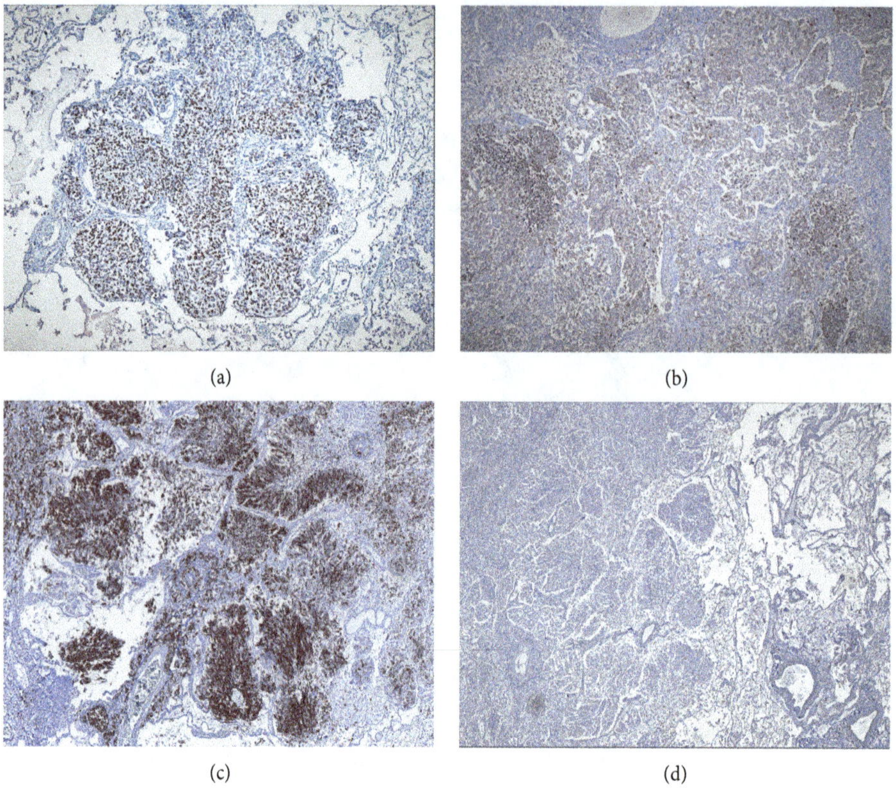

FIGURE 4: Immunohistochemistry evaluation of the lung surgical specimen. (a) 90% positive nuclear immunostaining for TTF-1 biomarker (IHC; 40X). (b) 85% positive cytoplasmic immunostaining for Napsin A biomarker (IHC; 40X). (c) Diffuse and intense membranous staining reaction for CK7 biomarker (IHC; 40X). (d) Negative immunostaining for CK20 biomarker (IHC; 40X).

neoplasms, the vast majority of cases of ADCs was positive for CK7, including lung (100%) and—in contrast—only a small percentage of cases of gastric ADC (28%) were CK7-positive [40]. Based on the differential pattern of CK staining reported in specialized literature, we decided to currently evaluate the CK expression in tissue samples of lung adenocarcinoma. In comparison with the mentioned studies, in the present case, the characteristic features of a positive stain for TTF-1 and Napsin A found in the lung tumor and the CK7+/CK20− confirmed the diagnosis of primary lung ADC and invalidated the hypothesis of a metastasis of gastric adenocarcinoma or another forms of lungs cancer.

Based on these results, the final diagnosis was synchronous MPMN composed of non-small-cell lung ADC, presenting a solid growth pattern, with secondary determination in the kidney and adrenal gland, and low grade/moderately differentiated gastric adenocarcinoma.

Our results suggest that patients with lung cancer should be counselled at the time of diagnosis about their increased risk of developing second cancers, including GC.

4. Conclusions

This is a case report of synchronous lung and gastric ADCs, with an aggressive evolution, in a male patient with smoking history. The gastric lesions were diagnosed only at autopsy and the lung tumors showed a solid growth pattern and were positive for TTF-1, Napsin A, CK7, and negative for CK20.

The increased incidence of multiple malignant tumors is a challenge for physicians; an early diagnosis is essential for the patient to be eligible for radical treatment, which thereafter shows an improved prognosis. Thorough medical monitorization of elderly males present or ex-smokers with lung cancer is recommended.

We also highlight the importance of the ancillary test to distinguish a primary tumor from a metastatic one because the diagnosis of the metastatic carcinoma of unknown origin can be very difficult and the determination of the primary site of the metastasis is a challenge to both oncologists and pathologists, potentially having important clinical and therapeutic consequences.

Authors' Contributions

All authors contributed to this work and commented on the manuscript at all stages, and the last version was approved for publication.

Acknowledgments

This research was performed in the Centre for Research and Development of the Morphological and Genetic Studies of Malignant Pathology-CEDMOG from of the "Ovidius" University of Constanţa, Romania.

References

[1] Z. Liu, C. Liu, W. Guo, S. Li, and O. Bai, "Clinical analysis of 152 cases of multiple primary malignant tumors in 15,398 patients with malignant tumors," *PLoS One*, vol. 10, no. 5, Article ID e0125754, 2015.

[2] S. Warren and O. Gates, "A survey of the literature and statistical study," *American Journal of Cancer*, vol. 16, pp. 1358–4142, 1932.

[3] D. N. Chirila, N. A. Turdeanu, N. A. Constantea et al., "Multiple malignant tumors," *Chirurgia*, vol. 108, no. 4, pp. 498–502, 2013.

[4] "SEER program code manual," 1998, https://seer.cancer.gov/tools/codingmanuals/historical.html.

[5] K. Kurishima, H. Satoh, K. Kagohashi et al., "Patients with lung cancer with metachronous or synchronous gastric cancer," *Clinical Lung Cancer*, vol. 10, no. 6, pp. 422–425, 2009.

[6] S. Hou, S. Zhou, Z. Qin et al., "Evidence, mechanism, and clinical relevance of the transdifferentiation from lung adenocarcinoma to squamous cell carcinoma," *American Journal of Pathology*, vol. 187, no. 5, pp. 954–962, 2017.

[7] J. R. Goldblum, D. S. Zander, and C. F. Farver, *Pulmonary Pathology: A Volume in the Series Foundations in Diagnostic Pathology*, Elsevier, Amsterdam, Netherlands, 2018.

[8] W. D. Travis, E. Brambilla, A. P. Burke, A. Marx, and A. G. Nicholson, *WHO Classification of Tumours of the Lung, Pleura, Thymus and Heart*, International Agency for Research on Cancer, Lyon, France, 4th edition, 2015.

[9] L. A. Byers and C. Michael Gay, *Pathobiology and Staging of Small Cell Carcinoma of the Lung*, Wolters Kluwer, Alphen aan den Rijn, Netherlands, 2019.

[10] A. Fisseler-Eckhoff and K. M. Müller, "Differential diagnosis of primary lung tumors and pulmonary metastases," *Verhandlungen der Deutschen Gesellschaft für Pathologie*, vol. 84, pp. 106–117, 2000.

[11] A. Jemal, F. Bray, M. M. Center, J. Ferlay, E. Ward, and D. Forman, "Global cancer statistics," *CA: A Cancer Journal for Clinicians*, vol. 61, no. 2, pp. 69–90, 2011.

[12] R. Sitarz, M. Skierucha, J. Mielko, J. Offerhaus, R. Maciejewski, and W. P. Polkowski, "Gastric cancer: epidemiology, prevention, classification, and treatment," *Cancer Management and Research*, vol. 10, pp. 239–248, 2018.

[13] D. Forman and V. J. Burley, "Gastric cancer: global pattern of the disease and an overview of environmental risk factors," *Best Practice and Research Clinical Gastroenterology*, vol. 20, no. 4, pp. 633–649, 2006.

[14] D. Lokuhetty, V. A. White, and R. Watanabe, *WHO Classification of Tumours-Digestive System Tumours*, International Agency for Research on Cancer, Lyon, France, 5th edition, 2019.

[15] F. Berlth, E. Bollschweiler, U. Drebber, A. H. Hoelscher, and S. Moenig, "Pathohistological classification systems in gastric cancer: diagnostic relevance and prognostic value," *World Journal of Gastroenterology*, vol. 20, no. 19, pp. 5679–5684, 2014.

[16] C. Shi, J. Berlin, and P. A. Branton, *Protocol for the Examination of Specimens from Patients with Carcinoma of the Stomach*, College of American Pathologists, Northfield, IL, USA, 2020.

[17] A. Qasrawi, M. A. Ghanimeh, S. Albadarin, and O. Yousef, "Gastric metastases from lung adenocarcinoma causing gastrointestinal bleeding," *ACG Case Reports Journal*, vol. 4, no. 1, p. e25, 2017.

[18] M. J. Kim, J. H. Hong, E. S. Park, and J. H. Byun, "Gastric metastasis from primary lung adenocarcinoma mimicking primary gastric cancer," *World Journal of Gastrointestinal Oncology*, vol. 7, no. 3, pp. 12–16, 2015.

[19] G. C. Cozaru, M. Aschie, A. F. Mitroi, G. I. Bălţătescu, A. A. Nicolau, and I. Poinăreanu, "Correlation between Her2 expression and clinic-pathological features of invasive gastric carcinoma," *The 26th European Congress of Pathology*, vol. 465, p. S146, 2014.

[20] G. I. Baltatescu, M. Aschie, M. Deacu et al., "The role of artificial intelligence for image analysis in surgical pathology," *Economics and Applied Informatics*, vol. 26, no. 2, pp. 41–48, 2020.

[21] H. Vidarsdottir, L. Tran, B. Nodin et al., "Comparison of three different TTF-1 clones in resected primary lung cancer and epithelial pulmonary metastases," *American Journal of Clinical Pathology*, vol. 150, no. 6, pp. 533–544, 2018.

[22] Y. Yamashita, T. Nagasaka, A. Naiki-Ito et al., "Napsin A is a specific marker for ovarian clear cell adenocarcinoma," *Modern Pathology*, vol. 28, no. 1, pp. 111–117, 2015.

[23] E. Cigna, A. Gradilone, V. Sorvillo, and N. Scuderi, "ABCB5 in peripheral blood of a patient affected by multiple primary malignancies," *Annali Italiani di Chirurgia*, vol. 82, pp. 49–53, 2011.

[24] L. L. Xu and K. S. Gu, "Clinical retrospective analysis of cases with multiple primary malignant neoplasms," *Genetics and Molecular Research*, vol. 13, no. 4, pp. 9271–9284, 2014.

[25] T. Papajík, M. Myslivecek, Z. Sedová et al., "Synchronous second primary neoplasms detected by initial staging F-18 FDG PET/CT examination in patients with non-hodgkin lymphoma," *Clinical Nuclear Medicine*, vol. 36, no. 7, pp. 509–512, 2011.

[26] B. W. Eom, H. J. Lee, M. W. Yoo et al., "Synchronous and metachronous cancers in patients with gastric cancer," *Journal of Surgical Oncology*, vol. 98, no. 2, pp. 106–110, 2008.

[27] C. S. Duchateau and M. P. Stokkel, "Second primary tumors involving non-small cell lung cancer: prevalence and its influence on survival," *Chest*, vol. 127, no. 4, pp. 1152–1158, 2005.

[28] E. Weisenberg, "Carcinoma-general. Pathology outlines.com website," 2020, https://www.pathologyoutlines.com/topic/stomachcarcinomageneral.html.

[29] J. Crawford, *The Gastrointestinal Tract. Pathologic Basis of Disease*, WB Saunders Co, Philadelphia, PA, USA, 1994.

[30] M. Ikeguchi, S. Ohfuji, A. Oka, S. Tsujitani, M. Maeda, and N. Kaibara, "Synchronous and metachronous primary malignancies in organs other than the stomach in patients with early gastric cancer," *Hepato-Gastroenterology*, vol. 42, no. 5, pp. 672–676, 1995.

[31] Y. Ikeda, M. Saku, H. Kawanaka, M. Nonaka, and K. Yoshida, "Features of second primary cancer in patients with gastric cancer," *Oncology*, vol. 65, no. 2, pp. 113–117, 2003.

[32] T. Ishida, G. Saitoh, R. Maruyama et al., "Survival following resection for lung cancer as a second primary cancer," *International Surgery*, vol. 80, no. 3, pp. 227–230, 1995.

[33] H. Kamiyama, T. Ikeya, K. Suda, K. Murai, K. Aoyama, and E. Hoshi, "Second primary digestive cancer after resection of lung cancer," *Surgery Today*, vol. 34, no. 7, pp. 577–580, 2004.

[34] D. S. Zander and C. F. Farver, *Pulmonary Pathology - Second Edition - a Volume in the Series Foundations in Diagnostic Pathology*, Elsevier, no. 535, , p. 534, 2018.

[35] Y. Zhang, J. Li, R. Wang et al., "The prognostic and predictive value of solid subtype in invasive lung adenocarcinoma," *Scientific Reports*, vol. 4, no. 1, p. 7163, 2014.
[36] M. Srodon and W. H. Westra, "Immunohistochemical staining for thyroid transcription factor-1: a helpful aid in discerning primary site of tumor origin in patients with brain metastases," *Human Pathology*, vol. 33, no. 6, pp. 642–645, 2002.
[37] D. Tacha, C. Yu, R. Bremer, W. Qi, and T. Haas, "A 6-antibody panel for the classification of lung adenocarcinoma versus squamous cell carcinoma," *Applied Immunohistochemistry and Molecular Morphology*, vol. 20, no. 3, pp. 201–207, 2012.
[38] S. Mukhopadhyay and A. L. A. Katzenstein, "Subclassification of non-small cell lung carcinomas lacking morphologic differentiation on biopsy specimens: utility of an immunohistochemical panel containing TTF-1, napsin A, p63, and CK5/6," *The American Journal of Surgical Pathology*, vol. 35, no. 1, pp. 15–25, 2011.
[39] B. M. Turner, P. T. Cagle, I. M. Sainz, J. Fukuoka, S. S. Shen, and J. Jagirdar, "Napsin A, a new marker for lung adenocarcinoma, is complementary and more sensitive and specific than thyroid transcription factor 1 in the differential diagnosis of primary pulmonary carcinoma: evaluation of 1674 cases by tissue microarray," *Archives of Pathology and Laboratory Medicine*, vol. 136, no. 2, pp. 163–171, 2012.
[40] P. Chu, E. Wu, and L. M. Weiss, "Cytokeratin 7 and Cytokeratin 20 expression in epithelial neoplasms: a survey of 435 cases," *Modern Pathology*, vol. 13, no. 9, pp. 962–972, 2000.

16

Pylephlebitis Associated with Inferior Mesenteric Vein Thrombosis Treated Successfully with Anticoagulation and Antibiotics in a 37-Year-Old Male

Mohamed Abdallah, Ahmad Gohar, Smitha Naryana Gowda, Hafez M. Abdullah, and Ali Al-hajjaj

Internal Medicine, University of South Dakota Sanford School of Medicine, Vermillion, SD 57069, USA

Correspondence should be addressed to Hafez M. Abdullah; dr.ammarabdullah@gmail.com

Academic Editor: Daniel C. Damin

Pylephlebitis is a condition in which there is septic thrombophlebitis of the portal-mesenteric venous system. It is a rare condition that usually arises as a complication of an intra-abdominal infection or inflammation. Being rare, it may be overlooked as a differential in cases of abdominal pain when the more common causes have been excluded. We present a case of a 37-year-old Hispanic male who presented with acute abdominal pain and loose stools. He was initially treated for acute gastroenteritis but his clinical condition deteriorated. He was eventually diagnosed with pylephlebitis with associated inferior mesenteric vein thrombosis. He was successfully treated with IV antibiotics and warfarin. Pylephlebitis should not be overlooked as a differential in an appropriate clinic setting as it has a high mortality rate.

1. Introduction

Pylephlebitis or portal vein septic thrombophlebitis, defined as suppurative thrombophlebitis of the portal-mesenteric venous system, is a very rare condition. It complicates less than 0.2% of all intra-abdominal infections with an estimated annual incidence of 0.37–2.7 cases per 100,000 inhabitants per year [1–3]. Inferior mesenteric vein thrombosis complicating pylephlebitis is exceedingly uncommon, complicating less than 2% of pylephlebitis cases [4]. Despite its rarity, portal vein thrombosis in the setting of intra-abdominal infection carries a high mortality, estimated to be more than 20% [1, 4]. Here, we report a rare case of pylephlebitis with associated thrombosis involving inferior mesenteric vein. The patient was managed with prolonged IV antibiotics and anticoagulation and made a successful recovery.

2. Case Presentation

A 37-year-old male presented to the emergency department with fever, vomiting, watery diarrhea, and diffuse abdominal pain for three days. His past medical history was significant for migraine headaches and alcohol abuse. He did not have a history of cirrhosis. He denied any blood in stools, rashes, neck stiffness, or recent travel. He worked as a construction worker and denied any sick contacts.

Physical examination was pertinent for tachycardia with a heart rate of 147 beats per minute, respiratory rate of 25 breaths per minute, temperature of 99.5°F, and oxygen saturation of 100% on room air. Blood pressure was 101/59 mmHg. The rest of his physical examination was unremarkable.

On laboratory workup, his hemoglobin was 15.3 g/dL (13.5–17.5 g/dL), white blood cells count was 2,900 cells/uL(4.5–11 K/uL), total bilirubin was 2.7 mg/dL (0.3–1.0 mg/dL), aspartate aminotransferase 152 U/L (13–39 U/L), alanine aminotransferase 167 U/L (4–33 U/L), alkaline phosphatase 174 U/L (34–104 U/L), lipase 68 U/L (11–82 U/L), prothrombin time 14.3 sec (11.8–14.9 sec), and aPTT 32.9 (24–36 sec).

A preliminary diagnosis of sepsis due to viral or bacterial gastroenteritis was made, and supportive management with intravenous (IV) fluids and antipyretics was initiated. However, his clinical condition deteriorated. On hospital day 5, he developed a fever of 102.5°F, chills and hypotension. White cell count rose to 17,200 cells/uL (4.5–11k cells/uL). Chest-X-ray, urinalysis, and abdominal ultrasound were unremarkable. An Ultrasound and MRCP only showed a small amount of fluid around the gallbladder. A HIDA scan was undertaken, which ruled out cholecystitis as the cause of the elevated liver enzymes and sepsis. Computed tomography (CT) of the abdomen and pelvis with intravenous contrast showed thickening and pericolonic stranding of descending colon and sigmoid colon, a large amount of portal venous gas, gas in the inferior mesenteric vein, and low attenuation filling defects of the inferior mesenteric vein (IMV) suggestive of septic thrombosis (Figures 1 and 2).

Meropenem 2 g every 8 hours was started for a presumable intra-abdominal bacterial infection. The patient's clinical condition improved over the following 48 hours. Blood cultures grew Bacteroides fragilis, Clostridium fragilis, and Fusobacterium necrophorum.

Given presence of concomitant bacteremia and inferior mesenteric vein thrombosis in light of coexisting colitis/diverticulitis, a diagnosis of pylephlebitis was made, and the patient was started on unfractionated heparin infusion in addition to the meropenem therapy.

The patients' clinical status improved over course of the following week with improvement of the abdominal pain and resolution of fever. The patient's transaminases started to trend down, and the patient was discharged home with IV ertapenem for one month and oral warfarin for anticoagulation. The liver enzymes normalized as the patient was followed up in the outpatient clinic. His abdominal symptoms resolved but his ESR remained elevated at 115 mm/hour, so CT abdomen was repeated which showed resolution of the portal vein gas but showed interval development of portal vein thrombosis and proximal superior mesenteric vein (Figure 3). Despite this radiologic progression, the patient's clinical status was improving as mentioned earlier. The case was discussed in a multidisciplinary team meeting involving hepatology, gastroenterology, hematology, and infectious disease teams. A decision was made to continue anticoagulation with Coumadin for a total 6 months duration and to do colonoscopy to evaluate for underlying inflammatory or neoplastic process beside the infectious process. Colonoscopy revealed sigmoid diverticulosis supporting diverticulitis as the etiology of pylephlebitis. The patient continued to follow-up in the clinic and has remained asymptomatic since then.

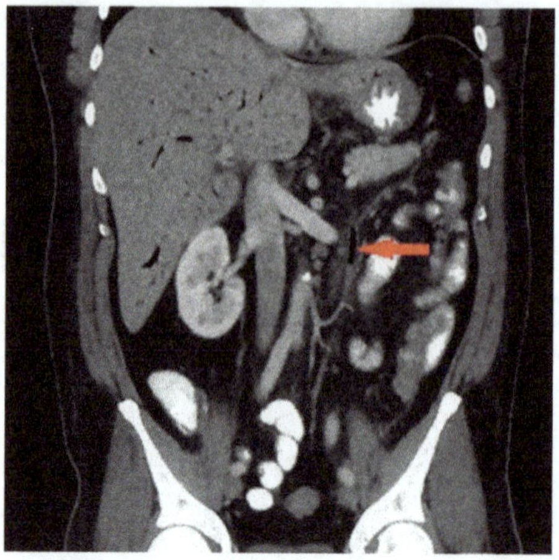

FIGURE 1: Computed tomography (CT) of the abdomen and pelvis with intravenous contrast showed gas in the inferior mesenteric vein.

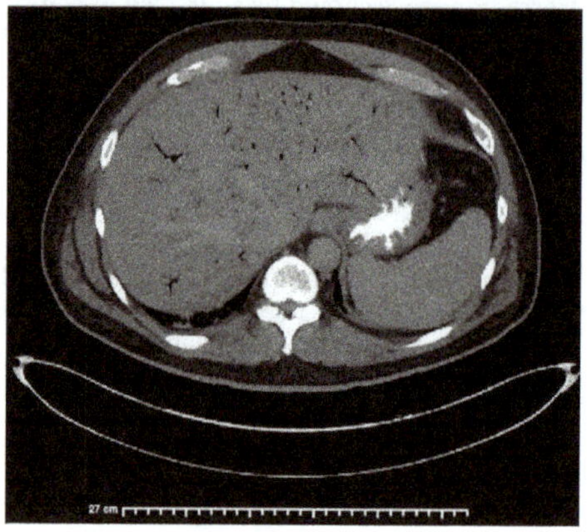

FIGURE 2: Computed tomography (CT) of the abdomen and pelvis with intravenous contrast showed a large amount of portal venous gas.

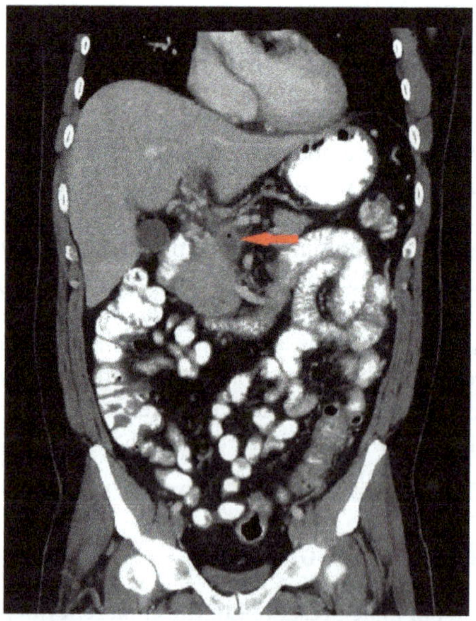

FIGURE 3: Computed tomography (CT) abdomen was repeated which showed resolution of the portal vein gas but showed interval development of portal vein thrombosis and proximal superior mesenteric vein.

3. Discussion

Pylephlebitis, first described in 1846 by Waller, is an uncommon yet serious condition that can complicate intra-abdominal infections [5]. A review of more than 100 published case reports of pylephlebitis from 1971 to 2009 showed that the mean age of presentation is 42.3 years. Acute pylephlebitis, which is diagnosed if symptoms start within 60 days of presentation, was seen in 81% of patients. Regarding clinical features, fever, abdominal pain, hepatomegaly, splenomegaly, transient, or permanent ascites are observed in 86%, 82%, 42%, 23%, and 21% of patients, respectively [4]. Leukocytosis is observed in 80% of patients, elevation of AST and/or ALT in 69%, alkaline phosphatase (ALP) and/or gamma-glutamyl transpeptidase (GGT) levels in 40%, total bilirubin in 55%, and anemia in 55% [4].

Diverticulitis is the most common etiology leading to pylephlebitis and is seen in 19–30% of patients, followed by pancreatitis (5–30%) and appendicitis (19%) [1, 4]. Associated conditions were recent abdominal surgery (19%), remote abdominal surgery in (18%), and immunosuppression (14%). Cultures from blood or other tissue were positive in 44–77% [1, 4]. In half of the patients, a polymicrobial infection is observed [4]. The most commonly isolated organisms are Bacteroides fragilis (27%), followed by Escherichia coli (22%) and Streptococcus spp (17%) [1, 4].

Diagnosis can be established through abdominal imaging using computerized tomography (CT), ultrasonography, or magnetic resonance imaging (MRI). However, the diagnostic modality of choice is intravenous contrast-enhanced CT, which can demonstrate thrombi (hypodense filling defects) and/or gas in the portal system (seen in 18% of cases) [6]. Unlike pneumobilia (the presence of gas in the biliary system), gas in the portal venous system extends to the hepatic periphery allowing differentiation between the two entities on imaging studies [6–8]. Complications of pylephlebitis include extension to the superior mesenteric vein (SMV) in 42%, thrombosis of the intrahepatic branches of PV (39%), liver abscesses (37%), splenic vein (12%), and inferior mesenteric vein thrombosis (2%). Of note, intestinal ischemia complicates up to 25% of patients with SMV thrombosis [4].

Management with antibiotics therapy is indicated in all patients. Anticoagulation therapy is controversial but has shown favorable outcomes, with more complete recanalization decreased mortality, compared to antibiotics therapy alone. Anticoagulation should be strongly considered in case of extension of the thrombosis to the mesenteric system, lack of response to monotherapy with antibiotics, persistence of fever, and the existence of thrombophilic condition [4, 9]. However, a case-by-case evaluation is recommended before offering anticoagulation [4]. Increased morbidity and mortality is observed in patients with significant comorbidities (liver transplantation, CRF, DM, burns, malignancies, and IBD), with sepsis and peritonitis being the most frequent causes of mortality [4].

4. Conclusions

Pylephlebitis is a condition in which there is septic thrombophlebitis of the portal-mesenteric venous system. It is a rare condition that usually arises as a complication of an intra-abdominal infection or inflammation. Being rare, it may be overlooked as a differential in cases of abdominal pain when more common causes have been excluded. It is treated with IV antibiotics and anticoagulation. Pylephlebitis should not be overlooked as a differential in an appropriate clinic setting as it has a high mortality rate.

References

[1] A. J. Choudhry, Y. M. K. Baghdadi, M. A. Amr, M. J. Alzghari, D. H. Jenkins, and M. D. Zielinski, "Pylephlebitis: a review of 95 cases," *Journal of Gastrointestinal Surgery*, vol. 20, no. 3, pp. 656-661, 2016.

[2] J. A. Chirinos, J. Garcia, M. L. Alcaide, G. Toledo, G. J. Baracco, and D. M. Lichtstein, "Septic thrombophlebitis," *American Journal of Cardiovascular Drugs*, vol. 6, no. 1, pp. 9–14, 2006.

[3] M. Belhassen-García, M. Gomez-Munuera, J. Pardo-Lledias et al., "Pylephlebitis: incidence and prognosis in a tertiary hospital," *Enfermedades Infecciosas y Microbiología Clínica*, vol. 32, no. 6, pp. 350–354, 2014.

[4] T. Kanellopoulou, A. Alexopoulou, G. Theodossiades, J. Koskinas, and A. J. Archimandritis, "Pylephlebitis: an overview of non-cirrhotic cases and factors related to outcome," *Scandinavian Journal of Infectious Diseases*, vol. 42, no. 11-12, pp. 804–811, 2010.

[5] R. J. Bolt, "Diseases of the hepatic blood vessels," in *Bockus Gastroenterology*, Chapter 169, WB Saunders, Philadelphia, PA, USA, 1985.

[6] W.-K. Lee, S. D. Chang, V. A. Duddalwar et al., "Imaging assessment of congenital and acquired abnormalities of the portal venous system," *Radiographics*, vol. 31, no. 4, pp. 905–926, 2011.

[7] R. M. Queiroz, F. D. C. Sampaio, P. E. Marques, M. A. Ferez, and E. M. Febronio, "Pylephlebitis and septic thrombosis of the inferior mesenteric vein secondary to diverticulitis," *Radiologia Brasileira*, vol. 51, no. 5, pp. 336-337, 2018.

[8] E. J. Balthazar and P. Gollapudi, "Septic thrombophlebitis of the mesenteric and portal veins: CT imaging," *Journal of Computer Assisted Tomography*, vol. 24, no. 5, pp. 755–760, 2000.

[9] J. F. Duffy, M. T. Millan, J. D. Schoetz, and C. R. Larsen, "Suppurative pylephlebitis and pylethrombosis: the role of anticoagulation," *The American Surgeon*, vol. 61, no. 12, pp. 1041–1044, 1995.

Protein Loss Enteropathy as an Initial Presentation of Gastric Epstein–Barr Virus Lymphoma

Bilal Niazi,[1] Saad Ali,[2] Sameh Elias,[1] and Michael Sciarra[2]

[1]*Department of Internal Medicine, HMH-Palisades Medical Center, North Bergen, NJ, USA*
[2]*Department of Gastroenterology, HMH-Palisades Medical Center, North Bergen, NJ, USA*

Correspondence should be addressed to Bilal Niazi; bniazi24@gmail.com

Academic Editor: Hirotada Akiho

Protein loss enteropathy (PLE) is a complex disease process that can result in potentially fatal protein losses. Gastrointestinal protein losses usually arise from damage to the gastrointestinal mucosa or from lymphatic obstruction. The goal of management is to identify and treat the underlying causes and maintain normal serum protein levels. Here, we present a patient with diarrhea and generalized edema, with decreased serum albumin and gamma-globulin levels, concerning for protein loss enteropathy. He was ultimately found to be positive for HIV infection, and his stool alpha-1 antitrypsin levels were diagnostic of protein loss enteropathy. His endoscopic and histologic evaluation revealed gastric Epstein–Barr virus-encoded small RNA- (EBER-) positive lymphoma. Though gastrointestinal lymphomas are known to cause PLE, this will be the first documented case of EBER-positive gastric lymphoma presenting with PLE. We hope to bring awareness to this unique presentation to aid in expedient diagnosis and treatment to avoid delays in treatment and potentially fatal outcomes.

1. Introduction

Diffuse edema and hypoalbuminemia are common initial presenting symptoms in protein loss enteropathy (PLE). PLE is a complicated and rare disease process that does not have a well-known incidence or prevalence [1]. PLE is usually due to gastrointestinal mucosal injuries or lymphatic obstructions. Mucosal injuries can occur from inflammatory bowel disease, infectious etiologies, or autoimmune causes [2]. Lymphatic obstruction can occur due to lymphangiectasias or lymphomas [2]. Risk factors for gastrointestinal lymphomas include immunodeficiency disorders such as HIV infection and other infections such as Epstein–Barr virus (EBV) and human herpesvirus-8 (HHV8) [3]. Here, we present a unique case of Epstein–Barr virus-encoded small RNA- (EBER-) positive lymphoma presenting as protein loss enteropathy in the setting of newly diagnosed HIV infection. This will be the first documented case of EBER-positive lymphoma presenting with PLE. We hope to bring awareness to this unique presentation of EBER-positive gastrointestinal lymphoma.

2. Case Report

We present a 38-year-old male presenting to the emergency department for generalized weakness, diarrhea, and leg swelling for one month. He was an immigrant and reported sexual encounters with multiple other males for many years. He had no known medical or surgical history. He denied tobacco or illicit drug use and only drank alcohol occasionally.

On initial examination, his vitals were unremarkable, though his physical exam was remarkable for cachexia and bilateral lower extremity edema. No oral thrush, rales/rhonchi, or skin lesions were noted. Initial lab work was significant for hypoalbuminemia <1.5 and positive HIV-1 antibody testing with a CD4 count of 104. Additionally, protein electrophoresis revealed decreased serum gamma globulins levels (0.8 g/dL) and increased stool alpha-1 antitrypsin clearance (695 mg/L). Stool cultures were positive for giardia lamblia infection. No evidence of pulmonary pathology was noted on chest X-ray. CT imaging of his chest, abdomen, and pelvis revealed scattered enlarged lymph

TABLE 1: The plateau of serum albumin levels.

	Hospital day 1	Hospital day 6	Hospital day 12	Hospital day 18	Hospital day 24	Hospital day 30	Hospital day 36 (death)
Albumin (g/dL)	<1.5	<1.5	1.7	1.9	1.9	2.6	2.1

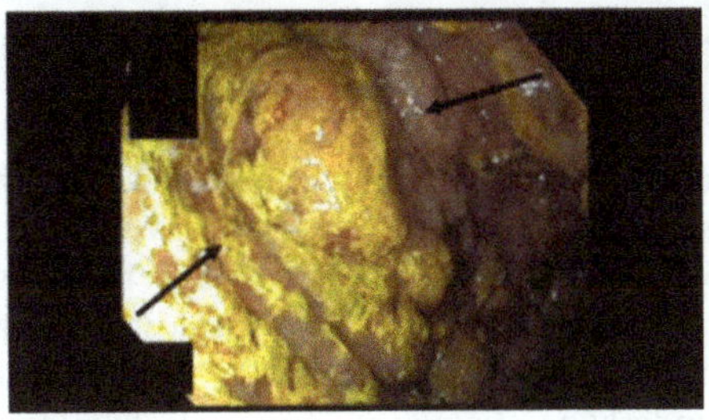

FIGURE 1: Esophagogastroduodenoscopy of the gastric mucosa reveals a suspected mass in the gastric mucosa, as highlighted by arrows, along with areas of inflammation. Imaging is limited by bile reflux. Image Credit: Michael Sciarra.

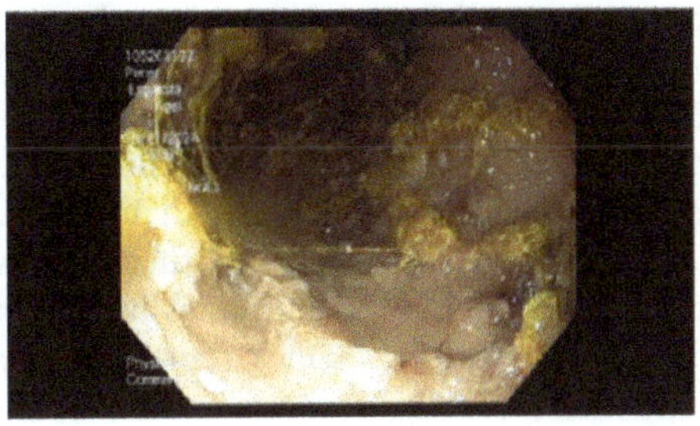

FIGURE 2: Esophagogastroduodenoscopy of gastric mucosa. The gastric body reveals active areas of inflammation. Image Credit: MichaelSciarra.

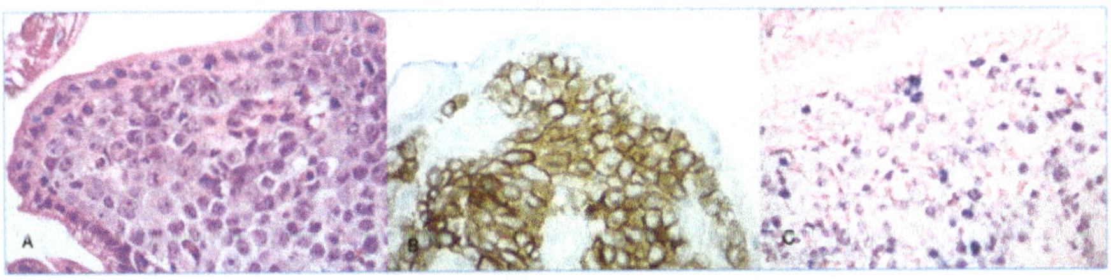

FIGURE 3: Histological evaluation of gastric mucosa. Slide (a): High-grade lymphoma seen under the gastric surface epithelium. Slide (b): Positive reactivity for CD30 with the use immunostaining. Slide (c): Tumor cells found to be positive for Epstein–Barr virus-encoded small RNA (EBER) with in situ hybridization. Image Credit: Kunchang Song.

nodes isolated to under his diaphragm. He was started on intravenous metronidazole, 30 grams of supplementary protein, and 190 grams of medium-chain triglycerides (MCT) daily for protein loss enteropathy (PLE) suspected to be due to giardia lamblia infection. His diarrhea progressively resolved by day 4 of metronidazole treatment without improvement of his serum albumin levels. The trend of serum albumin levels is given in Table 1. Subsequently, esophagogastroduodenoscopy was performed, which revealed a gastric mass with gastritis, as shown in Figure 1 and Figure 2. A gastric biopsy revealed immunophenotypic features consistent with primary effusion type high-grade Epstein–Barr virus- (EBV-) related CD30+ lymphoma, as shown in Figure 3. The proliferative Ki-67 index was found to be high at 99%.

His protein supplementation was progressively increased to 96 grams of protein daily without improvement of his albumin levels to any greater than 2.6. His hospital course was further complicated by deteriorating mental status, renal failure requiring hemodialysis, and acute liver failure. Initially, a chemotherapy regimen of etoposide, prednisone, vincristine, cyclophosphamide, doxorubicin, and rituximab was recommended for lymphoma treatment but ultimately held due to multiorgan failure. Ultimately, a decision was made to place the patient into hospice care, and he expired within 24 hours of hospice admission.

3. Discussion/Conclusion

Protein loss enteropathy is a complex disease process that can occur from insults to gastrointestinal mucosa and lymphatic obstruction. Mucosal erosions can occur from inflammatory bowel disease, intestinal tuberculosis, hypertrophic gastritis, eosinophilic gastritis, systemic lupus erythematosus, and infections such as *Giardia lamblia*, *Clostridium*, *Campylobacter*, *Salmonella*, and *Rotavirus* [2]. In comparison, lymphatic insults can occur from lymphangitis, lymphomas, lymphodysplasia, sarcoidosis, congestive heart failure, or restrictive pericarditis [2]. Protein loss enteropathy commonly presents with weight loss and generalized edema and is suspected in patients with low serum albumin and gamma globulin levels. It is confirmed with stool analysis revealing increased alpha-1 antitrypsin clearance levels [1, 4]. Our patient presented with weight loss, generalized edema, low serum albumin and gamma globulin levels, and an elevated alpha-1 antitrypsin stool clearance consistent with protein loss enteropathy.

PLE is managed by identifying the underlying etiology and initiating the appropriate treatment and nutritional supplementation with protein and medium-chain triglycerides [1]. Our patient was found to have a giardia lamblia infection and started on intravenous metronidazole. Colonoscopy was deferred as there was a likely clear etiology for his diarrhea. Additionally, his diet was supplemented with appropriate protein and MCT. His diarrhea resolved with metronidazole treatment which suggested resolution of giardia lamblia infection [5]. Despite the resolution of giardia lamblia infection and appropriate nutritional support, his albumin levels remained persistently low, suggesting an alternative etiology of PLE. Subsequently, esophagogastroduodenoscopy with biopsy revealed gastric EBER-positive lymphoma.

Primary gastrointestinal tract lymphomas are a known etiology of PLE and usually present with nausea, vomiting, weight loss, and even obstruction [6]. They represent <1% of all gastrointestinal tumors [7]. Risk factors for gastrointestinal lymphomas include celiac disease, immunosuppression, and infections such as *Helicobacter pylori* and Epstein–Barr virus [8, 9]. Our patient presented with weight loss and newly diagnosed HIV infection, consistent with known presentation and risk factors for lymphoma. Furthermore, his diagnosis was confirmed with the immunohistological evaluation of gastric mucosa, revealing EBER-positive lymphoma, consistent with stage II disease based on CT findings. PLE has not been previously described as a presentation of EBER-positive gastric lymphoma.

Epstein–Barr virus-encoded small RNA positivity has implicated a worse prognosis in certain lymphomas [10]. The underlying immunocompromised state of HIV infection leads to increased risk of Epstein–Barr virus. Epstein–Barr virus is known to have oncological properties and often associated with primary effusion lymphoma, as seen with our patient [11]. Diagnosis of the EBER-positive lymphoma subtype is made histologically with in situ hybridization of Epstein–Barr virus-encoded small RNA, and staging is established by the extent of lymph node involvement [12]. Treatment of EBER-positive lymphoma in the setting of HIV is primarily targeted with chemotherapy and HAART therapy for underlying HIV infection [11]. HIV infection, in particular, is associated with a 60–200 fold increased relative risk in non-Hodgkin lymphomas such as EBER-positive lymphomas [13]. Interestingly, HIV itself does not appear to carry oncologic transformation properties, and in vitro southern blot analyses of HIV-associated lymphomas have failed to detect HIV genes [14]. This suggests that the immunocompromised state and underlying oncologic properties of the infectious source play a more significant role in the progression of lymphomas rather than HIV infection itself.

The pathophysiology of PLE from lymphoma is poorly understood. As albumin is a water-soluble molecule, it diffuses freely across the gut interstitium against a pressure gradient in the intestinal lumen [2]. It is a valuable marker of protein loss as it has a slower turnover than other proteins and is the most affected protein [15]. In healthy people, enteric protein loss amounts to 1-2% of entire protein stores and less than 10% of albumin stores [16]. However, lymphoma can obstruct the lymphatic system, thereby disrupting the diffusion gradient of albumin from the intestinal lumen into the gut interstitium leading to enteric losses of protein.

Protein loss enteropathy is a rare disease complex that presents clinically with diarrhea, weight loss, and generalized edema. It is usually due to underlying pathology in gastrointestinal mucosa and lymphatic obstructions. Gastrointestinal lymphomas should be expediently ruled out as they remain a potentially fatal cause of PLE. PLE has not been previously described as an initial presentation of Epstein–Barr virus-encoded small RNA-positive gastric lymphomas. We hope that our unique case will bring awareness of PLE as an initial presentation for EBER-positive lymphoma.

Authors' Contributions

Bilal Niazi wrote the introduction, case presentation, discussion/conclusion, and literature review. Saad Ali, Michael Sciarra, and Sameh Elias assisted in revising the entire manuscript.

References

[1] N. D. S. Nagra, *Protein Losing Enteropathy*, StatPearls Publishing, Treasure Island, FL, USA, 2022.

[2] M. D. Craven and R. J. Washabau, "Comparative pathophysiology and management of protein-losing enteropathy," *Journal of Veterinary Internal Medicine*, vol. 33, no. 2, pp. 383–402, 2019.

[3] M. Olszewska-Szopa and T. Wróbel, "Gastrointestinal non-Hodgkin lymphomas," *Advances in Clinical and Experimental Medicine*, vol. 28, no. 8, pp. 1119–1124, 2019.

[4] M. J. A. M. Braamskamp, K. M. Dolman, and M. M. Tabbers, "Clinical practice. Protein-losing enteropathy in children: protein-losing enteropathy in children," *European Journal of Pediatrics*, vol. 169, no. 10, pp. 1179–1185, 2010.

[5] T. B. Gardner and D. R. Hill, "Treatment of giardiasis," *Clinical Microbiology Reviews*, vol. 14, no. 1, pp. 114–128, 2001.

[6] P. Ghimire, G.-Y. Wu, and L. Zhu, "Primary gastrointestinal lymphoma," *World Journal of Gastroenterology*, vol. 17, no. 6, p. 697, 2011.

[7] S. Ghai, J. Pattison, S. Ghai, M. E. O'Malley, K. Khalili, and M. Stephens, "Primary gastrointestinal lymphoma: spectrum of imaging findings with pathologic correlation," *RadioGraphics*, vol. 27, no. 5, pp. 1371–1388, 2007.

[8] Müller A. M. S., G. Ihorst, R. Mertelsmann, and M. Engelhardt, "Epidemiology of non-Hodgkin's lymphoma (NHL): trends, geographic distribution, and etiology," *Annals of Hematology*, vol. 84, no. 1, pp. 1–12, 2005.

[9] J. C. Peng, L. Zhong, and Z. H. Ran, "Primary lymphomas in the gastrointestinal tract: primary GI lymphomas," *Journal of Digestive Diseases*, vol. 16, no. 4, pp. 169–176, 2015.

[10] X. Gao, J. Li, Y. Wang, S. Liu, and B. Yue, "Clinical characteristics and prognostic significance of EBER positivity in diffuse large B-cell lymphoma: a meta-analysis," *PLoS One*, vol. 13, no. 6, Article ID e0199398, 2018.

[11] A. Noy, "Optimizing treatment of HIV-associated lymphoma," *Blood*, vol. 134, no. 17, pp. 1385–1394, 2019.

[12] M. D. Diamantidis, M. Papaioannou, and E. Hatjiharissi, "Primary gastric non-Hodgkin lymphomas: recent advances regarding disease pathogenesis and treatment," *World Journal of Gastroenterology*, vol. 27, no. 35, pp. 5932–5945, 2021.

[13] R. J. Biggar, R. E. Curtis, T. R. Cote, C. S. Rabkin, and M. Melbye, "Risk of other cancers following Kaposi's sarcoma: relation to acquired immunodeficiency syndrome," *American Journal of Epidemiology*, vol. 139, no. 4, pp. 362–368, 1994.

[14] D. M. Knowles, "Etiology and pathogenesis of AIDS-related non-Hodgkin's lymphoma," *Hematology-Oncology Clinics of North America*, vol. 17, no. 3, pp. 785–820, 2003.

[15] H. Takeda, K. Ishihama, T. Fukui et al., "Significance of rapid turnover proteins in protein-losing gastroenteropathy," *Hepato-Gastroenterology*, vol. 50, no. 54, 2003.

[16] P. N. Schmidt, S. Blirup-Jensen, P. J. Svendsen, and J. H. Wandall, "Characterization and quantification of plasma proteins excreted in faeces from healthy humans," *Scandinavian Journal of Clinical and Laboratory Investigation*, vol. 55, no. 1, pp. 35–45, 1995.

18

Gastric Signet-Ring Cell Carcinoma that Presented as an Elevated Lesion due to Fibromuscular Obliteration in the Lamina Propria

Yoshitsugu Misumi,[1] **Shin Ichihara**,[2] **Kouichi Nonaka**,[1] **Hiromi Onizuka**,[3] **and Yoji Nagashima**[3]

[1]*Department of Digestive Endoscopy, Tokyo Women's Medical University Hospital, 8-1, Kawada-cho, Shinjuku-ku, Tokyo 162-8666, Japan*
[2]*Department of Surgical Pathology, Sapporo-Kosei General Hospital, 8-5, Kita 3 Jouhigashi, Chu-o-ku, Sapporo, Hokkaido 060-0033, Japan*
[3]*Department of Surgical Pathology, Tokyo Women's Medical University Hospital, 8-1, Kawada-cho, Shinjuku-ku, Tokyo 162-8666, Japan*

Correspondence should be addressed to Yoshitsugu Misumi; yoshikft34@gmail.com

Academic Editor: Matteo Neri

The widespread use of *Helicobacter pylori* eradication therapy in recent years has reduced the *H. pylori* infection rate, indicating that gastric cancer cases diagnosed in the future may be *H. pylori*-naïve. The typical endoscopic presentation of signet-ring cell carcinoma, which accounts for the majority of *H. pylori*-naïve gastric cancer cases, is a discolored, flat, or depressed lesion; it is rarely presented as an elevated lesion. In this study, we treated a patient with elevated signet-ring cell carcinoma in an *H. pylori*-naïve stomach. Histopathological testing after endoscopic submucosal dissection showed proliferation of fibromuscular tissue in the tumor, which may have caused the formation of the elevated lesion.

1. Introduction

In the past, most cases of gastric cancer occurred in the stomach of people infected with *Helicobacter pylori* [1]. However, the widespread use of *H. pylori* eradication therapy in recent years has reduced the *H. pylori* infection rate, indicating that higher rates of *H. pylori*-naïve gastric cancer cases may be diagnosed in the future. *H. pylori*-naïve gastric cancer is broadly divided into three types: signet-ring cell carcinoma (SRCC), fundic gland-type gastric carcinoma, and foveolar-type gastric carcinoma [2]. Amongst these, SRCC reportedly accounts for over 90% of the cases [3].

The World Health Organization Classification of Tumors classifies all carcinomas consisting of discohesive cells arranged singly or in small clusters and lacking well-formed glands as poorly cohesive carcinoma. Cancer that mainly exhibits a signet-ring morphology is designated as SRCC [4]. Gastric SRCC is typically observed via endoscopy as a discolored lesion in the middle and lower gastric corpus of relatively young persons [3]. Upon gross inspection, most lesions can be seen as flat or flat-depressed, and elevated lesions are rare [5, 6]. However, a few reports of elevated undifferentiated gastric carcinoma mention its histopathological characteristics [5]. Here, we report a case of a small flat-elevated SRCC, which was curatively resected by endoscopic submucosal dissection (ESD), and discuss the pathology of its flat-elevated appearance.

2. Case Report

A 63-year-old female with no relevant medical history underwent upper gastrointestinal endoscopy for screening. She neither smoked nor drank alcohol and had no family history of malignancy. The patient's *H. pylori* serology result

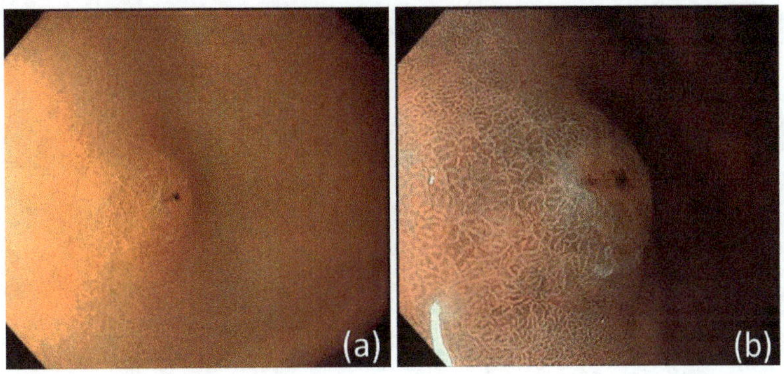

FIGURE 1: (a) A 5 mm poorly demarcated pale-red elevated lesion observed in the anterior wall of the antrum against the background of nonatrophic *H. pylori*-negative mucosa. (b) Swelling of the glandular structures is present, although the demarcation line is unclear.

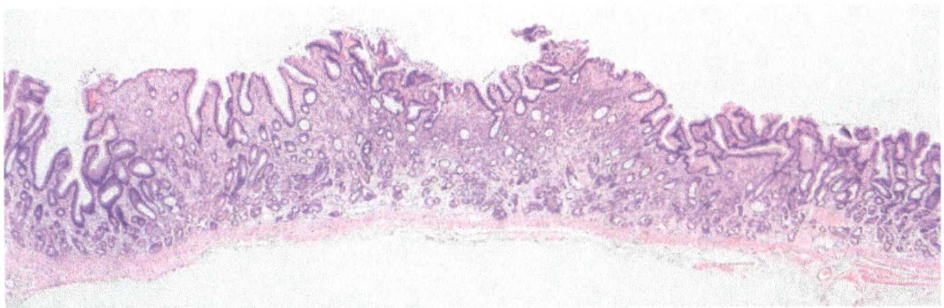

FIGURE 2: Cancer cells seen mainly invading the height of the glandular neck zone, with none in the deep mucosa. There is neither erosion of the surface epithelium nor any signs of tumor cell exposure on the surface. This is a flat-elevated lesion proliferating within the mucosa.

(IgG < 3) and fecal *H. pylori* antigen were negative. The patient had not undergone *H. pylori* eradication therapy.

Endoscopy revealed a 5 mm poorly demarcated pale-red elevated lesion with a slight depression at the top against the background of a nonatrophic *H. pylori*-negative mucosa (Figure 1). The demarcation line of the elevated lesion was also unclear under narrow-band imaging, but the swollen glandular structure of the elevated portion was clearly observed (Figure 1). The biopsy results of the elevated lesion confirmed that it was SRCC. As the lesion was small and neither thickened nor hard, it was diagnosed as intramucosal carcinoma. We finally assumed the lesion to be intramucosal gastric cancer composed of SRCC with 0-IIa + IIc according to the Paris classification; thus, endoscopic submucosal dissection was performed.

The resected specimen measured 28 × 18 mm and the lesion 8 × 5 mm. Histopathological investigations revealed signet-ring cell invasion at the tip of the elevated lesion and in the surrounding lamina propria. Layered cancer cells were mainly present at the height of the glandular neck zone; none were detected in the deep portion of the mucosa. In the areas where cancer cells were present, the foveolar epithelium of the surface layer showed mild hyperplasia and dilation of the intervening part between the crypts. However, there was no erosion of the surface epithelium, and no signs of direct tumor cell exposure on the surface. Hence, it was confirmed as a flat-elevated lesion proliferating within the mucosa with negative lymphovascular invasion and clear resection margins (Figure 2).

In the background mucosa surrounding the lesion, immunohistochemistry by anti-α-smooth muscle actin revealed thin muscular bundles in the lamina propria. Fibromuscular obliteration extended from the muscularis propria to the lamina propria, as if to support the mucosal structure, and thickened the mucosa (Figures 3 and 3). Furthermore, a similar phenomenon was demonstrated inside the cancerous lesion and seemed to support the superficial foveolar epithelium (Figure 3). The resection was concluded as curative, and upper gastrointestinal endoscopy follow-up was scheduled 12 months after the ESD.

3. Discussion

Gastric SRCC is usually flat or depressed; however, there are rare cases of elevated lesions that have been successfully resected [5]. Two causes of elevated lesions include upwards tumor growth into the gastric lumen and coexistent desmoplastic or fibrotic reaction [7]. However, neither of these reasons was applicable in the case we report here. Instead, a fibromuscular obliteration was observed both inside and outside the lesion. Fibromuscular obliteration is seen in conditions such as mucosal prolapse syndrome (MPS) of the rectum and occurs when smooth muscle bundles extend from the muscularis mucosa into the lamina propria [8]. As the patient exhibited strong peristalsis, which was so frequent that it was difficult to take clear pictures, it is possible that a previously slightly depressed lesion was pushed out by intense peristaltic movements that led to fibromuscular obliteration

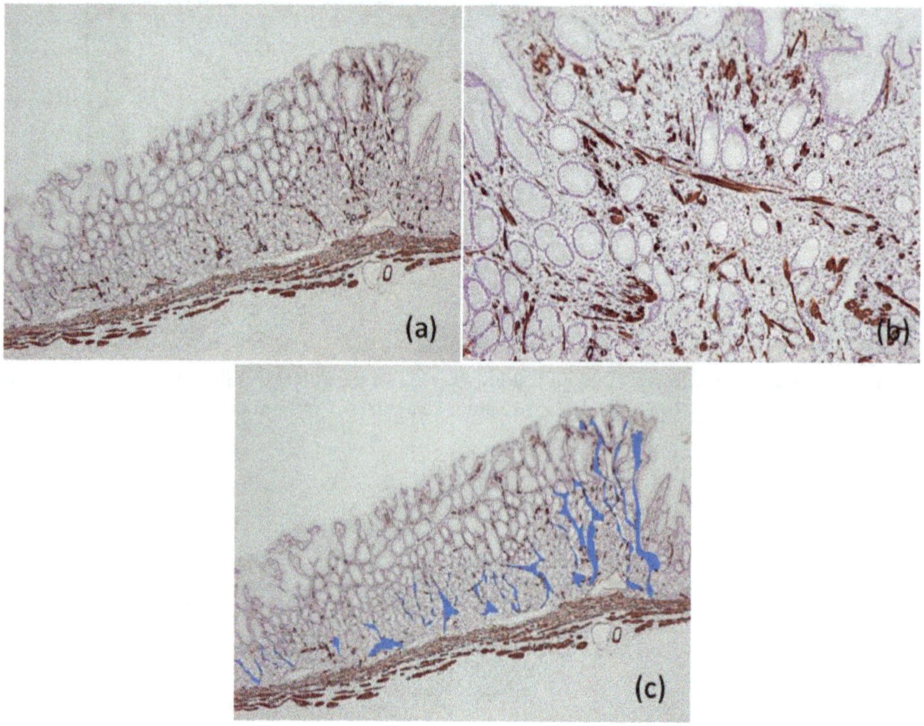

Figure 3: (a) Fibromuscular obliteration by α-smooth muscle myosin observed around the pyloric glands in the background mucosa surrounding the lesion; in places, this extends as if to support the foveolar epithelium. (b) Inside the lesion, fibromuscular obliteration seems to support the foveolar epithelium. (c) Schema representing fibromuscular obliteration. Fibromuscular obliteration is surrounded by blue paint.

of the lamina propria, consequently lifting the mucosa within the lesion to give it an elevated appearance. Additionally, the distribution of the SRCC in the present case was mostly limited to the glandular neck zone, and the absence of surface erosion indicated that no remarkable depression or step was formed, which may have also contributed to the observation of the lesion mainly as an elevation.

Although this report is just one case and further research is essential, we suggest the term "fibromuscular elevation" (FE) to describe the phenomenon by which fibromuscular obliteration, induced by peristalsis, elevates both tumor and nontumor tissue towards the luminal side. Similar to the present case, there is a report that the same "FE" phenomenon was observed in some differentiated adenocarcinoma [9]. Although this is a rare case, the possibility of undifferentiated carcinoma exhibiting FE should be considered when an elevated lesion is encountered in the antrum of an *H. pylori*-naïve stomach. In addition, it is difficult to differentiate the lesion from the raised erosions commonly seen in the antrum based on only endoscopic findings. Hence, a biopsy is mandatory when a single lesion is seen in the antrum.

Acknowledgments

The authors would like to thank Editage (https://www.editage.com) for English language editing.

References

[1] Y. Yamaoka, "Mechanisms of disease: *Helicobacter pylori* virulence factors," *Nature Reviews Gastroenterology & Hepatology*, vol. 7, no. 11, pp. 629–641, 2010.

[2] K. Yao, Y. Takaki, T. Matsui et al., "Clinical application of magnification endoscopy and narrow-band imaging in the upper gastrointestinal tract: new imaging techniques for detecting and characterizing gastrointestinal neoplasia," *Gastrointestinal Endoscopy Clinics of North America*, vol. 18, no. 3, pp. 415–433, 2008.

[3] Y. Yamamoto, J. Fujisaki, M. Omae, T. Hirasawa, and M. Igarashi, "Helicobacter pylori-negative gastric cancer: characteristics and endoscopic findings," *Digestive Endoscopy*, vol. 27, no. 5, pp. 551–561, 2015.

[4] G. Lauwers, F. Carneiro, D. Graham, M. Curado, S. Franceschi, and E. Montgomery, "WHO classification of tumours of the digestive system," in *Tumours of the Stomach: Gastric Carcinoma*, F. T. Bosman, F. Carneiro, R. H. Hruban et al., Eds., pp. 48–58, IARC, Lyon, France, 4th edition, 2010.

[5] Y. Shiratori, T. Ikeya, K. Suzuki, K. Nakamura, and K. Fukuda, "The rare case of elevated signet ring cell gastric carcinoma with Helicobacter pylori-naïve mucosa," *Clinical Journal of Gastroenterology*, vol. 13, no. 5, pp. 736–739, 2020.

[6] Y. Horiuchi, J. Fujisaki, N. Yamamoto et al., "Biological behavior of the intramucosal Helicobacter pylori-negative undifferentiated-type early gastric cancer: comparison with Helicobacter pylori-positive early gastric cancer," *Gastric Cancer*, vol. 19, no. 1, pp. 160–165, 2016.

[7] T. Hirano, S. Yamaguchi, H. Kusano et al., "Signet ring cell early gastric cancer presenting as an elevated lesion," *Gastroenterologia Japonica*, vol. 25, no. 5, pp. 625–629, 1990.
[8] M. Murata, M. Sugimoto, H. Ban et al., "Cap polyposis refractory to *Helicobacter pylori* eradication treated with endoscopic submucosal dissection," *World Journal of Gastrointestinal Endoscopy*, vol. 9, no. 10, pp. 529–534, 2017.
[9] M. Takita, K. Ohata, R. Inamoto et al., "Endoscopic and histological features of *Helicobacter pylori* - negative differentiated gastric adenocarcinoma arising in the antrum," *JGH Open*, vol. 5, no. 4, pp. 470–477, 2021.

19

Complete Radiologic Response of Metastatic Pancreatic Ductal Adenocarcinoma to Microwave Ablation Combined with Second-Line Palliative Chemotherapy

Hakon Blomstrand,[1] **Karin Adolfsson**,[2] **Per Sandström**,[3] **and Bergthor Björnsson**[3]

[1]*Department of Clinical Pathology and Department of Clinical and Experimental Medicine, Linköping University, 58183 Linköping, Sweden*
[2]*Department of Oncology, Ryhov County Hospital, 55305 Jönköping, Sweden*
[3]*Department of Surgery and Department of Clinical and Experimental Medicine, Linköping University, 58183 Linköping, Sweden*

Correspondence should be addressed to Bergthor Björnsson; bergthor.bjornsson@liu.se

Academic Editor: Shiro Kikuchi

Pancreatic ductal adenocarcinoma (PDAC) has a bleak prognosis, especially for the majority of patients diagnosed with metastatic disease. The primary option for palliative treatment is chemotherapy, and responses beyond first-line treatment are rare and typically short. Here, we report a case of a 63-year-old woman with PDAC in the head of the pancreas who was initially successfully treated by pancreaticoduodenectomy followed by adjuvant chemotherapy with gemcitabine. However, disease recurrence with liver and para-aortic lymph node metastases was detected only two months after the completion of adjuvant chemotherapy. First-line palliative chemotherapy with gemcitabine-nab/paclitaxel was commenced. The results were discouraging, with disease progression (liver and lung metastases) detected at the first evaluation; the progression-free survival was just two months (64 days). Surprisingly, the response to second-line palliative chemotherapy with 5-fluorouracil-oxaliplatin was excellent; in combination with the ablation of a liver metastasis, this treatment regimen resulted in a complete radiological response and an 11-month treatment-free interval with a sustained good performance status.

1. Background

Pancreatic ductal adenocarcinoma (PDAC) is the fourth leading cause of cancer-related death in Sweden and the USA [1, 2]. Initial symptoms are often nonspecific, and most patients are diagnosed with locally advanced pancreatic cancer (LAPC) and/or metastatic disease.

PDAC without distant metastasis is divided into resectable PDAC, borderline resectable pancreatic cancer (BRPC), and LAPC, largely dependent on the extent of vessel involvement [3]. For resectable PDAC without vessel involvement, the standard treatment is initial surgery with pancreaticoduodenectomy or distal resection, depending on tumour location, followed by single-agent adjuvant chemotherapy with 5-fluorouracil (5FU) or gemcitabine [4]. This subgroup of PDAC patients has the best outcome, but the frequency of recurrence is high, and long-term survival at five years is only 15–20% [5]. Adjuvant combination chemotherapy with gemcitabine-5FU appears to improve outcomes [6], and neoadjuvant chemotherapy is being evaluated in several ongoing trials [7]. For the BRPC subgroup with tumour infiltration of local major vessels (mainly the celiac trunk, superior mesenteric artery, and hepatic artery), the risk of microscopically positive resection margins (R1 resection) following surgery is substantial; therefore, combination chemotherapy and multimodal treatments (e.g., chemotherapy with sequential or concomitant radiotherapy) have been tested in numerous trials, but the results on the most effective strategy are contradictory (reviewed in [8]). The LAPC subgroup with extensive vessel engagement has a high risk of macroscopically positive resection margins (R2 resection), and surgery should not be considered unless conversion to BRPC is achieved during palliative treatment [9].

In nonresponding LAPC or primary metastatic disease, resection of the primary tumour is not possible or not indicated, respectively, and the treatment option is palliative care. According to current guidelines, the only treatment modalities for patients with this disease are chemotherapy and radiation therapy for severe and refractory pain [10, 11]. The prognosis of patients with metastatic pancreatic cancer is poor, with an expected five-year survival rate of 8% in Sweden [12]. Histological subtypes other than ductal adenocarcinoma are rare, and signet ring cell carcinoma appears to have a similar prognosis [13], while the colloid variant (mucinous noncystic adenocarcinoma) has a markedly better prognosis [14].

2. Case Presentation

A 63-year-old Swedish woman consulted her local health centre due to nausea, bright coloured stools, and 4 kg weight loss. Laboratory tests revealed elevated aminotransferases and bilirubinaemia, and the patient was referred to the local surgical department. Abdominal ultrasound and computed tomography (CT) of the abdomen and thoracic cavity revealed a tumour in the pancreatic head measuring 25 mm, a borderline enlarged lymph node in the liver hilum, and dilation of the pancreatic and common bile ducts but no evidence of distant metastases. CA19-9 was elevated to 2741 kU/L (<35 kU/L) (Figure 1). Internal bile duct drainage via endoscopic retrograde cholangiopancreatography (ERCP) failed; thus, the patient underwent percutaneous transhepatic cholangiography (PTC) drainage and was treated twice for cholangitis with intravenous antibiotics before undergoing surgery at the regional university hospital. The surgical procedure was a standard pancreaticoduodenectomy with an uneventful recovery. The patient was discharged to the local hospital on the fourth postoperative day (POD) and to the home on POD 15. The histopathological examination confirmed moderately to poorly differentiated PDAC. Although minor sections of the tumour had mucinous and signet ring cell-like histology, the diagnosis was not changed. Perineural and lymphovascular invasion was evident. Carcinoma involvement was seen in two pancreaticoduodenal lymph nodes out of a total of 20 examined lymph nodes. The tumour grade was pT3N1MX (Figure 2). Postoperative CA19-9 was 6 kU/L. Six months of adjuvant treatment with gemcitabine (intravenous infusions on days 1, 8, and 15 in a four-week cycle at 1000 mg/m^2) was initiated. The patient completed the entire treatment regimen, except the dose on cycle 4 day 15 due to *E. coli* septicaemia, which was successfully treated with antibiotics. At the evaluation at the end of adjuvant treatment, 7.5 months after surgery, there were no signs of radiological recurrence on CT; however, CA19-9 was increased to 229 kU/L.

After an additional two months of observation, CA19-9 increased to 3026 kU/L, and CT revealed one liver metastasis in segment 6 (Figure 3) and multiple enlarged para-aortic lymph nodes. The patient was treated with two full cycles of gemcitabine/nab-paclitaxel as first-line palliative chemotherapy

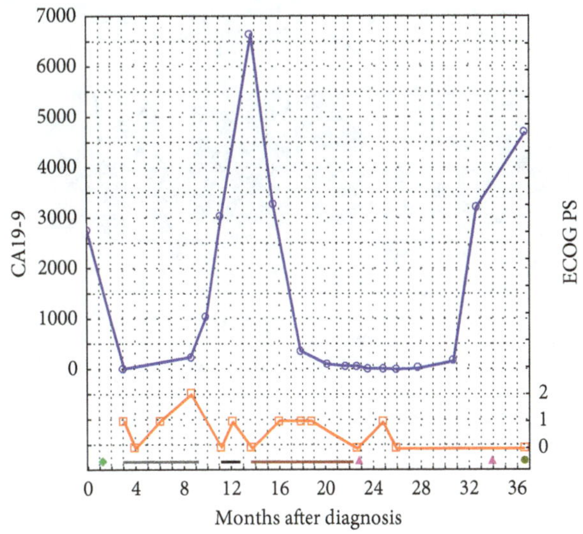

FIGURE 1: Variation over time in CA19-9 levels and the ECOG PS in relation to treatment. Abbreviations: ECOG, Eastern Cooperative Oncology Group; PS, performance status; Gem, gemcitabine; NabP, nab-paclitaxel; FLOX, bolus 5-FU plus oxaliplatin; FLIRI, bolus 5-FU plus irinotecan.

according to regional guidelines. The treatment was administered by intravenous infusions on days 1, 8, and 15 in a four-week cycle at 1000 mg/m^2 gemcitabine and 125 mg/m^2 nab-paclitaxel. The response was evaluated with positron emission tomography (PET)-CT, which revealed no change in the liver metastasis in segment 6 or in lymph nodes without uptake; however, a new paravertebral tumour with FDG uptake was detected in the lower right lobe of the lungs (Figures 4 and 5). CA19-9 was 6628 kU/L. The diagnosis was progressive disease, and second-line palliative 5FU-based chemotherapy was commenced. The first cycle was given as FLV (500 mg/m^2 5FU bolus plus 60 mg/m^2 leucovorin on days 1 and 2 in a two-week cycle) due to persistent chemotherapy-induced polyneuropathy (CIPN) from the first-line treatment. The CIPN decreased to CTCAE grade 1, allowing for the administration of FLOX (FLV plus the infusion of 85 mg/m^2 oxaliplatin on day 1 of the two-week cycle) from the second cycle. Repeated CT scans showed a partial response, and CA19-9 decreased to 44 kU/L during 17 cycles over a 9-month treatment period. The oxaliplatin dose was reduced because of CIPN and discontinued from cycle 14 due to an adverse drug reaction; drug hypersensitivity could not be ruled out. PET-CT and contrast-enhanced ultrasound of the liver showed a complete response in the thoracic cavity (Figure 6) and one 13-mm liver metastasis in segment 6 as the only remaining radiological evidence of disease.

Due to the earlier adverse reaction to oxaliplatin, persistent CIPN, and chemotherapy-related fatigue, continued palliative chemotherapy was difficult and had no curative potential. In part based on the patient's request, alternative

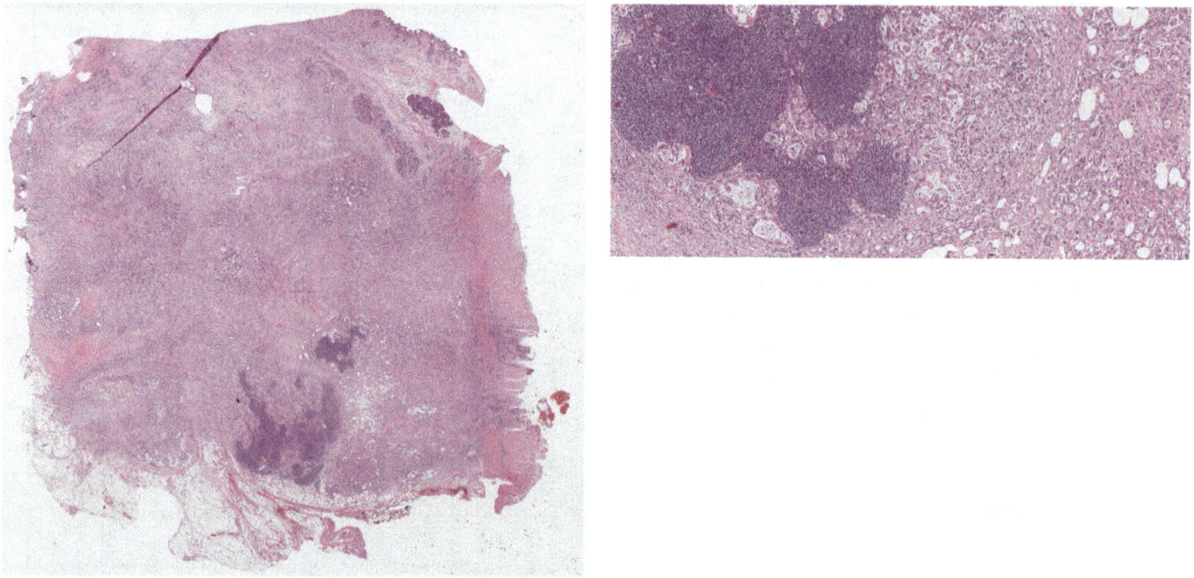

(a) (b)

Figure 2: Histologic haematoxylin- and eosin-stained paraffin section of the patient's primary tumour (a) and detailed image of lymphatic invasion and tumour morphology (b).

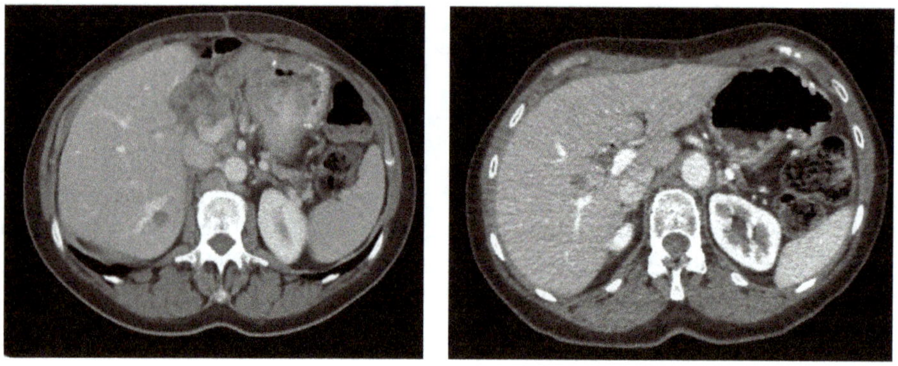

(a) (b)

Figure 3: Liver metastases: the lesion in segment 6 was treated with microwave ablation (a), and the lesion in segment 5 was treated with RFA (b).

treatment strategies were considered, and local treatment with microwave ablation (MWA) was offered after discussion at a multidisciplinary conference. The patient underwent MWA of the liver lesion 22 months after surgery for the primary tumour, and CA19-9 levels were normalized after MWA. Due to the presence of a postablation liver abscess, continued chemotherapy was contraindicated, and an active monitoring strategy was chosen. The patient was evaluated every second month and showed a slow increase in CA19-9 to 151 kU/L by 30 months after surgery for the primary tumour but no radiological evidence of relapse. CA19-9 further increased to 3182 kU/L after an additional 2 months, and PET-CT showed one liver metastasis in segment 5 measuring 15 mm (Figure 3) without additional dissemination; thus, the patient, after discussion at a multidisciplinary conference, underwent successful radiofrequency ablation (RFA) 33 months after surgery for the primary tumour.

At the next evaluation visit 3 months later (i.e., 36 months after primary surgery), a relapse was found both biochemically, with a further increase in CA19-9 to 4692 kU/L, and radiologically, with PET-CT showing three suspicious 4 to 8 mm lung metastases without FDG uptake and two metastases in the right liver lobe measuring 25 and 30 mm. Third-line palliative chemotherapy with FLIRI (FLV plus the intravenous infusion of 180 mg/m^2 irinotecan on day 1 in the two-week cycle) was started.

Except during the initial adverse event of a liver abscess following the MWA, which was successfully treated with antibiotics, the patient did not suffer from any side effects after local treatment. During the eleven-month relapse-free interval and until the start of third-line palliative chemotherapy with FLIRI, the patient reported a WHO performance status of 0. The patient experienced normal health and pursued physical activity and hobbies as before the cancer diagnosis.

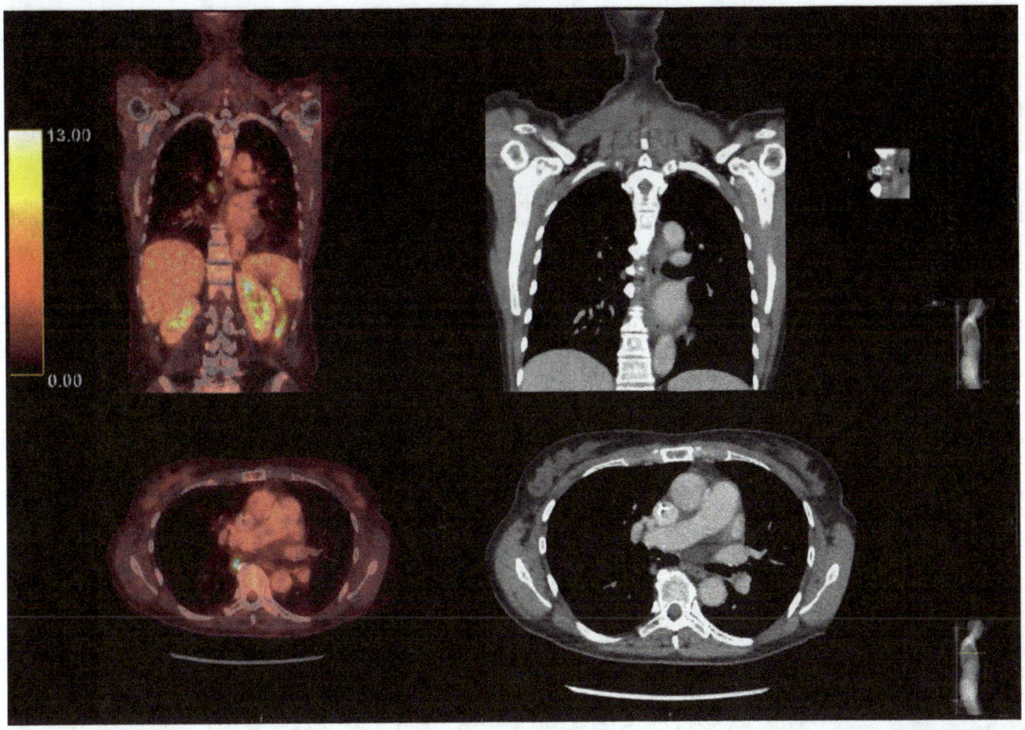

FIGURE 4: PET-CT evaluation of the response to first-line palliative chemotherapy showed disease progression with lung metastasis. PET-CT (left column) and CT (middle column) images. Top right inset: higher magnification image and measurement of the lesion. The SUVmax of the lesion was 9.7.

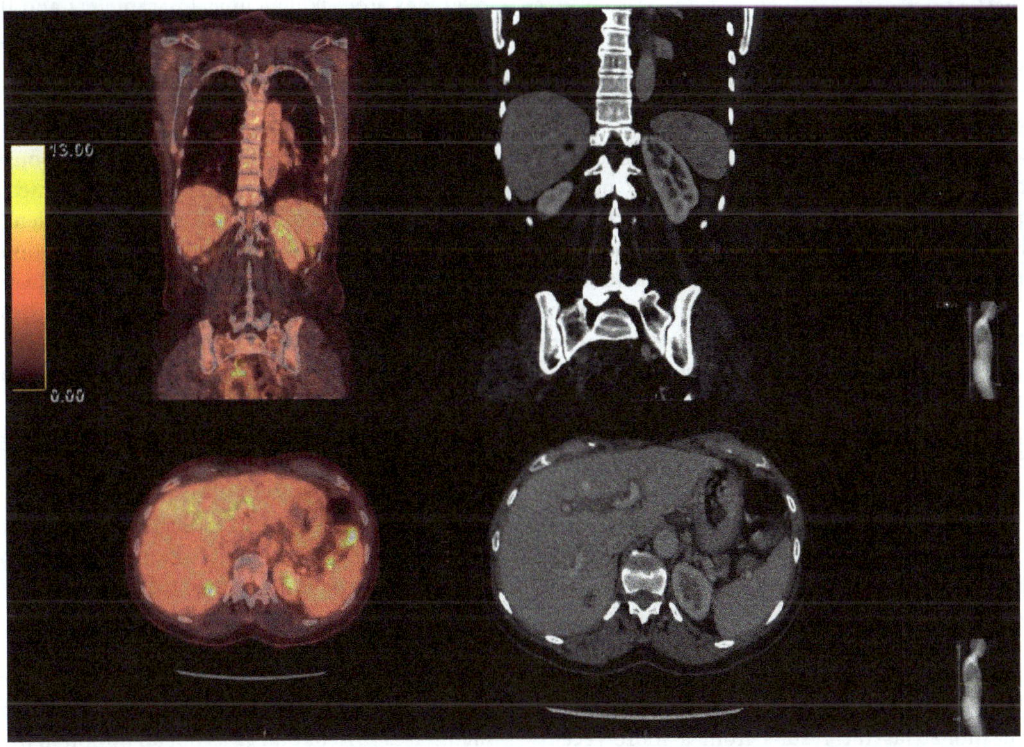

FIGURE 5: No change in the liver metastasis in segment 6 was observed upon evaluation of the response to first-line palliative chemotherapy. PET-CT (left column) and CT (right column) images. The SUVmax was 5.5 for the lesion and 3.1 for the surrounding liver.

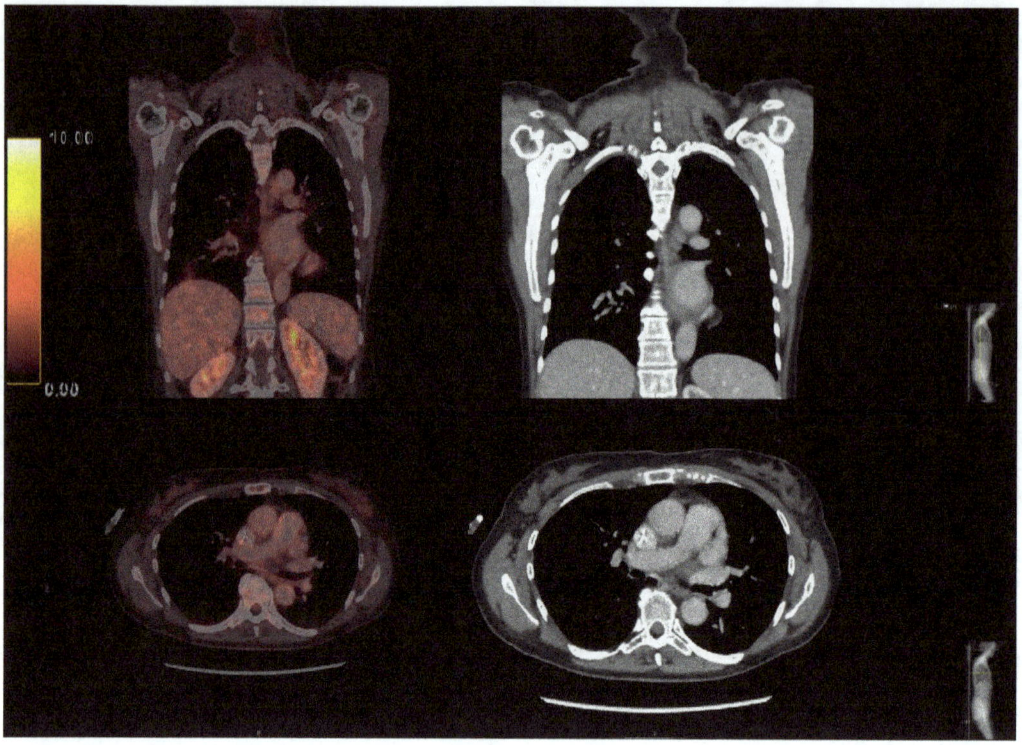

Figure 6: PET-CT images showing a complete radiological response of the lung metastasis. PET-CT (left column) and CT (right column) images.

3. Discussion

The frequently observed course of metastatic PDAC is rapid progression, but there is now a fairly good chance for a response to first-line palliative combination chemotherapy [15]; in the South East Region of Sweden, the median overall survival of this patient group is approximately 9 months [16]. Based on the results of the phase III MPACT trial [15], many guidelines advocate the use of gemcitabine-nab/paclitaxel as first-line palliative treatment in patients with metastatic PDAC and ECOG PS 0-1, as is the case in the South East Region of Sweden. This case illustrates that even in PDAC, some patients who are nonresponders to the recommended treatment do experience a response to alternative chemotherapy treatments, indicating the need for therapy-specific predictive factors to optimize oncologic treatment decision-making.

In treating patients with metastatic PDAC with second- or even third-line chemotherapy, there is a fine balance between patient frailty and drug toxicity. In Sweden, platinum-based combination chemotherapy (in this case, FLOX) is often offered to patients with a good performance status based on the survival benefit seen in previous small phase II studies and a phase III study [17]. These data have since been questioned as the results from a more recent phase III study were contradictory, with a shorter median OS in the platinum-based therapy (FOLFOX) group than in the FLV only group [18]. In addition, the objective response rate on second-line therapy is often less than 10% [19], indicating the importance of appropriate patient selection. As predictors of the outcome of individual chemotherapy regimens are lacking, clinical parameters and the ECOG or Karnofsky performance status are often used, and a nomogram to help choose the right patients for second-line treatment has been proposed [20].

With the abovementioned data in mind, this case illustrates an example of an exceptional response to second-line palliative chemotherapy. Although limited conclusions can be drawn from a single case, this patient had several prognostic factors associated with a poor outcome in the previously reported nomogram, such as liver metastasis, advanced age, and a very short duration of first-line chemotherapy. The factors that contributed to the therapeutic response in this patient are unknown, but the current report illustrates that second-line therapy can be effective and should be considered, even in motivated patients with multiple aggravating clinical factors.

In metastatic PDAC, clinical guidelines do not include surgery or local treatment modalities, which is in contrast to colorectal cancer, for which the surgical approach (with a curative intention) to liver and lung metastases is routine [21, 22]. For PDAC, the ablative modality of irreversible electroporation (IRE) has been evaluated as a first-line treatment for LAPC but has not shown a significant survival benefit [23]. IRE could theoretically be used for hilar liver metastases [24], but this was not an option in this case due to the location of the liver metastasis. Concerning the choice between RFA or MWA, data on hepatocellular carcinoma and colorectal liver metastases suggest similar efficacy, with a tendency towards better local control with MWA, especially in cases of large lesions [25, 26]. In the case presented herein, ablation of the liver metastasis was used in conjunction with chemotherapy and achieved an 11-month treatment-free interval without radiologically detectable disease and with a subjective and objective (WHO PS) good quality of life. The duration was far longer than expected, considering the unambiguous histopathological diagnosis of PDAC and the immediate progression on first-line palliative chemotherapy. This, together with the recurrence in another liver lobe and the absence of evidence for the curative potential of chemotherapy in metastatic PDAC, points towards an actual treatment effect of MWA. Though not possible in this case due to infectious complications of MWA, the effect could hypothetically have been prolonged by "adjuvant" chemotherapy, considering the previous response to second-line chemotherapy. However, as the overall intention was palliative, the value of the treatment-free period should not be underestimated.

The choice of a second liver ablation over chemotherapy was based on the treatment-free interval after the initial ablation, the good quality of life reported by the patient in the chemotherapy-free interval, and the radiological finding of a single new lesion in the liver.

4. Conclusion

This case illustrates that a treatment-free interval with a sustained good performance status can be achieved with second-line palliative chemotherapy in combination with the ablation of liver metastases in patients with pancreatic cancer and that local therapies should therefore be considered in select cases.

References

[1] R. L. Siegel, K. D. Miller, and A. Jemal, "Cancer statistics, 2017," *CA: A Cancer Journal for Clinicians*, vol. 67, no. 1, pp. 7–30, 2017.

[2] O. Bergman, *Cancerfondsrapporten*, M. Jaresand, Ed., The Swedish Cancer Society, Stockholm, Sweden, 2018.

[3] M. H. G. Katz, P. W. T. Pisters, J. E. Lee, and J. B. Fleming, "Borderline resectable pancreatic cancer: what have we learned and where do we go from here?" *Annals of Surgical Oncology*, vol. 18, no. 3, pp. 608–610, 2011.

[4] J. P. Neoptolemos, D. D. Stocken, C. Bassi et al., "Adjuvant chemotherapy with fluorouracil plus folinic acid vs gemcitabine following pancreatic cancer resection," *JAMA*, vol. 304, no. 10, pp. 1073–1081, 2010.

[5] S. Hishinuma, Y. Ogata, M. Tomikawa, I. Ozawa, K. Hirabayashi, and S. Igarashi, "Patterns of recurrence after curative resection of pancreatic cancer, based on autopsy findings," *Journal of Gastrointestinal Surgery*, vol. 10, no. 4, pp. 511–518, 2006.

[6] J. P. Neoptolemos, D. Palmer, P. Ghaneh et al., "ESPAC-4: a multicenter, international, open-label randomized controlled phase III trial of adjuvant combination chemotherapy of gemcitabine (GEM) and capecitabine (CAP) versus monotherapy gemcitabine in patients with resected pancreatic ductal adenocarcinoma," *Journal of Clinical Oncology*, vol. 34, no. 18_suppl, Article ID LBA4006, 2016.

[7] N. Silvestris, V. Longo, F. Cellini et al., "Neoadjuvant multimodal treatment of pancreatic ductal adenocarcinoma," *Critical Reviews in Oncology/Hematology*, vol. 98, pp. 309–324, 2016.

[8] N. Silvestris, O. Brunetti, E. Vasile et al., "Multimodal treatment of resectable pancreatic ductal adenocarcinoma," *Critical Reviews in Oncology/Hematology*, vol. 111, pp. 152–165, 2017.

[9] J. A. M. G. Tol, W. J. Eshuis, M. G. H. Besselink, T. M. van Gulik, O. R. C. Busch, and D. J. Gouma, "Non-radical resection versus bypass procedure for pancreatic cancer—a consecutive series and systematic review," *European Journal of Surgical Oncology (EJSO)*, vol. 41, no. 2, pp. 220–227, 2015.

[10] M. Ducreux, A. S. Cuhna, C. Caramella et al., "Cancer of the pancreas: ESMO Clinical Practice Guidelines for diagnosis, treatment and follow-up," *Annals of Oncology*, vol. 26, no. Suppl 5, pp. v56–v68, 2015.

[11] M. A. Tempero, M. P. Malafa, M. Al-Hawary et al., "Pancreatic adenocarcinoma, version 2.2017, NCCN clinical practice guidelines in oncology," *Journal of the National Comprehensive Cancer Network*, vol. 15, no. 8, pp. 1028–1061, 2017.

[12] O. Bergman, *Cancer I Siffror 2018*, E. Johansson, Ed., Socialstyrelsen, Stockholm, Sweden, 2018.

[13] M. Patel, "The impact of epidemiological factors and treatment interventions on survival in patients with signet ring cell carcinoma of the pancreas," *American Journal of Clinical Oncology*, vol. 41, no. 12, pp. 1176–1184, 2018.

[14] G. A. Poultsides, S. Reddy, J. L. Cameron et al., "Histopathologic basis for the favorable survival after resection of intraductal papillary mucinous neoplasm-associated invasive adenocarcinoma of the pancreas," *Annals of Surgery*, vol. 251, no. 3, pp. 470–476, 2010.

[15] D. D. Von Hoff, T Ervin, F. P Arena et al., "Increased survival in pancreatic cancer with nab-paclitaxel plus gemcitabine," *The New England Journal of Medicine*, vol. 369, no. 369, pp. 1691–1703, 2013.

[16] H. Blomstrand, U. Scheibling, C. Bratthäll, H. Green, and N. O. Elander, "Real world evidence on gemcitabine and nab-paclitaxel combination chemotherapy in advanced pancreatic cancer," *BMC Cancer*, vol. 19, no. 1, p. 40, 2019.

[17] H. Oettle, H. Riess, J. M. Stieler et al., "Second-line oxaliplatin, folinic acid, and fluorouracil versus folinic acid and fluorouracil alone for gemcitabine-refractory pancreatic cancer: outcomes from the CONKO-003 trial," *Journal of Clinical Oncology*, vol. 32, no. 23, pp. 2423–2429, 2014.

[18] S. Gill, Y.-J. Ko, C. Cripps et al., "PANCREOX: a randomized phase III study of fluorouracil/leucovorin with or without oxaliplatin for second-line advanced pancreatic cancer in patients who have received gemcitabine-based chemotherapy," *Journal of Clinical Oncology*, vol. 34, no. 32, pp. 3914–3920, 2016.

[19] O. E. Rahma, A. Duffy, D. J. Liewehr, S. M. Steinberg, and T. F. Greten, "Second-line treatment in advanced pancreatic cancer: a comprehensive analysis of published clinical trials," *Annals of Oncology*, vol. 24, no. 8, pp. 1972–1979, 2013.

[20] A. Vienot, G. Beinse, C. Louvet et al., "Overall survival prediction and usefulness of second-line chemotherapy in advanced pancreatic adenocarcinoma," *JNCI: Journal of the National Cancer Institute*, vol. 109, no. 10, 2017.

[21] P. M. Lykoudis, D. O'Reilly, K. Nastos, and G. Fusai, "Systematic review of surgical management of synchronous colorectal liver metastases," *British Journal of Surgery*, vol. 101, no. 6, pp. 605–612, 2014.

[22] Z. Sun and J. M. Thacker, "Contemporary surgical options for metastatic colorectal cancer," *Current Oncology Reports*, vol. 17, no. 4, p. 13, 2015.
[23] C. Månsson, R. Brahmstaedt, P. Nygren, A. Nilsson, J. Urdzik, and B.-M. Karlson, "Percutaneous irreversible electroporation as first-line treatment of locally advanced pancreatic cancer," *Anticancer Research*, vol. 39, no. 5, pp. 2509–2512, 2019.
[24] H. J. Scheffer, M. C. A. M. Melenhorst, A. M. Echenique et al., "Irreversible electroporation for colorectal liver metastases," *Techniques in Vascular and Interventional Radiology*, vol. 18, no. 3, pp. 159–169, 2015.
[25] A. Facciorusso, M. Di Maso, and N. Muscatiello, "Microwave ablation versus radiofrequency ablation for the treatment of hepatocellular carcinoma: a systematic review and meta-analysis," *International Journal of Hyperthermia*, vol. 32, no. 3, pp. 339–344, 2016.
[26] H. Takahashi, B. Kahramangil, E. Kose, and E. Berber, "A comparison of microwave thermosphere versus radiofrequency thermal ablation in the treatment of colorectal liver metastases," *HPB*, vol. 20, no. 12, pp. 1157–1162, 2018.

20

Gallbladder Agenesis without Additional Biliary Tracts Abnormality

Seyed Mostafa Meshkati Yazd,[1] Hamidreza Bayati,[2] Sara Sadat Nabavizadeh,[3] and Reza Shahriarirad[4]

[1]*Department of Surgery, Tehran University of Medical Sciences, Tehran, Iran*
[2]*Department of Surgery, Iran University of Medical Sciences, Tehran, Iran*
[3]*Student Research Committee, Shiraz University of Medical Sciences, Shiraz, Iran*
[4]*Thoracic and Vascular Surgery Research Center, Shiraz University of Medical Science, Shiraz, Iran*

Correspondence should be addressed to Reza Shahriarirad; r.shahriari1995@gmail.com

Academic Editor: Yoshifumi Nakayama

Background. Gallbladder agenesis (GA) is a very uncommon disorder of the biliary system. Diagnosis of GA can be difficult and may result in unnecessary procedures. In this case report, we will discuss our experience with an intraoperative accidental diagnosis of GA in a middle-aged woman that was effectively treated. *Case Presentation.* A 46-year-old woman presented with abdominal pain, nausea, vomiting, and intolerance to meals. Laparoscopic surgery was conducted based on sonographic imaging and a preliminary diagnosis of chronic cholecystitis. No gallbladder was seen during laparoscopy, and the patient was diagnosed as a case of GA. The laparoscopy was terminated, and the patient was referred for magnetic resonance cholangiopancreatography (MRCP) to confirm the diagnosis. Finally, endoscopic retrograde cholangiopancreatography (ERCP) and sphincterotomy were performed to alleviate symptoms. After one year of follow-up, the patient's overall condition is satisfactory and symptom-free. *Conclusion.* Our case exemplifies this common blunder. Therefore, we are reporting a case of GA discovered intraoperatively to increase surgeons' awareness and preparedness for this possible differential diagnosis and minimize unnecessary operational intervention.

1. Introduction

Gallbladder agenesis (GA) is a rare biliary system anatomical abnormality with an incidence rate of 0.01–0.075%. It is characterized by the absence of the gall bladder or cystic duct [1]. The actual incidence rate is unclear because most afflicted people present with no symptoms, and many are found inadvertently during unrelated procedures or autopsy [2]. Nonetheless, 50% of individuals may develop gallbladder pathology symptoms such as pain in the right upper quadrant, nausea or vomiting, intolerance to fatty foods, dyspepsia, and jaundice [3]. As a result, it becomes challenging to distinguish GA from other biliary illnesses. The disease's rarity and difficulty in preoperative diagnosis is a challenging issue that may result in unnecessary surgical intervention, a high risk of iatrogenic damage, and increased morbidity [4].

The following is a case report of a patient who presented with symptoms of biliary system involvement and was confirmed as GA during laparoscopy.

2. Case Presentation

We present the case of a recently treated 46-year-old woman with no significant medical history who came to the emergency department with approximately ten months of right upper quadrant pain described as sharp, intermittent, radiating to the back, and associated with nausea and vomiting. The pain was exacerbated by fatty meals without any change in bowel habits or urine symptoms. She denied having any additional medical conditions or a

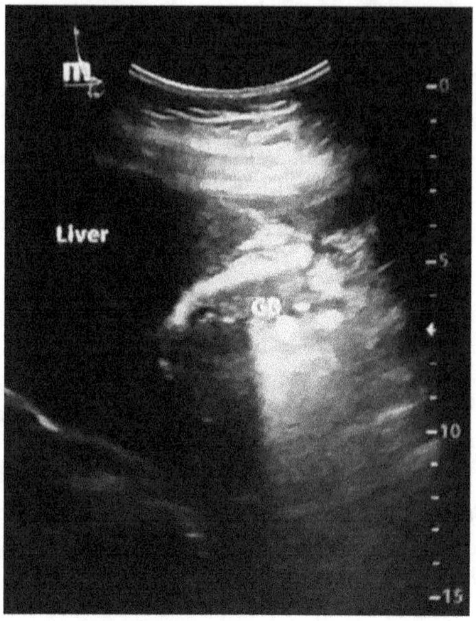

FIGURE 1: Scleroatrophic (shrunken) gallbladder with a normal biliary tree at abdominal ultrasonography.

family history of gastrointestinal problems. On physical examination, she exhibited normal vital signs, minor abdominal pain in the upper abdomen, and no significantly abnormal routine laboratory data. Her baseline metabolic profile was normal, including an unremarkable liver function test.

The patient underwent an abdominal ultrasound in the right upper quadrant, revealing features consistent with chronic cholecystitis and a scleroatrophic (shrinking) gallbladder, or in other words, contracted and shrunken in size, which made it not visible during the ultrasonographic imaging test. The biliary tree was normal. At the same time, there was no sonographic evidence of Murphy's sign, gallbladder wall thickening (2 mm), pericholecystic fluid, or intra or extrahepatic biliary duct dilatation (Figure 1).

According to the clinical and radiological findings, laparoscopic cholecystectomy was performed with the preliminary diagnosis of chronic cholecystitis.

Intraoperatively, the gallbladder could not be visualized from the junction of the left and right hepatic ducts until it disappeared behind the second part of the duodenum. There was no evidence of a gall bladder, cystic duct, or cystic artery (Figure 2 and supplementary file 1).

We concluded the operation at the laparoscopic level to avoid any unintended damage. Subsequently, on the first postoperative day, we performed magnetic resonance cholangiopancreatography (MRCP), which demonstrated normal liver structure, normal intrahepatic bile ducts, and slight dilatation of the common bile duct (CBD), with the absence of gallbladder (Figure 3). The patient underwent endoscopic retrograde cholangiopancreatography (ERCP) and sphincterotomy one day later to improve the remaining symptoms, based on the possibility of biliary tract dyskinesia. After treatment, the patient's symptoms alleviated over the next month, and the patient is still symptom-free one year later.

3. Discussion

GA, known as congenital absence of the gall bladder, is a rare developmental defect that affects less than one in every 6500 live births [5]. To our knowledge, Lemery et al. described the first case of GA in 1701. Since then, a few similar clinical cases have been recorded in the English medical literature. Along with its rarity, the disease's comparable symptoms and indistinguishable ultrasound imaging from other biliary illnesses contribute to its delayed identification [1, 3, 6].

The diagnosis is significantly delayed in most cases, resulting in adverse consequences from the unnecessary operation [7–9]. Our case exemplifies this common blunder. Therefore, we are reporting a case of GA discovered intraoperatively to increase surgeons' awareness and preparedness for this possible differential diagnosis and minimize unnecessary operational intervention. Differential diagnoses such as bile duct stenosis, Oddi sphincter stenosis, the presence of gallstones or sludge in the bile ducts, or bile duct dyskinesia are considered in these conditions.

Abdominal ultrasonography of the right upper quadrant is the standard initial assessment for patients presenting with biliary system involvement symptoms. Despite ultrasonography's high sensitivity for diagnosing biliary system diseases, GA cannot be reliably distinguished from a shrunken, constricted gallbladder, which may be accompanied by hyperechogenic shadows that were mistaken for chronic cholecystitis or cholelithiasis [10, 11]. Based on our patient's presence of biliary-related symptoms, we performed preoperative abdominal sonography, which revealed a scleroatrophic gallbladder with a normal biliary tree, increasing the suspicion of chronic cholecystitis. To avoid this common mistake, according to Malde's 2010 diagnostic and management algorithm for GA, in the absence of the WES triad (visualization of the gallbladder wall, stone echo, and acoustic shadow) and the presence of a contracted sclerotic gallbladder, additional imaging should be obtained before

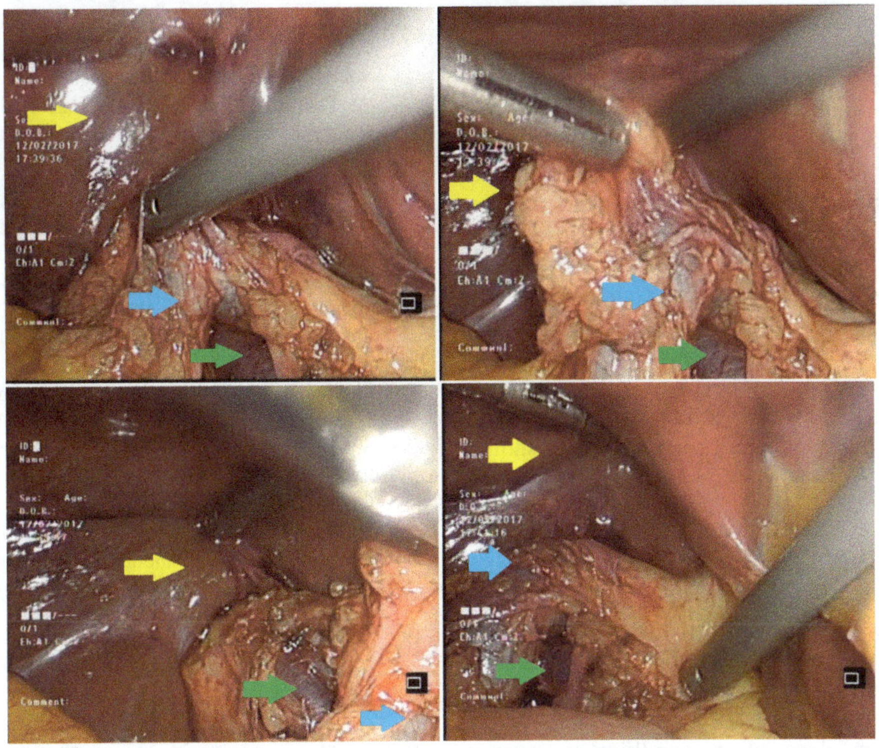

FIGURE 2: Intraoperative figures demonstrating liver (yellow arrow), common bile duct (blue arrow), and portal vein (green arrow).

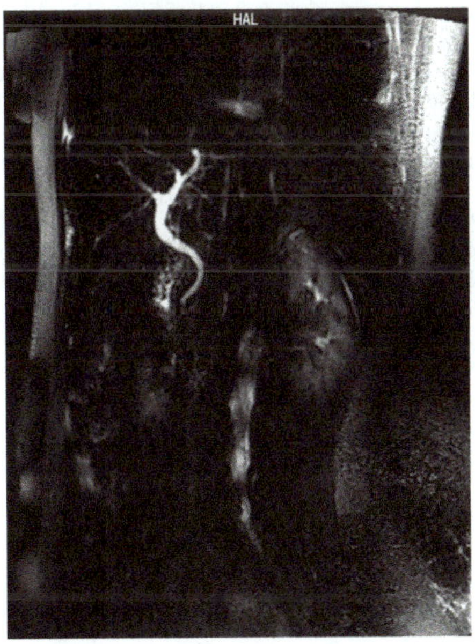

FIGURE 3: Magnetic resonance cholangiopancreatography during first-day postoperation, demonstrating normal intrahepatic bile ducts and slight dilation of common bile duct with an absence of gallbladder.

operative intervention to improve the accuracy of the diagnosis [11].

In the case of an intraoperative diagnosis of GA, the surgeon must rule out an ectopic gallbladder by exploring the ectopic gallbladder's most common sites. This procedure requires extensive surgical investigation, which increases the risk of biliary damage and the need for open surgery conversion. Most authors agree that if the gallbladder is not visible during laparoscopy, it is more beneficial to discontinue further surgical exploration and confirm the diagnosis with a comprehensive postoperative radiologic examination [12, 13].

MRCP is often considered the preferred diagnostic method. This noninvasive imaging technique allows a comprehensive evaluation of the biliary system. MRCP is the optimum imaging approach, since it accurately identifies GA before and after surgery and when ultrasonography is inconclusive and ruling out the possibility of an ectopic gallbladder. Additionally, computed tomography (CT) scanning and ERCP can be performed to determine GA. However, nonvisualization of the gallbladder is frequently attributed to a blocked cystic duct, anatomic differences, or technical errors, with GA being the least likely cause; therefore, they are preferred to be used as postoperative modalities if GA is suspected at laparoscopy [11, 14, 15]. After determining the possibility of GA during the laparoscopic procedure in our patient, we aborted the procedure and performed an MRCP to confirm the diagnosis. The results of MRCP dispelled our doubts about the biliary system's anatomical structure. It is worth mentioning that with the improvement of modern diagnostic imaging such as ultrasonography, CT, or MRI, diagnosing or at least suspecting GA has become less challenging. However, our experience regarding this case is that in cases with symptoms of biliary colic and an ultrasound report of chronic cholecystitis including contraction or shrunken gallbladder during preoperative evaluations, while ultrasound evidence was questionable, we recommend further evaluation with noninvasive imaging instruments associated with the gallbladder and bile ducts, including MRCP. Also, considering the possibility of GA in centers with limited imaging equipment and tertiary centers necessitates further evaluation and halting surgical interventions until a more precise diagnosis is achieved.

Due to the rarity of GA, there are no defined diagnosis and management guidelines. In individuals with mild to moderate symptoms, most experts recommend conservative therapy employing smooth muscle relaxants. Additionally, sphincterotomy should be performed in severe cases [3, 16]. In this case, she underwent ERCP and subsequent sphincterotomy due to the severity of the symptoms and failure to respond to muscle relaxants. Since patients with GA without biliary tract abnormality usually do not have biliary colic symptoms, the possibility of biliary tract dyskinesia should be considered.

4. Conclusion

GA is a rare congenital biliary defect that commonly resembles the clinical and radiologic features of more common biliary illnesses, demanding unnecessary surgical procedures. This situation may be averted in most cases by increasing surgeons' knowledge of this condition and proper use of radiologic techniques. In the event of a not visualized gallbladder in the ultrasound, a conservative strategy with follow-up imaging and preoperative MRCP is recommended. Furthermore, additional procedures should be avoided in cases detected during laparoscopy to prevent the morbidity associated with conversion to open surgery.

Authors' Contributions

S. M. and H. B. made the ultimate diagnosis of the case and carried out the therapeutic measures. R. S. and S. N. collected the data and drafted the manuscript. All authors read and approved the final version of the manuscript.

References

[1] A. A. Mohammed and S. H. Arif, "Gallbladder agenesis: an accidental finding during laparotomy for hepatic tumor," *International Journal of Surgery Case Reports*, vol. 82, Article ID 105875, 2021.

[2] H. Kabiri, O. H. Domingo, and C. D. Tzarnas, "Agenesis of the gallbladder," *Current Surgery*, vol. 63, no. 2, pp. 104–106, 2006.

[3] I. Ben Ismail, S. Rebii, H. Zenaidi, and A. Zoghlami, "Gallbladder agenesis in the elderly: a diagnostic challenge," *The Pan African Medical Journal*, vol. 37, p. 259, 2020.

[4] Y. Takano, M. Hoshino, S. Iriyama et al., "Gallbladder agenesis with hepatic impairment: a case report," *BMC Pediatrics* vol. 18, no. 1, p. 360, 2018.

[5] M. C. Salazar, K. E. Brownson, G. S. Nadzam, A. Duffy, and K. E. Roberts, "Gallbladder agenesis: a case report," *Yale Journal of Biology and Medicine*, vol. 91, no. 3, pp. 237–241, 2018.

[6] U. Baltazar, J. Dunn, S. Gonzalez-Diaz, and W. Browder, "Agenesis of the gallbladder," *Southern Medical Journal*, vol. 93, no. 9, pp. 914-915, 2000.

[7] A. Rajkumar and A. Piya, "Gall bladder agenesis: a rare embryonic cause of recurrent biliary colic," *The American Journal of Case Reports*, vol. 18, pp. 334–338, 2017.

[8] S. B. Turkel, V. Swanson, and P. Chandrasoma, "Malformations associated with congenital absence of the gall bladder," *Journal of Medical Genetics*, vol. 20, no. 6, pp. 445–449, 1983.

[9] M. A. Cabajo Caballero, J. C. Martin del Olmo, J. I. Blanco Alvarez, and R. Atienza Sanchez, "Gallbladder and cystic duct absence," *Surgical Endoscopy*, vol. 11, no. 5, pp. 483-484, 1997.

[10] T. M. Grandhi and S. M. El-Rabaa, "Agenesis of the gall bladder and cystic duct: laparoscopic diagnosis," *The Internet Journal of Gastroenterology*, vol. 4, no. 1, 2005.

[11] S. Malde, "Gallbladder agenesis diagnosed intra-operatively: a case report," *Journal of Medical Case Reports*, vol. 4, p. 285, 2010.

[12] S. Balakrishnan, T. Singhal, S. Grandy-Smith, and S. El-Hasani, "Agenesis of the gallbladder: lessons to learn," *JSLS: Journal of the Society of Laparoendoscopic Surgeons*, vol. 10, no. 4, pp. 517–519, 2006.

[13] N. Gotohda, S. Itano, S. Horiki et al., "Gallbladder agenesis with no other biliary tract abnormality: report of a case and review of the literature," *Journal of Hepato-Biliary-Pancreatic Surgery*, vol. 7, no. 3, pp. 327–330, 2000.

[14] A. Pierro, M. Martucci, G. Maselli, and A. Farchione, "Agenesis of the gallbladder with the presence of a small dysmorphic cyst: role of magnetic resonance cholangiopancreatography," *Journal of Clinical Imaging Sciences*, vol. 2, p. 17, 2012.

[15] V. Fiaschetti, G. Calabrese, S. Viarani, G. Bazzocchi, and G. Simonetti, "Gallbladder agenesis and cystic duct absence in an adult patient diagnosed by magnetic resonance cholangiography: report of a case and review of the literature," *Case Reports in Medicine*, vol. 2009, Article ID 674768, 4 pages, 2009.

[16] C. M. Wilcox, "Sphincter of oddi dysfunction Type III: new studies suggest new approaches are needed," *World Journal of Gastroenterology*, vol. 21, no. 19, pp. 5755–5761, 2015.

21

Transhepatic Insertion of Percutaneous Endoscopic Gastrostomy Tube

Zaid Imam[1] **and C. Roberto Simons-Linares**[2]

[1]*Department of Internal Medicine, William Beaumont Hospital, Royal Oak, MI, USA*
[2]*Gastroenterology and Hepatology Department, Digestive Diseases Institute, Cleveland Clinic, Cleveland, OH, USA*

Correspondence should be addressed to C. Roberto Simons-Linares; robertosimons@outlook.com

Academic Editor: Yoshifumi Nakayama

Inadvertent injury to interposing organs during percutaneous endoscopic gastrostomy (PEG) tube placement is a feared complication of this common and generally safe procedure. Transhepatic PEG insertion is likely an underrepresented complication which may be identified incidentally on imaging or present with life-threatening conditions such as sepsis or massive bleeding. Use of ultrasound in patients with known hepatomegaly may possibly help avoid this complication. We hereby report a case of transhepatic PEG insertion, one of 16 only other cases published in the literature, and review the characteristics of the previous reported cases.

1. Introduction

Enteral feeding is the preferred nutrition route for all patients with a functional gastrointestinal (GI) tract as it preserves the tract's physical and functional integrity [1, 2]. Gastrostomy and jejunostomy tubes are the preferred modality for administering enteral nutrition in patients unable to maintain enough oral intake to meet their metabolic needs [3]. PEG placement is preferred over surgical laparoscopic gastrostomy (SLG) placement as risks of general anesthesia are avoided with the former, and a lower risk of minor complications is reported with PEG placement [4].

PEG placement is a generally safe and well-tolerated procedure [5, 6]. Contraindications to PEG placement include severe ascites or coagulopathy, shock, sepsis, abdominal wall infection at the planned gastrostomy site, peritonitis, anatomical, and functional disorders of gastric emptying, and organ interposition [7]. Minor complications related to PEG placement include cutaneous PEG site infections, stomal leakage, and PEG tube dislodgement or obstruction. Life-threatening or severe complications are rare and include gastric perforation, peritonitis, vascular or organ trauma, metastatic tumor spread, necrotizing fasciitis, and buried bumper syndrome [7]. Traversing the liver is an extremely rare but very serious complication of PEG tube placement with only 16 previous case reports in the literature [8–20]. We report a case of transhepatic insertion of a PEG tube in a 92-year-old female incidentally discovered on imaging and review the literature on this complication.

2. Case Presentation

A 92-year-old African American female with past medical history significant for toxic megacolon for which she underwent a colectomy with an end ileostomy five years prior was admitted to the hospital for failure to thrive for several months. She had no history of dementia or liver disease, and extensive evaluation revealed no etiology for her condition besides poor intake. A decision to supplement her nutrition enterally was made. She underwent a PEG tube placement after a successful trial of nasogastric feeding.

During her PEG tube placement, her upper endoscopy demonstrated no gastric pathology. A pull method with transillumination was used to insert the PEG tube into position. No immediate complications were noted, and the patient was discharged home.

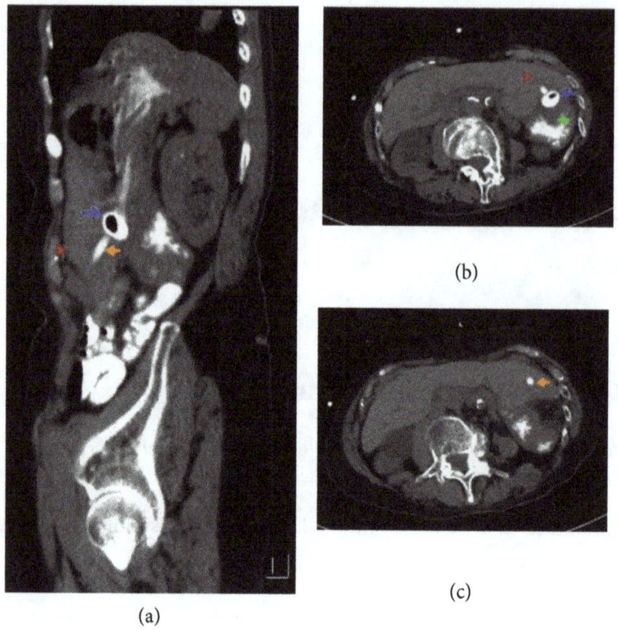

Figure 1: (a–c) Computed tomography of the abdomen demonstrating transhepatic insertion of the PEG tube. Blue arrow: retention balloon in the stomach, orange arrow: PEG tube crossing the left liver lobe, green arrow: stomach, and red arrow: left lobe of the liver.

Two weeks later, she presented with fatigue and abdominal discomfort. On examination, her vital signs were stable, her mucous membranes dry, and her ileostomy and PEG sites were normal. Her initial labs demonstrated a normal white cell count, a hemoglobin of 10.6 g/dl (10.7 g/dl pre-procedure), aspartate aminotransferase of 74 U/L (58 U/L pre-procedure), alanine aminotransferase of 74 U/L (28 U/L before procedure), alkaline phosphatase of 108 U/L (30 U/L before procedure), blood urea nitrogen of 128 mg/dl, and creatinine of 2.45 mg/dl (baseline of 1.2 mg/dl). Intravenous hydration was initiated, and a computed tomography (CT) of the abdomen with oral contrast was obtained which incidentally showed that the PEG tube coursed through the left hepatic lobe with no extravasation of enteric contrast or adjacent hematoma (Figure 1). Given the patient's hemodynamic stability, absence of leak or hematoma, and the need to maintain enteral access given dehydration, a decision to keep the PEG tube in place was done with plans for removal if further complications arose. The PEG tube flushed with no difficulty and was used for enteral nutrition during the patient's inpatient stay.

3. Discussion

Gastrostomies can be performed under endoscopic, fluoroscopic, or laparoscopic guidance. The former two techniques avoid complications of general anesthesia and hence are preferred to laparoscopic gastrostomy [5]. A "pull" technique is most commonly used for endoscopic placement of gastrostomy tubes. An alternative technique, the "push" method involves anchoring the stomach prior to PEG insertion with T-fasteners, and the gastrostomy tube is inserted transabdominally rather than transorally.

A comprehensive review of the English literature on inadvertent transhepatic or intrahepatic placement of PEG tubes revealed sixteen other cases, summarized in Table 1. All PEG tubes were inserted using the pull technique except for one. Most of the cases involved insertion through the left hepatic lobe which is expected anatomically. Nine cases (56.3%) complained of abdominal pain, one case (6.25%) presented with tube malfunction, and five cases (31.3%) were discovered incidentally. Three cases (18.8%) had associated bleeding, two of which required liver laceration repairs. Five cases (31.3%) underwent laparotomy. Laparotomy findings included presence of a gastrohepatic fistula in 2 cases, complete intrahepatic migration in 1 case, and a liver laceration in 2 cases. No cases reported hepatic necrosis, a theoretical worrisome complication. The incidence of transhepatic or intrahepatic placement of PEG tubes is likely underreported as most patients report abdominal pain at the PEG site postprocedurally that is frequently attributed to postprocedural abdominal wall pain rather than an ominous complication.

The patient reported had no theoretical risk factors for inadvertent hepatic injury that have been suggested such as hepatomegaly or obesity [20]. A mild otherwise unexplained transaminitis (>2 times upper limit of normal) was detected with no hemoglobin drop. A high suspicion index is needed to detect this complication, and complaints of abdominal pain with transaminitis or hemoglobin changes in a patient even several weeks from a PEG tube placement should warrant careful evaluation for PEG tube-related complications among other pathologies. It is also prudent to evaluate for hepatomegaly with physical examination prior to PEG insertion, and to consider using an ultrasound to evaluate for the presence of interposed liver tissue during PEG placement if hepatomegaly is noted. Additionally, the use of a "push" technique with the use of an anchoring system pulls the stomach closer to the abdominal wall which could displace the left lobe of the liver and hence result in a lower risk of

TABLE 1: Summary of cases of inadvertent transhepatic and intrahepatic PEG placement in the literature.

Author (year)	Age (years)/ sex	Indication	Placement technique	Presentation	Diagnosis	Management	Outcome
Stealatto et al (1987) [8]	NR	Gastric decompression; enterocutaneous fistula; perforated sigmoid colon	Pull technique	Incidental	Not reported	No intervention performed to PEG	Died of multiorgan failure 9 days following PEG placement
Stealatto et al (1987) [8]	NR	Gastrointestinal disconnection; subtotal gastrectomy with intra-abdominal sepsis	Pull technique	Incidental	Not reported	No intervention performed to PEG	Gut disconnection resolved and PEG removed
Stealatto et al (1987) [8]	NR	Chronic small bowel obstruction; short gut syndrome	Pull technique	Incidental	Not reported	No intervention performed to PEG	Discharged with PEG tube
Chaer et al (2003) [9]	78, F	Oropharyngeal cancer	Pull technique	Tube malfunction 2.5 months following PEG placement	Computed tomography: intrahepatic PEG	Laparotomy for PEG removal	No long-term complications reported
Gubler et al (2005) [10]	59, M	Nasopharyngeal cancer	Pull technique	Abdominal pain	Ultrasound: PEG tube along the left liver lobe	10-day course of analgesics	Asymptomatic at 6-month follow-up
Gubler et al (2005) [10]	81, F	Esophageal cancer	Pull technique	Abdominal discomfort 1 week following PEG placement	Ultrasound: PEG tube along the left liver lobe edge	3-week course of analgesics	Died at 6 weeks secondary to respiratory failure, thought not PEG-related
Wiggins et al (2007) [11]	61, F	Prolonged mechanical ventilation	Pull technique	Abdominal pain, hypotension 8 hours after procedure	Computed tomography: PEG tube in the left hepatic lobe with 10.1 subcapsular hematoma	Laparotomy: tube removal, repair of liver laceration, and new PEG insertion	Died in 3 months secondary to respiratory failure, thought not PEG-related
Burke et al (2009) [12]	33, M	Intracranial hemorrhage	Pull technique	Fever, chills, and transaminitis 7 weeks after PEG placement	Computed tomography: PEG tube button outside stomach near liver	Antibiotics, laparotomy for tube removal	Long-term outcome not reported
Shaw et al (2009) [13]	35, M	Enteral nutrition in critically ill patient	Pull technique	Abdominal pain 2 days following procedure	Computed tomography: PEG tube inserted through the left liver lobe	Removed 3 months later. No immediate complications reported.	Long-term outcome not reported
Fyock et al (2009) [14]	34, F	Failure to thrive	Not reported	Abdominal tenderness, massive hemorrhage through PEG site	Computed tomography: PEG inserted through the liver	Laparotomy and liver laceration repair	No long-term complications reported
Poggi et al (2013) [15]	56, F	Hypopharyngeal cancer	Pull technique	Abdominal pain, few hours following procedure, mild transaminitis, leukocytosis	Computed tomography: PEG tube inserted through the left liver lobe	Analgesia and antibiotics for few days. PEG removed 4 months later with no complications	Long-term outcome not reported
Mercky et al (2014) [16]	55, F	Squamous cell cancer of the tongue	Pull technique	Abdominal pain 1 week after placement	Computed tomography: intrahepatic PEG placement	Removed. No immediate complications.	No complications at 3-month follow-up

Table 1: Continued.

Author (year)	Age (years)/ sex	Indication	Placement technique	Presentation	Diagnosis	Management	Outcome
Bichille et al (2014) [17]	57, F	Dysphagia	Pull technique	Incidental, spiked fever of 100.3 F that was drug induced	Computed tomography: PEG tube inserted through the liver	Removed after 1 week. No immediate complications	Long-term outcome not reported
Harta et al (2015) [18]	44, NR	Hypopharyngeal cancer	Pull technique	Abdominal pain, 4 days after placement	Ultrasound: PEG tube in the left hepatic lobe, hepatomegaly	PEG removal and site closure. Reinsertion 1 week later	No immediate complications, long-term outcome not reported
Atalaia-Martins et al (2017) [19]	55, M	Metastatic nasopharyngeal carcinoma	Pull technique	Abdominal pain 1 year after placement	Computed tomography: PEG migrated into the liver with extensive metastasis	Laparotomy and removal of PEG tube	Long-term outcome not reported. No immediate complications
Chhaparia et al (2018) [20]	78, F	Postcardiac arrest, ischemic stroke	Pull technique	Incidental, imaging done to rule out colonic perforation	Computed tomography: PEG in hepatic segment 3, associated 4 cm hematoma	No intervention performed	Died on day 3 of discharge. Thought unrelated to PEG.

M: male, F: female, NR: not reported.

inadvertent transhepatic insertion, supported by the scarcity of this complication being reported with the "push" technique.

In summary, transhepatic insertion of a PEG tube is a serious complication carrying significant morbidity, evidenced by around one-third of patients having to undergo laparotomies as part of the complication's management. Treatment options include keeping the PEG tube in place if it remains functional and no life-threatening complications are noted, or immediate removal if a life-threatening complication such as severe hemorrhage occurs. Concerns with immediate removal would include forming a gastrohepatic fistula. On the other hand, keeping the PEG tube carries the risks of possible migration reported by two cases, and further difficulties with removal. No clear guidelines exist on the management of this complication, and further research is needed to explore the optimal treatment. It seems reasonable, nevertheless, if a transhepatic PEG tube insertion occurs with no hemodynamic changes, significant symptoms, or lab abnormalities, closely observe the patient and continue using the PEG tube.

Authors' Contributions

Imam and Simons-Linares have participated equally in preparing the manuscript.

Supplementary Materials

The video legends for the supplementary materials are as follows: Video 1: sagittal computed tomography of the abdomen and pelvis demonstrating transhepatic passage of the percutaneous endoscopic gastrostomy (PEG) tube. Video 2: axial computed tomography of the abdomen and pelvis demonstrating transhepatic passage of the percutaneous endoscopic gastrostomy (PEG tube). (*Supplementary Materials*)

References

[1] C.-P. Heidegger, P. Darmon, and C. Pichard, "Enteral vs. parenteral nutrition for the critically ill patient: a combined support should be preferred," *Current Opinion in Critical Care*, vol. 14, no. 4, pp. 408–414, 2008.

[2] S. A. Mcclave, J. K. Dibaise, G. E. Mullin, and R. G. Martindale, "ACG clinical guideline: nutrition therapy in the adult hospitalized patient," *American Journal of Gastroenterology*, vol. 111, no. 3, pp. 315–334, 2016.

[3] P. Mendiratta, J. M. Tilford, P. Prodhan, K. Curseen, G. Azhar, and J. Y. Wei, "Trends in percutaneous endoscopic gastrostomy placement in the elderly from 1993 to 2003," *American Journal of Alzheimer's Disease and Other Dementiasr*, vol. 27, no. 8, pp. 609–613, 2012.

[4] J. Bravo, E. Ide, A. Kondo et al., "Percutaneous endoscopic versus surgical gastrostomy in patients with benign and malignant diseases: a systematic review and meta-analysis," *Clinics*, vol. 71, no. 3, pp. 169–178, 2016.

[5] M. Itkin, M. H. DeLegge, J. C. Fang et al., "Multidisciplinary practical guidelines for gastrointestinal access for enteral nutrition and decompression from the Society of Interventional Radiology and American Gastroenterological Association (AGA) Institute, with endorsement by Canadian Interventional Radiological Association (CIRA) and cardiovascular and Interventional Radiological Society of Europe (CIRSE)," *Gastroenterology*, vol. 141, no. 2, pp. 742–765, 2011.
[6] T. Hucl and J. Spicak, "Complications of percutaneous endoscopic gastrostomy," *Best Practice and Research Clinical Gastroenterology*, vol. 30, no. 5, pp. 769–781, 2016.
[7] A. A. Rahnemai-Azar, A. A. Rahnemaiazar, R. Naghshizadian, A. Kurtz, and D. T. Farkas, "Percutaneous endoscopic gastrostomy: indications, technique, complications and management," *World Journal of Gastroenterology*, vol. 20, no. 24, pp. 7739–7751, 2014.
[8] T. A. Stellato and M. W. L. Gauderer, "Percutaneous endoscopic gastrostomy for gastrointestinal decompression," *Annals of Surgery*, vol. 205, no. 2, pp. 119–122, 1987.
[9] R. A. Chaer, D. Rekkas, J. Trevino, R. Brown, and N. J. Espat, "Intrahepatic placement of a PEG tube," *Gastrointestinal Endoscopy*, vol. 57, no. 6, pp. 763–765, 2003.
[10] C. Gubler, S. M. Wildi, and P. Bauerfeind, "Liver injury during PEG tube placement: report of two cases," *Gastrointestinal Endoscopy*, vol. 61, no. 2, pp. 346–348, 2005.
[11] T. F. Wiggins, R. Kaplan, and M. H. DeLegge, "Acute hemorrhage following transhepatic PEG tube placement," *Digestive Diseases and Sciences*, vol. 52, no. 1, pp. 167–169, 2007.
[12] D. T. Burke and A. I. Geller, "Peritonitis secondary to the migration of a trans-hepatically-placed percutaneous endoscopic gastrostomy tube: a case report," *Archives of Physical Medicine and Rehabilitation*, vol. 90, no. 2, pp. 354–357, 2009.
[13] J. Shaw and K. Casey, "A PEG tube through the liver," *The American Journal of Gastroenterology*, vol. 104, no. 5, pp. 1323-1324, 2009.
[14] C. J. Fyock and S. R. Kethu, "PEG placement causing liver perforation," *Journal of Clinical Gastroenterology*, vol. 43, no. 4, p. 385, 2009.
[15] G. Poggi, B. Montagna, and P. D. Cesare, "Transhepatic percutaneous endoscopic gastrostomy," *Open Journal of Gastroenterology*, vol. 03, no. 02, pp. 87-88, 2013.
[16] P. Mercky, A. Goffic, and P. Ah-Soune, "Transhepatic endoscopic gastrostomy," *Endoscopy*, vol. 46, no. S 01, p. E385, 2014.
[17] T. Bichile, T. Aung, and J. Vainder, "A rare complication of PEG tube placement," *Practical Gastroenterology*, vol. 38, no. 9, 2014.
[18] T. Herta, M. Hecker, F. van Boemmel, A. Hoffmeister, and T. Karlas, "Sonographic diagnosis of transhepatic placement of a percutaneous endoscopic gastrostomy (PEG) tube," *Endoscopy*, vol. 47, no. 1, pp. E453–E454, 2015.
[19] C. Atalaia-Martins, S. Barbeiro, P. Marcos, I. Gil, and I. Cotrim, "Intrahepatic migration of gastrostomy tube after inadvertent transhepatic PEG placement," *ACG Case Reports Journal*, vol. 4, no. 1, p. e76, 2017.
[20] A. Chhaparia, M. B. Hammami, J. Bassuner, and C. Hachem, "Trans-hepatic percutaneous endoscopic gastrostomy tube placement: a case report of A rare complication and literature review," *Gastroenterology Research*, vol. 11, no. 2, pp. 145–149, 2018.

22

A Rare Case of Disseminated *Mycobacterium avium-intracellulare* Presenting as Proctitis

Chukwunonso Chime[1,2] **Peter Bhandari**[2] **Masooma Niazi**[3] **and Harish Patel**[1,2]

[1]*Division of Gastroenterology, BronxCare Hospital Center a Clinical Affiliate of Mt Sinai Health Systems and Academic Affiliate of Icahn School of Medicine, Bronx, NY 10457, USA*
[2]*Department of Medicine, BronxCare Hospital Center a Clinical Affiliate of Mt Sinai Health Systems and Academic Affiliate of Icahn School of Medicine, Bronx, NY 10457, USA*
[3]*Department of Pathology, BronxCare Hospital Center a Clinical Affiliate of Mt Sinai Health Systems and Academic Affiliate of Icahn School of Medicine, Bronx, NY 10457, USA*

Correspondence should be addressed to Chukwunonso Chime; cchime@bronxleb.org

Academic Editor: Engin Altintas

Mycobacterium avium intracellulare (MAI) infections are common in *Human Immuno-deficiency Virus* (HIV) positive patients. MAI infection can have localized or disseminated presentation, patients with low CD4 count presenting with disseminated infection. Fever, abdominal pain, diarrhea, and weight loss are generally the presenting symptoms of disseminated MAI. We present a rare case of a patient with HIV and low CD4 count presenting with proctitis as manifestation of disseminated MAI infection. A 25 year-old-man with HIV came to the emergency room (ER) with complaints of intermittent rectal bleeding for two months. His CD4 count was less than 20 cells/μL. He was MSM (men having sex with men) and has receptive anal intercourse with men. His stool work-up was unrevealing for infectious etiology. Swabs for gonorrhea and chlamydia were negative. Colonoscopy revealed erythematous, congested, friable rectal mucosa with two superficial ulcers. Biopsies of the ulcer were positive for acid fast staining bacteria and the culture grew MAI. His blood culture was negative for growth of acid-fast bacteria (AFB). However, liver biopsy performed for elevated alkaline phosphatase of 958 units/L revealed noncaseating granuloma. Gastro-duodenoscopy with duodenal biopsy did not reveal any mucosal abnormality. He was managed as with disseminated MAI infection using clarithromycin, ethambutol, and rifabutin in addition to HAART therapy. Interval Colonoscopy in 20 months showed resolution of rectal ulcer. The gut is often involved in patients with disseminated MAI infection, with the duodenum being the most common site. MAI infection should be suspected as possible etiology for proctitis in HIV positive patient with low CD4 count, as proctitis, though infrequent can be the sole presentation for disseminated MAI infection in patients with HIV and low CD4 count.

1. Introduction

The association between *Mycobacterium avium intracellulare* (MAI) and acquired immune deficiency syndrome (AIDS) was identified in the 1980's [1]. Immune compromise status in general is a risk factor for acquiring MAI infection. The epidemic of MAI is concurrent to the AIDS epidemic [2] with a low CD4 count being a risk factor for acquiring MAI infection [3]. With advent of Highly Active Anti-Retroviral Therapy (HAART) there has been a control of MAI epidemic, however, nonadherence to HAART can decrease the CD4 count and hence increase susceptibility to MAI infection [4]. The occurrence of MAI infection is relatively late in the course of the natural history of Human Immuno-deficiency Virus (HIV) infection [5] and with improvement in life expectancy in the era of HAART, there can be an increased frequency of MAI infections [5, 6].

MAI infection can present as a localized disease or a disseminated presentation, patients with AIDS being more prone to disseminated infection. Blood stream infection, lymph nodes, and liver infections are common in patients with disseminated MAI. Gastrointestinal manifestations are also common in patients with systemic MAI infections, the duodenum being the most common organ to be involved [7]. We present

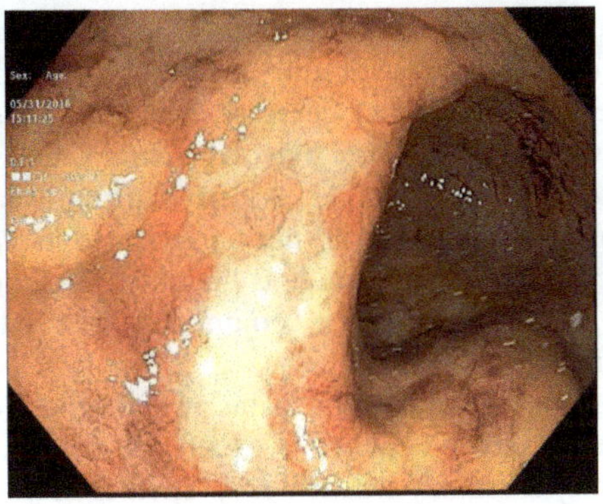

Figure 1: Rectal mucosal with ulcerations.

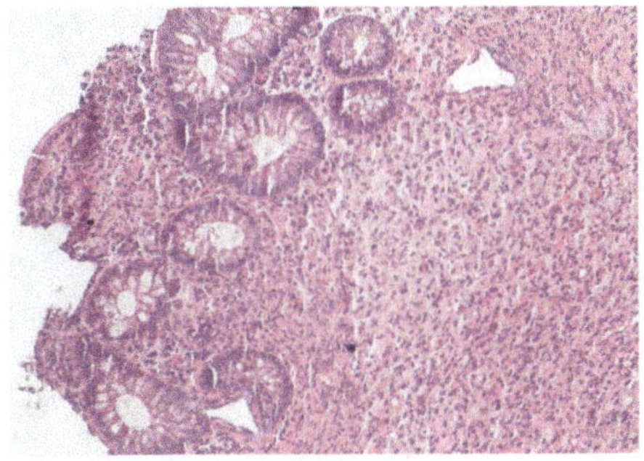

Figure 2: Rectal biopsy showing diffuse expansion of lamina propria with infiltration by lymphohistiocytic cells. (*H* and *E*, magnification ×200).

a case of a young male with AIDS presenting with proctitis and diagnosis of the disseminated MAI, successfully treated with triple combination therapy.

2. Case Presentation

A 25-year-old male presented to the emergency room (ER) with complaints of rectal bleeding, described as bright red blood on formed stool, for 2 months. His medical co-morbid condition includes a 7-year history of Human Immuno Deficiency Virus (HIV) infection, nonadherence to Highly Active Retroviral Therapy (HAART) with a CD4 count <20 cells/μL and HIV viral load of 151,257 copies/mL. He is MSM (men having sex with men) and has receptive anal intercourse with men. He reported remote treatment for Genital Herpes. In the ER, his vitals were within normal limits and physical examination was unremarkable except for minimal right upper quadrant tenderness upon palpation and numerous tender perirectal ulcerations. Rectal examination revealed normal sphincter tone with empty but tender rectal vault. There was no peripheral lymphadenopathy.

Laboratory investigations showed haemoglobin of 10.4 g/dL, leukocyte count of 3.1 K cells/μL, platelet count of 339 K cells/μL, aminotransferase levels 3X ULN, total bilirubin levels of 7.0 mg/dL with conjugated bilirubin of 5.2 mg/dL, serum lactate dehydrogenase of 327 unit/L, serum gamma glutamyl transferase of 414 units/L, and alkaline phosphatase of 958 unit/L. Stool work up was negative for *Cryptosporidium*, *Cryptococcal* antigen, *Clostridium difficile*, *Cyclospora*, *Microsporidium*, and *Isospora*. No Ova and parasites isolated from stool studies. Blood cultures for regular pathogens acid-fast bacteria (AFB) were negative. Patient was admitted and colonoscopy performed to further identify the cause of rectal bleeding revealed diffusely erythematous, congested, friable rectal mucosa with two superficial ulcers (Figure 1). Biopsies were taken of the rectal mucosa as well as normal appearing proximal colon and terminal ileum. Rectal swabs were negative for chlamydia and gonorrhea. Pathology for rectal biopsy revealed AFB positive organism (Figures 2 and 3) and culture revealed growth of *Mycobacterium avium-intracellulare (MAI)* organisms. During this clinical course, he had an unremarkable upper endoscopy and was started on clarithromycin 500 mg BID, ethambutol 1200 mg QD, and rifabutin 300 mg QD in addition to HAART therapy.

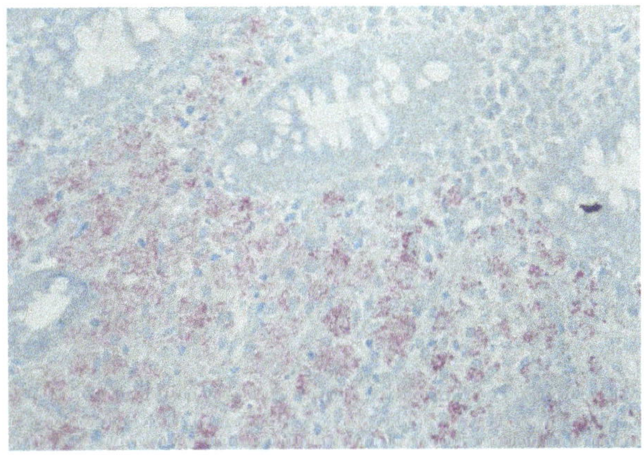

Figure 3: Rectal biopsy: acid fast staining showing sheets of macrophages packed with bundles of acid-fast bacilli, characteristic of *Mycobacterium avium intracellulare*. (Acid fast stain, magnification ×400).

Clinical presentation was highly suspected for disseminated MAI infection. Given negative blood culture, we further pursued evaluation of elevated alkaline phosphatase and performed liver biopsy. Pathology was reported to have necrotizing granulomas composed of lymphohistiocytic collections (Figure 4), highly suggestive of MAI infection. This confirmed our diagnosis of disseminated MAI. Patient was on and off the recommended regimen, flexible sigmoidoscopy after a short course of interrupted treatment again demonstrated similar initial findings in the rectum (Figure 5) but a follow up colonoscopy 20 months after diagnosis showed healing of rectal mucosa with negative biopsies for MAC. There was also a decreasing trend of alkaline phosphatase while on treatment, with last reported value of 218 unit/L.

3. Discussion

Nontuberculous Mycobacteria (NTM) are environmental organisms that are opportunistic in nature and under favorable conditions, cause a wide range of diseases ranging from pulmonary to disseminated infections, with the former being the most common [8]. Immune suppression is the typical predisposing factor and includes patients with HIV/AIDS, using

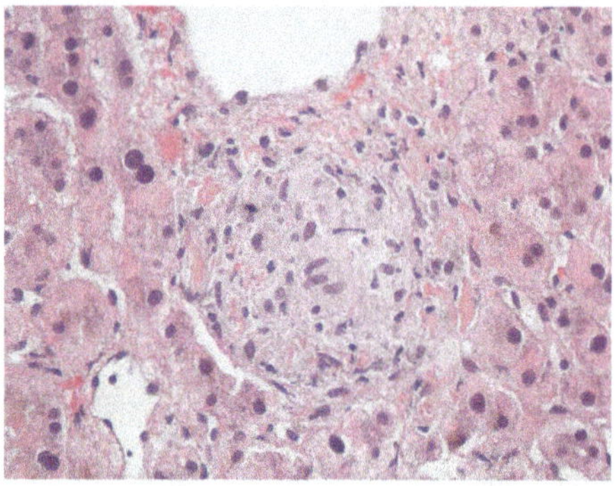

Figure 4: Liver biopsy with nonnecrotizing granuloma. Composed of lymphohistiocytic collections. (*H* and *E*, magnification ×400).

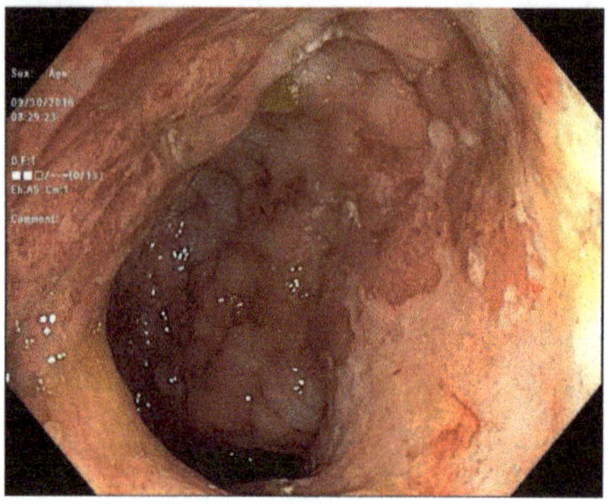

Figure 5: Friable rectal mucosa with edema (2 months after initiation of MAI treatment).

immunosuppressive therapy and undergoing solid organ or haematologic transplant [9]. A CD4 count below 50 cells/μL presents the highest risk for NTM infection and there has been suggestion of a genetic predisposition determined by human leukocyte antigen (HLA) class [10]. In the context of immune suppression, the vast majority of NTM cases are still *Mycobacterium avium complex* (MAC) but several factors lead to increased recognition of other species like *M. fortuitum*, *M. abscessus*, *M. chelonae*, and *M. haemophilium*, these include host factors and improved laboratory diagnostics [9]. In the United States, Tuberculosis (TB) has been overtaken by NTM as the predominant cause of mycobacterial lung disease [11].

Proctitis can be from infectious or noninfectious etiology. In MSM (men having sex with men) population, proctitis presents as sexually transmitted disease with gonorrhea being the most common infection [12]. MAI related proctitis is an uncommon presentation and it is not considered to be a sexually transmitted disease. Localized and disseminated disease are the two presentations of MAC in patients infected with HIV with the latter declining with increasing use of HAART [13]. Disseminated MAC present with malabsorption, rectal bleeding and loose stool when the gastrointestinal tract is involved [14], with the duodenum being the most commonly involved location in a case series [7]. In patients with advanced AIDS, MAI is one of the most common etiology of hepatic opportunistic infection [15]. It has a varied clinical manifestation ranging from granulomatous liver disease to presentation of a liver mass [16]. The increase in alkaline phosphatase in our patient appears to arise from MAI induced granulomatous liver disease and with anti-microbial management for MAI, there was an interval decrease in alkaline phosphatase levels. Liver involvement is a sign of disseminated MAI infection. Once diagnosis of MAC is derived from liver biopsy, endoscopic work-up is usually not warranted to start anti-microbial treatment. Hence, there is literature to opine on the rates of rectal infection in conjunction with liver MAI involvement.

In general, cultures are the mainstay of diagnosis of infection with MAI. Blood cultures are preferred in disseminated cases as they are highly sensitive [13]. There is a role for stool culture in early diagnosis of patients with disseminated disease, especially in cases with confirmed gastrointestinal involvement, with sensitivity and specificity as high as 86% and 99% respectively [7, 17]. In our patient, stool culture was largely negative and did not reveal any opportunistic pathogen. Upper endoscopy and colonoscopy can aid in visual identification of any abnormalities in the mucosa and result in tissue specimens that can be stained and directly observed for acid fast bacilli present in the setting of noncaseating granuloma as was the case in our index patient. In patients with MAI colitis, erythema, friability, and ulcerations are commonly seen endoscopic findings [14], these were also noted in our patient and shown in Figures 1 and 5 above. A case of MAI presenting with severe gastrointestinal bleeding in a non HIV patient, diagnosed with colonoscopy with biopsy specimens staining positive for acid fast organisms, was described by Nguyen et al. [18].

In a nonHIV patient with extrapulmonary MAI, given that lack of consensus on the duration of treatment, a minimum duration of 6 months is usually adopted, meanwhile the pulmonary cases are tailored towards treatment for 12 months after sputum cultures have remained negative [19]. The main stay of treatment for MAI is with dual therapy comprising of ethambutol and macrolides, especially in patient with AIDS [13]. Some special circumstances that warrant a third agent include elevated mycobacterial burden, lack of antiretroviral therapy and patients with advanced immune compromise [20]. The preferred third agent is usually Rifabutin but other choices could be amikacin or fluroquinolones like moxifloxacin and levofloxacin, these combinations are typically used for at least 12 months, preferably for minimum of 6 months after sustained CD4 count above 100 cells/μL [20].

Our patient was started on triple therapy, issues were encountered during his treatment course given his poor adherence. But after 20 months of therapy, he had clinical and endoscopic cure of his MAI proctitis. He is currently on treatment for the MAI, concurrent with his HAART given that his CD4 count is still not at target.

4. Conclusion

Disseminated MAI with gastrointestinal involvement should always be considered as a cause of lower gastrointestinal bleeding, in patients with immune compromise. The findings, including friability, and ulcerations, are nonspecific and can be seen in other clinical entities that include but are not limited to inflammatory bowel disease and cytomegalovirus colitis, both of which are commonly seen with immune deficiency. Biopsy with special stains helps to identify MAI as the causative organism. Treatment will depend on immune status and location, with extra pulmonary cases like our index case requiring at least 12 months of treatment. Given the correlation between this opportunistic pathogen and low CD4 count in the HIV patients, concurrent treatment with HAART is also warranted.

Authors' Contributions

All authors have reviewed the literature and contributed to manuscript drafting. Chukwunonso Chime and Peter Bhandari were responsible for the revision of the manuscript for important intellectual content. Masooma Niazi has reviewed patient slides and legends for the pathology figures. Harish Patel has critical reviewed manuscript and figures. All authors issued final approval for the version to be submitted.

References

[1] J. A. Havlik Jr., C. R. Horsburgh, B. Metchock, P. P. Williams, S. A. Fann, and S. E. Thompson, "Disseminated *Mycobacterium avium* complex infection: clinical identification and epidemiologic trends," *Journal of Infectious Diseases*, vol. 165, no. 3, pp. 577–580, 1992.

[2] C. R. Horsburgh and R. M. Selik, "The epidemiology of disseminated nontuberculous mycobacterial infection in the acquired immunodeficiency syndrome (AIDS)," *American Review of Respiratory Disease*, vol. 139, no. 1, pp. 4–7, 1989.

[3] J. Chiu, "Treatment of disseminated *Mycobacterium avium* complex infection in AIDS with amikacinethambutol, rifampin, and ciprofloxacin. California collaborative treatment group," *Annals of Internal Medicine*, vol. 113, no. 5, p. 358, 1990.

[4] C. Fortin and D. Rouleau, "Cerebral *Mycobacterium avium* abscesses: late immune reconstitution syndrome in an HIV-1-infected patient receiving highly active antiretroviral therapy," *The Canadian Journal of Infectious Diseases & Medical Microbiology*, vol. 16, no. 3, pp. 187–189, 2005.

[5] C. R. Horsburgh, "*Mycobacterium avium* complex infection in the acquired immunodeficiency syndrome," *The New England Journal of Medicine*, vol. 324, no. 19, pp. 1332–1338, 1991.

[6] J. Hoy, A. Mijch, M. Sandland, L. Grayson, R. Lucas, and B. Dwyer, "Quadruple-drug therapy for *Mycobacterium avium-intracellulare* bacteremia in AIDS Patients," *Journal of Infectious Diseases*, vol. 161, no. 4, pp. 801–805, 1990.

[7] J. R. Gray and L. Rabeneck, "Atypical mycobacterial infection of the gastrointestinal tract in AIDS patients," *The American Journal of Gastroenterology*, vol. 84, no. 12, pp. 1521–1524, 1989.

[8] L. Zhang, W. M. Lin, H. Li et al., "Hepatic nontuberculous mycobacterial granulomas in patients with cancer mimicking metastases: an analysis of three cases," *Quantitative Imaging in Medicine and Surgery*, vol. 9, no. 6, pp. 1126–1131, 2019.

[9] E. Henkle and K. L. Winthrop, "Nontuberculous mycobacteria infections in immunosuppressed hosts," *Clinics in Chest Medicine*, vol. 36, no. 1, pp. 91–99, 2015.

[10] E. Naik, S. LeBlanc, J. Tang, L. P. Jacobson, and R. A. Kaslow, "The complexity of HLA class II (DRB1, DQB1, DM) associations with disseminated *Mycobacterium avium* complex infection among HIV-1-seropositive whites," *Journal of Acquired Immune Deficiency Syndromes*, vol. 33, no. 2, pp. 140–145, 2003.

[11] D. R. Prevots, P. A. Shaw, D. Strickland et al., "Nontuberculous mycobacterial lung disease prevalence at four integrated health care delivery systems," *American Journal of Respiratory and Critical Care Medicine*, vol. 182, no. 7, pp. 970–976, 2010.

[12] J. D. Klausner, R. Kohn, and C. Kent, "Etiology of clinical proctitis among men who have sex with men," *Clinical Infectious Diseases*, vol. 38, no. 2, pp. 300–302, 2004.

[13] J. A. Gonzales Zamora and C. Milikowski, "Proctitis caused by *Mycobacterium avium-intracellulare* in an HIV-infected patient," *Diseases*, vol. 6, no. 2, p. 36, 2018.

[14] C. Keller, S. Kirkpatrick, K. Lee, M. Paul, I. C. Hanson, and M. Gilger, "Disseminated *Mycobacterium avium* complex presenting as hematochezia in an infant with rapidly progressive acquired immunodeficiency syndrome," *The Pediatric Infectious Disease Journal*, vol. 15, no. 8, pp. 713–715, 1996.

[15] J. C. Price and C. L. Thio, "Liver disease in the HIV-infected individual," *Clinical Gastroenterology and Hepatology*, vol. 8, no. 12, pp. 1002–1012, 2010.

[16] M. Bonacini, "Hepatobiliary complications in patients with human immunodeficiency virus infection," *The American Journal of Medicine*, vol. 92, no. 4, pp. 404–411, 1992.

[17] T. J. Hellyer, I. N. Brown, M. B. Taylor, B. W. Allen, and C. S. F. Easmon, "Gastro-intestinal involvement in *Mycobacterium avium*-intracellulare infection of patients with HIV," *Journal of Infection*, vol. 26, no. 1, pp. 55–66, 1993.

[18] H. N. Nguyen, D. Frank, S. Handt et al., "Severe gastrointestinal hemorrhage due to *Mycobacterium avium* complex in a patient receiving immunosuppressive therapy," *The American Journal of Gastroenterology*, vol. 94, no. 1, pp. 232–235, 1999.

[19] D. E. Griffith, T. Aksamit, B. A. Brown-Elliott et al., "An official ATS/IDSA statement: diagnosis, treatment, and prevention of nontuberculous mycobacterial diseases," *American Journal of Respiratory and Critical Care Medicine*, vol. 175, no. 4, pp. 367–416, 2007.

[20] J. E. Kaplan, J. E. Kaplan, C. Benson et al., "Guidelines for prevention and treatment of opportunistic infections in HIV-infected adults and adolescents: recommendations from CDC, the national institutes of health, and the HIV medicine association of the infectious diseases society of America," *MMWR Recommendations and Reports*, vol. 58, no. RR-4, pp. 1–207, 2009, Quiz CE1-4.

23

Malabsorption Syndrome due to Intestinal Amyloidosis as Presentation of Renal Cell Carcinoma

Filipe Bessa, Pedro Gaspar, Pedro Antunes Meireles, Maria Inês Parreira, Juliana Serrazina Pedro, Marisa Teixeira da Silva, João Meneses, Rui Victorino, and Catarina Mota

Clínica Universitária de Medicina II, CHLN-Hospital de Santa Maria, Lisbon, Portugal

Correspondence should be addressed to Filipe Bessa; jfbessa.sze@gmail.com

Academic Editor: Haruhiko Sugimura

Renal cell carcinoma accounts for approximately 3% of adult malignancies. Designated in the literature as "the great masquerader," the great diversity of clinical manifestations is associated with the several paraneoplastic syndromes that potentially accompany it. Paraneoplastic amyloidosis is described in about 3–8% of cases, only exceptionally as an initial manifestation, with uncommon gastrointestinal involvement. A rare case of malabsorption by intestinal amyloidosis is presented as initial manifestation of renal cell carcinoma, emphasizing the need for early recognition of these paraneoplastic conditions.

1. Introduction

Renal cell carcinoma (RCC) originates in the renal cortex, accounting for approximately 3% of adult malignancies and 90–95% of the primary tumors of the kidney [1]. It appears as the 6th most frequent tumor in the Europe, with an incidence of 12.4 new cases per 100,000 inhabitants [2]. The diagnosis is more common between the seventh and eighth decades of life and slightly more frequent in men (M : F, 3 : 2) [3].

The frequent absence of symptoms in the early stages makes the diagnosis usually incidental, with around 25% of patients being asymptomatic [1, 3]. The classic triad of hematuria, flank pain, and palpable abdominal mass is rarely detected, presents only in 10–15% of cases, and is usually a sign of advanced disease [3]. On the contrary, the earlier manifestations may include paraneoplastic syndromes, which arise as a result of the production of several hormones and cytokines by the tumor or adjacent tissues responsible for modulation of the immune system and endocrine dysregulation of the kidney [3]. Among them, the most frequent are hypertension, constitutional symptoms, and hypercalcemia present in 40%, 20–30%, and 10–20% of the cases, respectively [1, 4].

Amyloid A amyloidosis (AA amyloidosis) results from the extracellular deposition of fibrils composed of fragments of the serum apolipoprotein amyloid A, an acute-phase reagent produced by hepatocytes. It appears as a complication of chronic inflammatory diseases such as rheumatoid arthritis and inflammatory bowel disease, chronic infections such as tuberculosis or syphilis, and tumors. As a paraneoplastic syndrome, AA amyloidosis has been described secondarily to renal cell carcinoma, non-Hodgkin's lymphoma, and, less frequently, bladder tumors and gastrointestinal stromal tumors [5, 6].

The clinical manifestations of AA amyloidosis depend on the extent and location of fibers deposition, with amyloid deposits found mostly in the kidney (80% of cases) and, at latter stages of the disease, in the heart and nervous system [7–9]. Gastrointestinal involvement by amyloid deposition in the *muscularis mucosae*, close to the vasculature and nerve plexus, is particularly infrequent [10, 11].

The authors describe a rare case of malabsorption due to intestinal amyloidosis as presentation of renal cell carcinoma.

2. Case Presentation

A 60-year-old man, with a previous history of hypertension and smoking habits (30 pack-years), was hospitalized with a four-month history of asthenia and weight loss of 20% of total body weight, associated with diarrhea and epigastric discomfort in the month before admission. No other complaints were registered.

Physical examination revealed marked cachexia (BMI 15.5 kg/m^2), pallor and dehydration, blood pressure 105/62 mmHg, heart rate 72/min, and respiratory rate 20/min. There were no rashes or skin lesions or palpable lymphadenopathies. Cardiovascular and pulmonary examination was normal. The abdomen was excavated, painful at lower quadrants palpation, and without palpable masses. The limbs exhibited muscle mass atrophy. The remaining examination was unremarkable.

The blood tests revealed normochromic microcytic anemia with a hemoglobin of 12.3 g/dL, leukocytosis ($22,5 \times 10^9$/L) with neutrophilia ($19,8 \times 10^9$/L), thrombocytosis (901×10^9/L), elevated C-reactive protein (17.11 mg/dL), renal injury with creatinine of 5.5 mg/dL, urea of 329 mg/dL, hyponatremia of 124 mmol/L, and compensated metabolic acidosis. Renal ultrasound showed a massive solid mass in the left kidney with 12 cm of greater axis. The abdominal computed tomography (CT) revealed on the left kidney, centered to the lower two-thirds, a neoformative mass with heterogeneous enhancement, and some areas of liquefaction, for which the greater dimensions were $10.5 \times 11.7 \times 8.5$ cm longitudinal, anteroposterior, and transversal axis, respectively (Figure 1). It was assumed as the initial hypothesis primary kidney tumor with cachexia/malabsorption syndrome secondary to paraneoplastic syndrome.

During hospitalization, severe anorexia was observed with reduced ingestion, general malaise, and diffuse abdominal discomfort, 8 to 10 diarrheal discharges per day with fatty and bloody content and foamy urine. The remaining investigation revealed hypoalbuminemia of 1.9 g/dl and hypocalcaemia of 7.1 mg/dl, suggesting malabsorption and nephrotic range proteinuria (3 g/24 h). Considering the location and size of the renal tumor and the clinical evolution, with gastrointestinal involvement presenting as malabsorption syndrome and nephrotic-like renal involvement, it was considered the hypothesis of renal cell carcinoma with paraneoplastic amyloidosis. Colonoscopy was performed, showing a diffusely edematous mucosa, some areas with loss of vascular pattern and erythema/spontaneous hemorrhage. The anatomopathological examination of colon biopsies revealed deposits of amyloid substance of predominant subepithelial and perivascular location (Figure 2), and immunohistochemical staining with antibodies specific for the major amyloid precursors (AA, immunoglobulin L chains of κ or λ type, antitransthyretin) showed positivity only for AA fibrils (Figure 3).

During the investigation, the patient presented with nosocomial pneumonia and was started on empirical antibiotic therapy with piperacillin-tazobactam. The clinical evolution was unfavorable, with refractory septic shock and death on the 8th day of hospitalization.

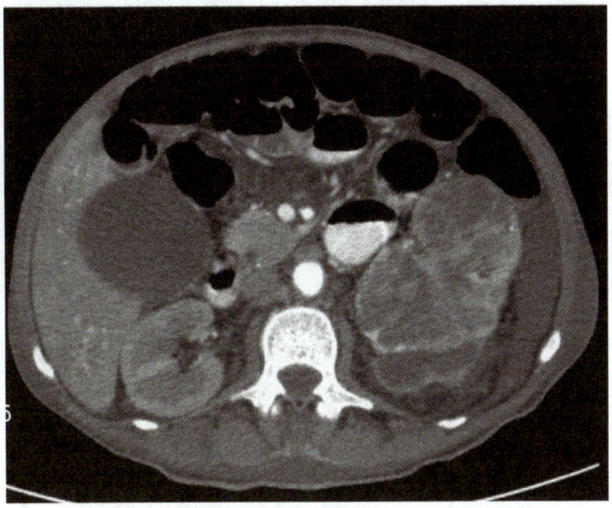

Figure 1: Computed axial tomography of the abdomen with intravenous administration of iodinated contrast: centered on the lower two-thirds of the left kidney, neoformative mass with heterogeneous enhancement, and some areas of liquefaction with greater longitudinal anteroposterior and transversal axis evaluated as $10.5 \times 11.7 \times 8.5$ cm, respectively.

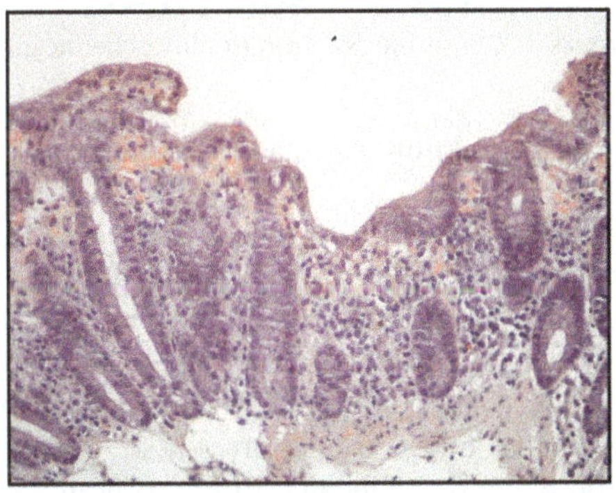

Figure 2: Colon biopsy. Fragment of mucosa from the distal portion of the intestine with conserved general architecture. Deposits of amyloid substance predominantly subepithelial and perivascular, positive for Congo red staining.

3. Discussion

Typically, RCC remains clinically silent for a long period of the disease course, due in part to the retroperitoneal location of the affected organ [1, 12]. Local symptoms arise only when the tumor is of an adequate size to deflect or invade adjacent structures. The palpable abdominal mass, hematuria, and low back pain triad occurs only in 10–15% of patients, and when present, it is a sign of advanced disease [1]. Notwithstanding, the individual components of this triad are more frequent: hematuria is the most common clinical presentation and is present in 40–60% of cases; flank pain involves distension of the renal capsule and is present in 40%

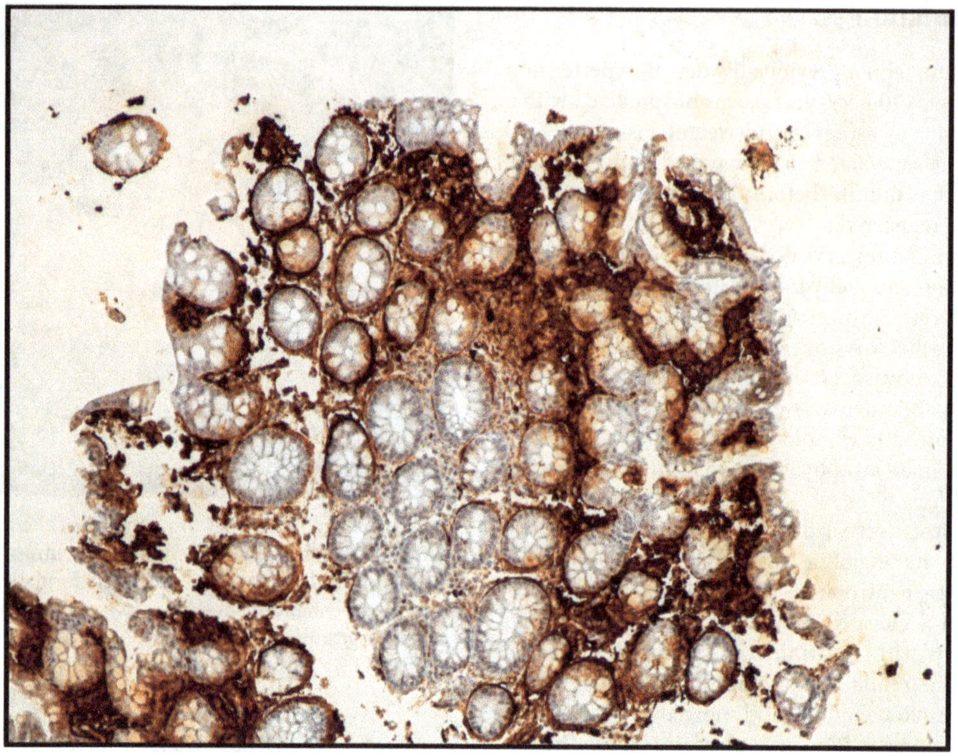

FIGURE 3: Colon biopsy. Immunohistochemical characterization of amyloid substance deposits, positive for AA amyloid.

of cases; palpable abdominal mass is found in one-third of patients [1].

Commonly known in the literature as "The Great Masquerader," RCC is recognized for its frequent association with multisystem paraneoplastic syndromes (10–40% of cases), which require recognition of a wide variety of symptoms [4]. In about one-third of the cases, constitutional symptoms are the first presentation of RCC. Fever occurs in 20–30% of patients, reflecting tumor production of inflammatory cytokines, such as interleukin-6. Tumor production of TNF-α alters adipocyte metabolism, clinically resulting in asthenia, cachexia, and weight loss in 66% of patients [13]. Hypercalcemia is one of the most common paraneoplastic syndromes, occurring in about 20% of patients [14]. RCC is still the malignancy most frequently associated with ectopic erythropoietin production (EPO), which occurs in 66% of patients, resulting in erythrocytosis in only 8% of them [1, 15].

AA amyloidosis is a paraneoplastic syndrome rarely associated with RCC (3–8% of cases) although several autopsies have suggested that RCC is the solid malignancy that most often causes AA amyloidosis, accounting for 25–42% of cases of solid tumors with secondary amyloidosis [1, 6, 8, 16]. It is characterized by multisystem extracellular deposition of amyloid fibrils derived from cleavage fragments of the *N*-terminal portion of serum amyloid protein A [7, 17]. The clinical manifestations of AA amyloidosis depend on the extent and location of fibers deposition. Amyloid deposits are found mostly in the kidney (80% of cases), possibly resulting in proteinuria, nephrotic syndrome, and renal injury. Although amyloid deposits are common in the liver and spleen, their clinical relevance is significantly lower in the earlier stages of disease. Cardiac involvement, with restrictive cardiomyopathy associated with heart failure, and neurological involvement occur at a terminal stage of the disease in <2% of cases [7–9]. Involvement of the gastrointestinal tract by AA amyloidosis, such as the case the authors present, is uncommon. Amyloid fibers are deposited in the *muscularis mucosae* of the gastrointestinal tract, near the vasculature and nerve plexus, which increases blood vessel friability, delays peristalsis, and decreases compliance of the intestinal wall, resulting in myopathy and neuromuscular dysfunction [10, 11]. The presence of amyloid in the gastric mucosa mainly determines clinically nausea, vomiting, hematemesis, and epigastric pain. The small intestine is, in the gastrointestinal tract, the organ most affected by amyloid deposits, with associated malabsorption, diarrhea, steatorrhea, hemorrhage, or obstruction. In the colon, amyloid deposition may macroscopically resemble aspects of inflammatory bowel disease, ischemic colitis, or colorectal cancer and may lead to major complications such as stenosis, bleeding, obstruction, and perforation [10, 11, 18].

The first association between amyloidosis and renal cell carcinoma was described by Ask-Up-mark in 1940 [8]. We found in the literature 19 cases of AA amyloidosis secondary to RCC [6]. Amyloid deposits are documented in the kidney, gastrointestinal tract, retroperitoneum, liver, spleen, adrenal glands, conjunctiva, and upper respiratory tract mucosa. Renal involvement was the most common presentation of AA amyloidosis. Of the 19 published cases, 14 had amyloid deposits in the kidney, with associated hematuria, nephrotic syndrome, and acute renal injury [6]. Amyloidosis with gastrointestinal involvement was found in four of the nineteen cases, resulting in diarrhea, abdominal discomfort, and weight loss. As inaugural presentation of RCC, gastrointestinal amyloidosis is reported in only two cases.

It has been shown that RCC-associated paraneoplastic syndromes are not a marker of advanced disease or poor prognosis, usually remitting with tumor removal. Early recognition of the symptoms associated with these conditions is, therefore, of particular importance and may provide early diagnosis and treatment. Paraneoplastic amyloidosis is only exceptionally an initial manifestation, with uncommon intestinal involvement. A rare case of malabsorption due to intestinal paraneoplastic amyloidosis is presented as initial manifestation of renal cell carcinoma.

References

[1] K. Sachdeva and J. Abel, "Renal cell carcinoma," *Emedic*, vol. 49, 2020.

[2] J. Ferlay, E. Steliarova-foucher, J. Lortet-tieulent et al., "Cancer incidence and mortality patterns in Europe: estimates for 40 countries in 2012," *European Journal of Cancer*, vol. 49, no. 6, pp. 1374–1403, 2013.

[3] F. Calais da Silva, "Recomendações clínicas no tratamento do carcinoma de células renais," 2015.

[4] G. S. Palapattu, B. Kristo, and J. Rajfer, "Paraneoplastic syndromes in urologic malignancy: the many faces of renal cell carcinoma," *Reviews in Urology*, vol. 4, no. 4, pp. 163–170, 2002.

[5] B. P. Hazenberg, Van Gameren II, J. Bijzet, P. L. Jager, and M. H. van Rijswijk, "Diagnostic and therapeutic approach of systemic amyloidosis," *The Netherlands Journal of Medicine*, vol. 62, no. 4, pp. 121–128, 2004.

[6] A. Babu, H. Lachmann, T. Pickett, P. Boddana, and L. Ludeman, "Renal cell carcinoma presenting as AA amyloidosis: a case report and review of the literature," *CEN Case Reports*, vol. 3, no. 1, pp. 68–74, 2014.

[7] D. Real de Asua, J. M. Galvan, M. T. Filigghedu, D. Trujillo, R. Costa, and J. Cadinanos, "Systemic AA amyloidosis: epidemiology, diagnosis, and management," *Clinical Epidemiology*, vol. 23, no. 6, pp. 369–377, 2014.

[8] J. G. Azzopardi and T. Lehner, "Systemic amyloidosis and malignant disease," *Journal of Clinical Pathology*, vol. 7, no. 19, pp. 539–548, 1966.

[9] H. J. Lachmann, H. J. B. Goodman, J. A. Gilbertson et al., "Natural history and outcome in systemic AA amyloidosis," *The New England Journal of Medicine*, vol. 23, no. 356, pp. 2361–2371, 2007.

[10] S. Petre, I. A. Shah, and N. Gilani, "Review article: gastrointestinal amyloidosis-clinical features, diagnosis and therapy," *Alimentary Pharmacology & Therapeutics*, vol. 23, no. 27, pp. 1006–1016, 2008.

[11] K. Rowe, J. Pankow, F. Nehme, and W. Salyers, "Gastrointestinal Amyloidosis: review of the literature," *Cureus*, vol. 9, no. 5, pp. 1–6, 2017.

[12] K. Rowe, "Renal cell cancer treatment (PDQ®)-patient version," 2017.

[13] T. Tsukamoto, Y. Kumamoto, N. Miyao, N. Masumori, A. Takahashi, and M. Yanase, "Interleukin-6 in renal cell carcinoma," *Journal of Urology*, vol. 148, no. 6, pp. 1778–1782, 1992.

[14] O. J. Nielsen, "Overview of cancer-related hypercalcemia: epidemiology and etiology," *Seminars in Oncology*, vol. 17, pp. 3–9, 1990.

[15] O. J. Nielsen, F. Jespersen, and M. Hilden, "Erythropoietin-induced secondary polycythemia in a patient with a renal cell carcinoma," *APMIS*, vol. 23, no. 96, pp. 688–694, 1988.

[16] W. S. G. M. McDougal, "Clinical signs and symptoms of renal cell carcinoma," *Comprehensive Textbook of Genitourinary Oncology*, vol. 139, pp. 154–159, 1995.

[17] A. Tennent, D. J. Evans, and M. B. Pepys, "Demonstration of Amyloid A protein and Amyloid P component in deposits of systemic amyloidosis associated with renal adenocarcinoma," *The Pathological Society of Great Britain and Ireland*, vol. 139, pp. 159–166, 1983.

[18] U. Syed, R. A. Ching Companioni, H. Alkhawam, and A. Walfish, "Amyloidosis of the gastrointestinal tract and the liver," *European Journal of Gastroenterology & Hepatology*, vol. 28, no. 10, pp. 1109–1121, 2016.

24

Report of a Misleading Case of the Superior Mesenteric Artery Syndrome

Amir Mohammad Salehi,[1] **Hossain Salehi**,[2] **Maryam Hasanzarrini**,[3] **and Elham Khanlarzadeh**[4]

[1]*School of Medicine, Hamadan University of Medical Sciences, Hamadan, Iran*
[2]*Gastroenterology Ward, Farhikhtegan Hospital, Azad University of Medical Sciences, Tehran, Iran*
[3]*Hepatology of Hamadan University of Medical School, Hamadan, Iran*
[4]*Department of Community Medicine, School of Medicine Hamadan University of Medical Sciences, Hamadan, Iran*

Correspondence should be addressed to Elham Khanlarzadeh; khanlarzadeh800@yahoo.com

Academic Editor: Matteo Neri

Superior mesenteric artery syndrome (SMAS), which is also known as the cast syndrome, Wilkie's syndrome, or chronic duodenal ileus, is a specific type of duodenal obstruction characterized by the obstruction of the inferior part of the duodenum due to its compression between the superior mesenteric artery (SMA) and the aorta. This problem is usually resulting from loss of the mesenteric fat pad. The present report describes a case of SMAS who was an 18-year-old woman presenting with weight loss and postprandial pain. The patient was initially diagnosed with *Helicobacter pylori* infection and underwent antibiotic therapy. However, the related symptoms did not resolve. Finally, she was ordered a CT scan, which led to the diagnosis of SMAS.

1. Introduction

Superior mesenteric artery syndrome (SMAS) was first described in 1861 by Carl von Rokitansky. Afterward, Wilkie spelled out its detailed clinical and pathophysiological characteristics, naming the condition as the chronic duodenal ileus [1]. SMAS is a problem of the upper gastrointestinal (GI) tract resulting from a life-threatening duodenal compression that mainly presents itself with rapid and significant weight loss, with the most prominent symptoms including early satiety, postprandial pain, and bile reflux [2]. The diagnosis is usually challenging, particularly in young patients and infants. The suitable approach for SMAS diagnosis is controversial because the symptoms are not always relevant or consistent with the radiological findings. Moreover, in several cases, symptoms are not fully resolved after the treatment [1]. Therefore, the problem is usually underdiagnosed or misdiagnosed with other anatomical or motility-related causes of the duodenal obstruction [3].

2. Case Report

Our case report describes an 18-year-old female patient who presented to our clinic about 6 months ago with severe epigastric pain, nausea, heartburn, regurgitation, and weight loss (about 5 kg). Her epigastric pain had a colic nature and did not radiate to other parts of the abdomen, the regurgitation content included bile secretions, and there was no report of dysphagia. Moreover, she had no history of malignancy, trauma, burn, malabsorption, spinal cord injury, neurological diseases, or long-term hospitalization. No significant finding was reported in the physical examination except abdominal distention without any evidence of tenderness or hyperactive bowel sounds. The patients underwent endoscopy, revealing antral erythema and mild to moderate gastritis. Eventually, she was diagnosed with *Helicobacter pylori* infection using gastric biopsy and was prescribed a one-month course of antibiotic therapy.

However, there was no symptom alleviation. After one month, the patient presented to our clinic for the second time with the same symptoms. Therefore, she was rehospitalized and underwent abdominal and pelvic CT scan with IV contrast (Figures 1 and 2). According to the CT findings, the proximal part of the duodenum was dilated, and the angle between the aorta and SMA was about 8 degrees. A consultation with the surgery service was ordered for the patient to confirm the diagnosis of SMAS. Due to the severity of epigastric pain and severe reduction of the angle between the aorta and SMA, the patient was then transferred to the surgery ward and underwent laparoscopic duodenojejunostomy. Following abdominal insufflation, a laparoscope was introduced into the peritoneal cavity, which showed the dilation of the proximal duodenum. However, the jejunum seemed to be normal. Afterward, 3 additional trocars were placed. After retraction of the transverse colon, the Treitz ligament was identified, and SMA was noted to be prominent and lying across the distal duodenum, which was collapsed. A duodenojejunostomy was performed. Then, a side-to-side anastomosis was made. Moreover, the methylene blue test did not show any leakage. The patient responded to the surgery dramatically. Four days after the surgery, she could consume oral fluids and then start a regular diet.

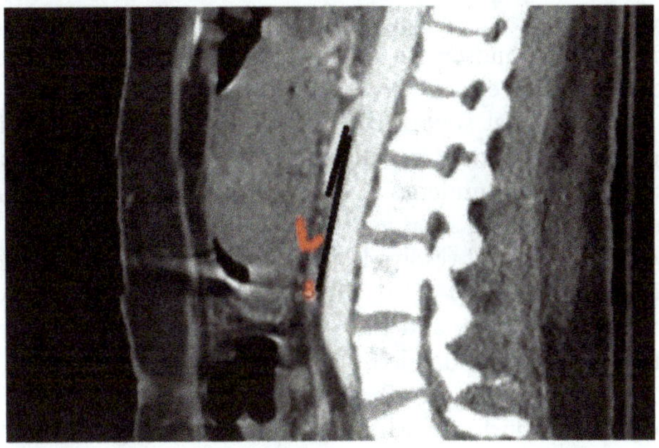

Figure 1: CT sagittal view showing an angle of 8 degrees between the superior mesenteric artery and aorta.

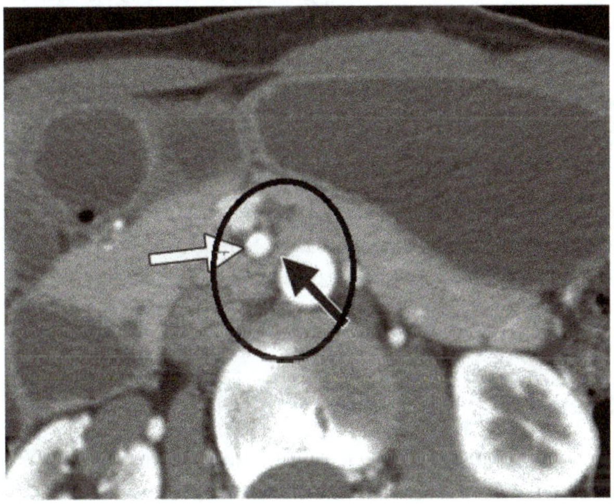

Figure 2: CT scan (axial view) with duodenal compression (black arrow) between the aorta and superior mesenteric artery (white arrows).

3. Discussion

The third part of the duodenum is confined to the mesenteric root and SMA anteriorly, while its posterior part touches the aorta and spine. The angle between the SMA and aorta is about 25–60 degrees, while the duodenum lies in a cavity between these two arteries with a diameter of 10–28 mm. In the SMAS, the angle is reduced to 6–15 degrees, decreasing the cavity diameter to 2–8 mm. Therefore, the descending duodenum appears dilated in the CT scan and is compressed between the aorta and SMA. Other common causes of the SMAS include ectopic origin of the SMA, superior and abnormal location of the Treitz ligament, the presence of a short Treitz ligament, and loss of the retroperitoneal fat, which usually surrounds the SMA and aorta like a cushion [1, 4, 5]. Up to now, about 400 cases of SMAS have been reported [2], with a higher prevalence in women compared to men [3]. According to the studies, the symptoms are usually developed in the acute form of the disease, which can be observed in 0.13%–0.3% of the barium series studies of the upper GI [1].

Most cases of SMAS are associated with severe, debilitating diseases leading to excessive weight loss, such as malignancies, malabsorption syndromes, AIDS [6], trauma, burn [5, 7], bariatric surgery [8], spinal cord injury, paraplegia [9], substance abuse [10], and anorexia nervosa [11], while the syndrome has also been reported in the conditions leading to mild weight loss, such as reconstructive surgery for scoliosis treatment [12], celiac axis compression syndrome [13], and nutcracker syndrome [14].

The symptom severity depends on the underlying cause and obstruction severity. In mild cases, only postprandial pain and early satiety may be reported, while patients with severe SMAS may develop nausea, weight loss, and the symptoms of bile reflux. It is usually believed that the symptoms may resolve when a given patient lies in the lateral decubitus or prone positions as these positions remove the pressure from the mesentery and SMA, widening the space between the SMA and aorta. However, the present patient did not report this phenomenon [1]. The physical examination findings are usually nonspecific and include abdominal distension, succussion splash, and increased bowel sounds. Laboratory findings can be nonspecific as well. However, the patients experiencing severe vomiting or regurgitation may develop significant electrolyte abnormalities, including metabolic alkalosis [15]. Delayed diagnosis of the problem may lead to dangerous complications, such as gastrointestinal perforation, gastric pneumatosis, portal venous gas, formation of a bezoar caused by the duodenal obstruction, electrolyte abnormalities, or deaths [15, 16].

Conservative treatment includes nasogastric tube placement to alleviate the duodenal pressure and treating the electrolyte abnormalities, such as metabolic alkalosis. In patients suffering from severe obstruction, nutritional support using a nasojejunal feeding tube can be necessary to help the patient gain weight [17]. In adult patients with mild disease and children whose disease is probable to be acute, the conservative treatment is usually successful if combined with nutritional support. However, nutritional support is not usually sufficient in patients with chronic disease. These patients should undergo electrolyte abnormality resolution and feeding using a nasogastric tube for a short time. If the symptoms are not resolved, various surgical options should be considered [7, 17, 18], including duodenojejunostomy, gastrojejunostomy, and the Strong's procedure, where the Treitz ligament is divided to free the duodenum from the aortomesenteric space. The preferred surgical option is the duodenojejunostomy, which is performed using the transabdominal or laparoscopic approaches. However, the laparoscopic procedure has recently replaced the transabdominal approach [3]. This procedure is the treatment of choice due to its high chance of success and low possibility of complications, such as ulcers [19].

Authors' Contributions

A. M. Salehi and E. Khanlarzadeh conceptualized and designed the study. H. Salehi provided administrative support. M. Hasanzarrini and H. Salehi involved in provision of study materials or patients. All authors contributed to write the article and approved the manuscript.

References

[1] R. Singal, P. Sahu, M. Goel et al., "Superior mesenteric artery syndrome: a case report," *North American Journal of Medical Sciences*, vol. 2, no. 8, pp. 392–394, 2010.

[2] R. C. Shukla and R. Pathak, "Superior mesenteric artery syndrome: case report," *Nepal Medical College Journal*, vol. 10, no. 2, pp. 144-145, 2008.

[3] N. Van Horne and J. P. Jackson, *Superior Mesenteric Artery Syndrome*, StatPearls, Treasure Island, FL, USA, 2020.

[4] F. Lippl, C. Hannig, W. WeiB, H. D. Allescher, M. Classen, and M. Kurjak, "Superior mesenteric artery syndrome: diagnosis and treatment from the gastroenterologist's view," *Journal of Gastroenterology*, vol. 37, no. 8, pp. 640–643, 2002.

[5] T. Gebhart, "Superior mesenteric artery syndrome," *Gastroenterology Nursing*, vol. 38, no. 3, pp. 189–193, 2015.

[6] R. Stümpfle, A. Wright, and J. Walsh, "Superior mesenteric artery syndrome in an HIV positive patient," *Sexually Transmitted Infections*, vol. 79, no. 3, pp. 262-263, 2003.

[7] J. M. Reckler, H. M. Bruck, A. M. Munster, P. W. Curreri, and B. A. Pruitt, "Superior mesenteric artery syndrome as a consequence of burn injury," *The Journal of Trauma, Injury, Infection, and Critical Care*, vol. 12, no. 11, pp. 979–985, 1972.

[8] D. Goitein, D. J. Gagne, P. K. Papasavas et al., "Superior mesenteric artery syndrome after laparoscopic roux-en-y gastric bypass for morbid obesity," *Obesity Surgery*, vol. 14, no. 7, pp. 1008–1011, 2004.

[9] I. Laffont, D. Bensmail, C. Rech, G. Prigent, G. Loubert, and O. Dizien, "Late superior mesenteric artery syndrome in paraplegia: case report and review," *Spinal Cord*, vol. 40, no. 2, pp. 88–91, 2002.

[10] J. B. Barnes and M. Lee, "Superior mesenteric artery syndrome in an intravenous drug abuser after rapid weight loss," *Southern Medical Journal*, vol. 89, no. 3, pp. 331–334, 1996.

[11] J. A. Sours and L. J. Vorhaus, "Superior mesenteric artery syndrome in anorexia nervosa: a case report," *American Journal of Psychiatry*, vol. 138, pp. 519-520, 1981.

[12] F. Zadegan, T. Lenoir, O. Drain et al., "Superior mesenteric artery syndrome following correction of spinal deformity: case report and review of the literature," *Revue de chirurgie orthopedique et reparatrice de l'appareil moteur*, vol. 93, no. 2, pp. 181–185, 2007.

[13] C.-K. Tseng, W. B. Su, H. C. Lai et al., "Superior mesenteric artery syndrome caused by celiac axis compression syndrome: a case report and review of the literature," *European Journal of Gastroenterology and Hepatology*, vol. 20, no. 6, pp. 578–582, 2008.

[14] M. Inal, B. Unal Daphan, and M. Y. Karadeniz Bilgili, "Superior mesenteric artery syndrome accompanying with nutcracker syndrome: a case report," *Iranian Red Crescent Medical Journal*, vol. 16, no. 10, 2014.

[15] J. E. Lim, G. L. Duke, and S. R. Eachempati, "Superior mesenteric artery syndrome presenting with acute massive gastric dilatation, gastric wall pneumatosis, and portal venous gas," *Surgery*, vol. 134, no. 5, pp. 840–843, 2003.

[16] M. A. Fuhrman, D. M. Felig, and M. E. Tanchel, "Superior mesenteric artery syndrome with obstructing duodenal bezoar," *Gastrointestinal Endoscopy*, vol. 57, no. 3, p. 387, 2003.

[17] N. D. Merrett, R. B. Wilson, P. Cosman, and A. V. Biankin, "Superior mesenteric artery syndrome: diagnosis and treatment strategies," *Journal of Gastrointestinal Surgery*, vol. 13, no. 2, pp. 287–292, 2009.

[18] V. Biank and S. Werlin, "Superior mesenteric artery syndrome in children: a 20-year experience," *Journal of Pediatric Gastroenterology and Nutrition*, vol. 42, no. 5, pp. 522–525, 2006.

[19] M. S. Makary, A. Patel, A. M. Aquino, and S. K. Chamarthi, "Clinical and radiologic considerations for idiopathic superior mesenteric artery syndrome," *Cureus*, vol. 9, no. 11, 2017.

25

Two Cases of Atraumatic Chylous Ascites Characterized by Hypotriglyceridemia and Partially Managed with an Oral Fat-Free Elemental Diet

Michihiro Kamigaki, Satoko Kunita, Makoto Nakano, Miwako Tanaka, Shinya Aoki, Katsutoshi Tsuga, Hiroyuki Ito, and Hideo Matsuura

Department of Internal Medicine, Saiseikai Kure Hospital, 2-1-13 Sanjo, Kure City, Hiroshima Prefecture 737-0821, Japan

Correspondence should be addressed to Michihiro Kamigaki; kamigaki@saiseikai-kure.jp

Academic Editor: Hideto Kawaratani

Most cases of chylous ascites occur after surgery, but it also develops in nonoperative cases, although rarely. Such cases are often difficult to treat. In this study, we treated 2 cases of atraumatic chylous ascites, which were controlled by combining diuretic treatment with an oral fat-free elemental diet (Elental®, EA Pharma Co., Ltd., Tokyo, Japan). Elental can provide oral nutrition compatible with a lipid-restricted diet, which may be useful for control of chylous ascites. We report on these cases, including literature review-based considerations.

1. Introduction

Chylous ascites is characterized by the accumulation of triglyceride (TG)-rich peritoneal fluid with a milky appearance due to intestinal tract and the mesentery leakage [1]. Most cases of chylous ascites occur after surgery [1–3], and the proportion of nonsurgical cases is low. The most frequent causes of nonsurgical chylous ascites include malignancies (25%), liver cirrhosis (16%), and tuberculosis (15%) [4, 5]. Chylous ascites may be treated by ligation of broken lymphatic vessels after surgery. It is generally recommended to place a central venous catheter in a fasting patient as a means of delivering total parenteral nutrition (TPN) and bypassing the intestinal tract [2, 4, 6]. However, parenteral nutrition together with an oral fat-free elemental diet have reportedly been used as initial treatments for chylous ascites [7, 8]. As there are cases where TPN cannot be used for some reason, elemental diet can also be an option for such cases. Here we present two cases of atraumatic chylous ascites, which were controlled by combining diuretic treatment with an elemental diet. In both cases, the patients provided informed consent.

2. Case Presentations

2.1. Case 1. An 83-year-old man with a medical history of high blood pressure and a gastric ulcer complained of epigastralgia and symptoms of jaundice, and was admitted to our hospital for observation. He was diagnosed with hepatic portal cholangiocarcinoma. Given the patient's age and the progression of the lesion, radical curative resection was considered too difficult. Eventually, he was discharged after undergoing an endoscopic biliary stent placement procedure (Figure 1).

At an outpatient clinic, the patient began chemotherapy with gemcitabine and ascitic fluid gradually accumulated. Therefore, the patient was administered combination oral diuretic therapy with furosemide 20 mg/day and spironolactone 25 mg/day. Ascitic fluid continued to increase with chemotherapy and the patient's activities of daily living also declined, necessitating hospitalization for further examination.

The patient's height was 172 cm and his weight was 60 kg. His blood pressure 128/64 mmHg, and his pulse 96/min. The patient displayed abdominal distension, and intestinal peristaltic sound was heard. Blood test findings are shown in Table 1.

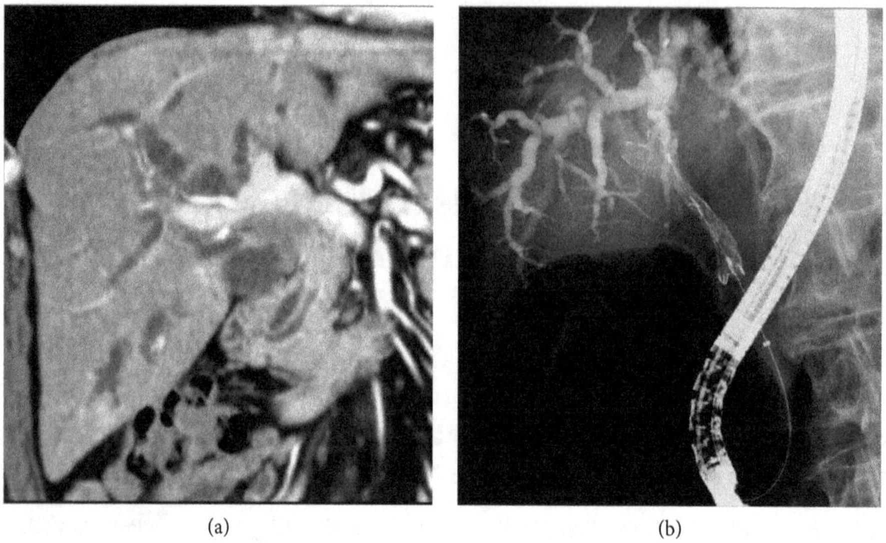

FIGURE 1: The stenosis and contrast effect are recognized in the bile duct of the hepatic portal. Expansion of bilateral intrahepatic bile duct is admitted upstream of stenosis (a). ERCP was performed and a metallic stent was placed in the left and right hepatic bile ducts (b).

An abdominal computed tomography (CT) image showed a large accumulation of ascitic fluid, and a test puncture revealed its milky appearance, and was indicative of chylous ascites (Figure 2).

The ascitic fluid was culture-negative, and cytology showed Class V of the Papanicolaou classification. In a biochemical examination of the ascites, TP (total protein) was lower but TGs were higher (Table 1). Because it was slightly lower than the definition provided by Wallis [9], we judged it as chylous ascites with a relatively low TG concentration. Initially, we reduced the NaCl and lipid content of the patient's diet to 5 g and 60 g per day, respectively, and continued treatment with furosemide and spironolactone, but we observed almost no decrease in ascetic fluid. Therefore, we stopped using medium-chain TGs (MCT) and reformulated the patient's diet to make it fat-restricted (1400 kcal, lipid 40 g per day) and added a single portion per day of Elental (300 kcal/80 g).

Elental was given orally and no side effects such as vomiting or diarrhea occurred.

Seven days after the change in diet, the patient's body weight decreased from 58 to 54 kg and his abdominal circumference decreased from 88 to 84 cm (Figure 3).

Chemotherapy was subsequently resumed at the outpatient clinic with tegafur/gimeracil/oteracil (TS-1). The ascitic fluid did not resolve completely but was attenuated by comparison with baseline status when managed via the oral administration of an elemental diet for approximately 1 month.

TABLE 1: Laboratory findings on admission (Case 1).

WBC	2700	/μl	Glu	96	mg/dl
RBC	342	$\times 10/^4 \mu$l	Na	142	mEq/l
Hb	10.1	g/dl	K	4.2	mEq/l
Plt	16.7	$\times 10/^4 \mu$l	Cl	107	mEq/l
T-Bil	0.6	mg/dl	T-cho	144	mg/dl
AST	29	IU/l	TG	47	mg/dl
ALT	20	IU/l			
LDH	177	IU/l		Ascites	
ALP	399	IU/l	TP	0.8	g/dl
γ-GTP	41	IU/l	LDH	37.0	IU/l
AMY	50	IU/l	Na	139.7	mEq/l
TP	6.5	g/dl	K	3.8	mEq/l
Alb	2.9	g/dl	Cl	111.3	mEq/l
BUN	9.9	mg/dl	Glu	133	mg/dl
Cre	0.54	mg/dl	TG	48	mg/dl
CEA	92.1	ng/ml	Bacterial culture; negative		
CA19-9	<2.0	U/ml	Cytology; Class V		

Abbreviations: WBC: whole blood cell count, RBC: red blood cell count, Hb: hemoglobin, Plt: platelet count, T-Bil: total-value bilirubin, AST: aspartate transferase, ALT: alanine transaminase, LDH: lactate dehydrogenase, ALP: alkaline phosphatase, γ-GTP: gamma-glutamyl transferase, AMY: amylase, TP: total protein, Alb: albumin, BUN: blood urea nitrogen, CRE: creatinine, CEA: carcinoembryonic antigen, CA 19-9: cancer antigen 19-9, Glu: glucose, Na: sodium, K: potassium, Cl: chlorine, T-cho: total cholesterol, TG: triglycerides.

2.2. Case 2. An 82-year-old man with a history of cerebral infarction sequelae and dementia of the Alzheimer's type was treated for 2 weeks with antibiotics after a diagnosis of mesenteric panniculitis. One month after discharge from the hospital, the patient gained weight and experienced fatigue, upon which he visited the hospital. He was diagnosed with ascites, pleural effusion, and pericardial effusion, and he was then readmitted to the hospital.

The patient's height was 163 cm and his weight was 59.5 kg. There was no noise in the heart sound. Abdominal distension and lower leg edema were observed. Blood test findings were somewhat low (Table 2).

An abdominal CT image showed a large amount of ascites (Figure 4(a)), and a test puncture revealed its milky appearance. A bacterial culture of the ascites was negative, and cytology showed it to be Class I of the Papanicolaou classification.

Initially, we placed the patient on a fat-restricted diet (1400 kcal and lipid 40 g per day), furosemide 10 mg/day, and a single dose of elemental diet, Elental, but

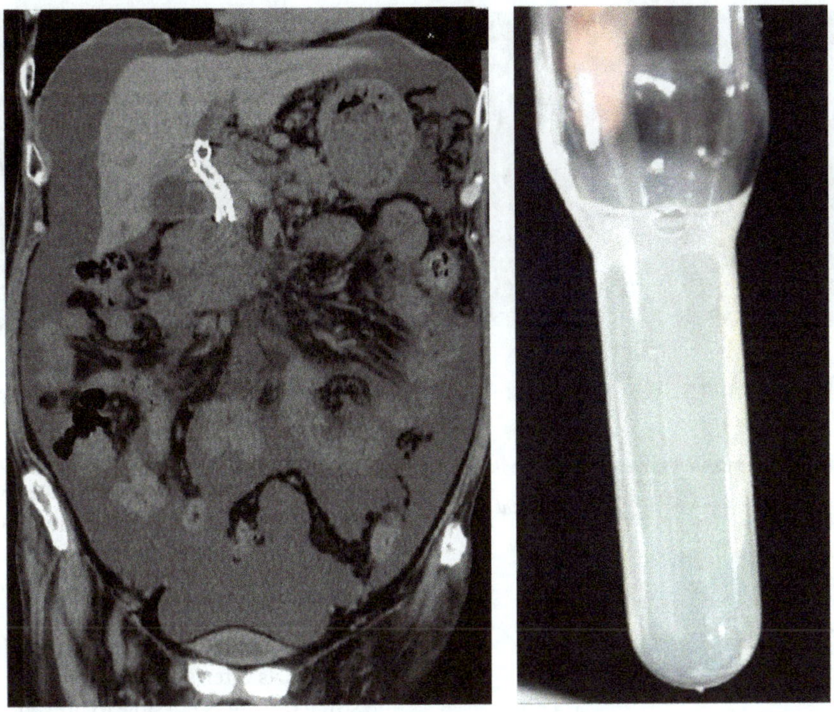

(a) (b)

FIGURE 2: A large amount of ascites was stored in the abdominal CT (a). Harvested ascites (b).

TABLE 2: Laboratory findings on admission (Case 2).

WBC	6000	/μl	Na	136	mEq/l
RBC	346	×10/⁴μl	K	3.5	mEq/l
Hb	10.0	g/dl	Cl	107	mEq/l
Plt	24.6	×10/⁴μl	T-cho	166	mg/dl
T-Bil	0.27	mg/dl	TG	57	mg/dl
AST	15	IU/l			
ALT	9	IU/l		Ascites	
LDH	187	IU/l	TP	0.8	g/dl
ALP	358	IU/l	LDH	28.0	IU/l
γ-GTP	50	IU/l	Na	139.6	mEq/l
AMY	64	IU/l	K	3.4	mEq/l
TP	6.2	g/dl	Cl	116.5	mEq/l
BUN	13.9	mg/dl	Glu	193	mg/dl
Cre	1.53	mg/dl	TG	71	mg/dl
CEA	<0.5	ng/ml	Bacterial culture; negative		
Glu	113	mg/dl	Cytology; Class I		

Abbreviations: WBC: whole blood cell count, RBC: red blood cell count, Hb: hemoglobin, Plt: platelet count, T-Bil: total-value bilirubin, AST: aspartate transferase, ALT: alanine transaminase, LDH: lactate dehydrogenase, ALP: alkaline phosphatase, γ-GTP: gamma-glutamyl transferase, AMY: amylase, TP: total protein, BUN: blood urea nitrogen, CRE: creatinine, CEA: carcinoembryonic antigen, Glu: glucose, Na: sodium, K: potassium, Cl: chlorine, T-cho: total cholesterol, TG: triglycerides.

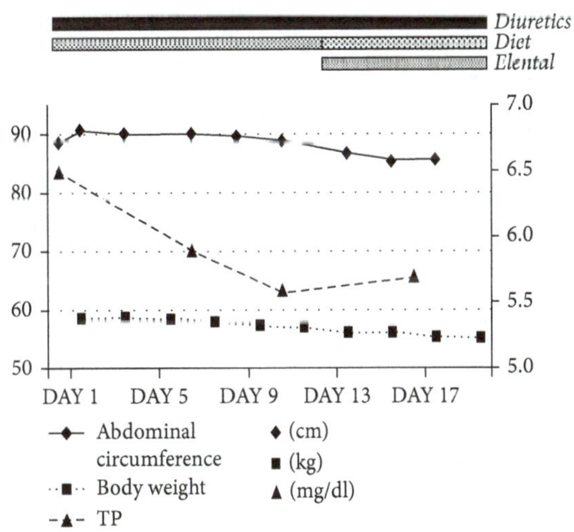

FIGURE 3: The body weight and abdominal girth decreased with the fat-restricted diet and the diuretic, Elental. At the same time, serum TP trended upward. TP, total protein.

improvements in weight and waist circumference were poor. Oral administration of Elental did not cause any side effects.

After that, we stopped the fat-restricted diet and increased the amount of Elental to 3 times a day. In addition, peripheral parenteral nutrition was administered by infusion. The patient's body weight then decreased from 62 to 53 kg in 25 days, and his abdominal girth improved from 90 to 70 cm (Figure 5).

After that, we restarted the patient on a fat-restricted diet at 900 kcal divided into morning and evening, and lipid at 20 g/day, and the patient also consumed 2 bottles of Elental daily at noon.

Ultimately, oral nutrition and a small amount of diuretic administered orally resulted in better control of weight and abdominal girth. Abdominal CT also showed a marked improvement in ascites (Figure 4(b)). He was discharged from the hospital and continued treatment on an outpatient basis.

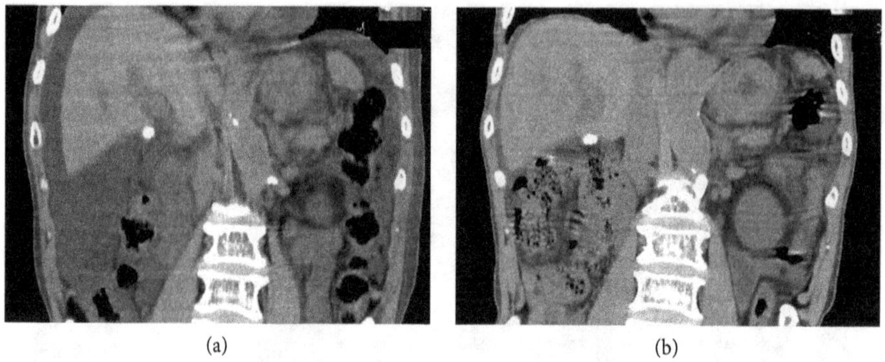

FIGURE 4: Abdominal CT showed massive storage of ascites (a) and a decrease in ascites after treatment (b).

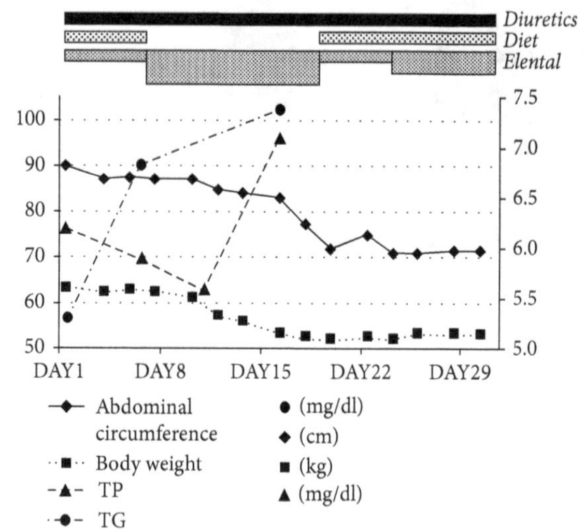

FIGURE 5: The body weight and abdominal girth decreased with the fat-restricted diet, the diuretic, and elental. At the same time, serum TG and TP increased.

3. Discussion

Chylous ascites has a milky appearance and contains an abundant amount of TG, which leaches from the intestinal tract and the mesentery [1]. TGs ingested from meals are absorbed from the small intestine and flow into the portal vein via the lymph duct. However, if the lymphatic vessels in the abdominal cavity rupture and if TGs and lymph leak into the abdominal cavity from the collapsed site, chylous ascites occurs [1, 2, 10, 11]. If left untreated, the patient's general condition may deteriorate due to malnutrition and reduction of immunity. Therefore, appropriate treatment is necessary.

The causes of ascites are diverse, but the frequency of encountering chylous ascites is small. According to the report of Press et al., chylous ascites is found at a frequency of one case in 20,000 hospital cases, and of one case in 11,589 cases after intraperitoneal surgery [3]. It is a very rare condition. Most cases of chylous ascites occur after surgery [1], and the proportion of nonsurgical cases is low. It is said that malignancies (25%), liver cirrhosis (16%), and tuberculosis (15%) are among the most frequent causes of nonsurgical chylous ascites [4, 5]. Case 1 had bile duct cancer, and it was presumed that chylous ascites resulted from periportal lesion or peritoneal splenic lesion infiltrating the lymph duct [11].

In Case 2, mesenteric panniculitis spreading to lymph vessels was presumed to have caused the chylous ascites. In both cases, it was difficult to locate the site of failure in the lymphatic vessels using CT scans.

Chylous ascites may be treated by ligation of broken lymphatic vessels after surgery. However, by circumventing the intestinal tract, it is possible to prevent TGs from leaking into the abdominal cavity from the broken lymphatic vessels. First, it is recommended that primary management of chylous ascites should involve the placement of a central venous catheter in a fasting patient to provide TPN while bypassing the intestinal tract [2, 4, 6].

Secondary considerations may include MCTs and octreotide which have been mentioned as supplementary treatments. Since MCTs do not pass through the lymphatic system, but rather are absorbed directly into the portal vein according to several reports, MCTs do not increase lymph flow [2, 12, 13]. However, the response rate is less than 50%. Octreotide, a somatostatin analog, inhibits gut hormone secretion and exocrine secretions such as gastric juice, pancreatic juice, and bile. Octreotide treatment leads to control of nutrient absorption from the digestive tract, gastrointestinal motility, and secretion of lymph, which in turn promotes repair of the lymphatic system [5, 12]. However, the treatment of chylous ascites with octreotide is not covered by the current medical insurance plan in Japan.

Both patients in this report were elderly. The first patient had cancer with a poor prognosis, and the second patient had dementia such that there was a high risk of his pulling out the central venous catheter. In both cases, there were strong reasons to continue oral intake. To preserve quality of life, we treated the patients with an oral diet (fat-restricted diet and an elemental diet) before resorting to TPN via a central venous catheter.

There have been reports that parenteral nutrition and an oral fat-free elemental diet have been used as initial treatments for chylous ascites [7, 8]. In the patients in our report, although complete disappearance of ascites was not reached according to the imaging, weight, and abdominal girth decreased and quality of life improved.

In Case 1, blood TP improved from 5.6 to 5.7 mg/dl in 7 days. In Case 2, we were able to track improvements such as blood TG at 57–102 mg/dl in 18 days and TP at 5.6–7.1 mg/dl in 7 days.

Typical chylous ascites is defined as TG > 200 mg/dl [1, 3]. However, there are reports that set the cutoff value at ≥110 mg/dl [3], and those that report TG concentration in ascites as 2–8 times the serum TG concentration [5, 14]. Serum TG concentration was relatively low in the 2 cases at our hospital. We presumed that the ascites TG concentrations were low due to the fact that these cases were atraumatic and that the serum TG concentrations were low due to aging and malnutrition. According to the classification in the report by Wallis [9], cases with relatively low concentration of ascites TG are defined as pseudo-chylous ascites. In addition, according to the report of Cardenas and Chopra [15], such cases are considered as atypical chylous ascites. However, the treatment method for cases with a relatively low ascites TG concentration has not been discussed until our report.

Elental is an enteral high calorie nutritional supplement with amino acids. Elental was created in the process of developing easy-to-absorb food for astronauts and was then applied for medical use. It is administered to patients with poor oral intake, patients with hypoproteinemia and patients requiring nutritional management after surgery or for Crohn's disease to give the intestines respite for healing [16]. A preparation with a lower lipid concentration is also frequently used for conditions such as chronic or acute pancreatitis [17, 18]. Nakayama and colleagues reported on a patient who developed chylous ascites 3 weeks after surgery for advanced rectal cancer; the ascites disappeared 7 weeks after initiation of Elental at 30 kcal/kg/day [8].

The two patients in this report had nonpostoperative, atraumatic chylous ascites. Among cases of chylous ascites, such cases are relatively rare. Atraumatic chylous ascites like these two cases may be difficult to treat by ligation of broken lymphatic vessels. The site of rupture of lymphatic vessels is unclear. The original disease makes it difficult to cure the broken site. Because of these two reasons, chylous ascites of our patients may have been managed only partially.

Elental was chosen because the patients had two needs: continuation of oral nutrition intake and fat restriction. Both patients showed good control of both weight and abdominal circumference by approximately 1–3 weeks after starting Elental. In the meantime, we observed serum TG and TP improvement.

It is unknown whether a specific type of chylous ascites can be managed with an oral elemental diet and a specific TG concentration. Furthermore, the amount and the period of use have not yet been defined. In order to clarify these points, future cases must be studied.

4. Conclusion

Fat restriction with Elental was provided with concurrent oral nutrition. Elental could be useful as a treatment option for chylous ascites.

References

[1] S. A. Al-Busafi, P. Ghali, M. Deschenes, and P. Wong, "Chylous ascites: evaluation and management," *ISRN Hepatology*, vol. 2014, Article ID 240473, 10 pages, 2014.

[2] O. O. Aalami, D. B. Allen, and C. H. Organ Jr., "Chylous ascites: a collective review," *Surgery*, vol. 128, no. 5, pp. 761–778, 2000.

[3] O. W. Press, N. O. Press, and S. D. Kaufman, "Evaluation and management of chylous ascites," *Annals of Internal Medicine*, vol. 96, no. 3, pp. 358–364, 1982.

[4] Q. Ui Ain, Y. Bashir, and S. Johnston, "Idiopathic chylous ascites simulating acute appendicitis: a case report and literature review," *International Journal of Surgery Case Reports*, vol. 29, pp. 189–192, 2016.

[5] G. D'amata, M. Rega, V. Viola, V. Bove, P. Simeone, and G. Baiano, "Chyloperitoneum associated with idiopathic pancreatitis: case report and review of the literature," *Giornale di Chirurgia—Journal of Surgery*, vol. 37, no. 4, pp. 167–170, 2016.

[6] J. F. Lippey and T. L. Yong, "Chyle leak following biliary pancreatitis," *Journal of Surgical Case Reports*, vol. 2014, no. 7, p. 52, 2014.

[7] Y. Cao, W. Yan, L. Lu et al., "Parenteral nutrition combined with rice soup can be a safe and effective intervention for congenital chylous ascites," *Asia Pacific Journal of Clinical Nutrition*, vol. 25, no. 3, pp. 631–635, 2016.

[8] G. Nakayama, D. Morioka, T. Murakami, H. Takakura, Y. Miura, and S. Togo, "Chylous ascites occurring after low anterior resection of the rectum successfully treated with an oral fat-free elemental diet (Elental®)," *Clinical Journal of Gastroenterology*, vol. 5, no. 3, pp. 216–219, 2012.

[9] R. L. M. Wallis, "Chylous and pseudo-chylous ascites," *Proceedings of the Royal Society of Medicine*, vol. 6, no. 1, pp. 136–142, 1913.

[10] S. Akbulut, D. Yilmaz, S. Bakir, E. Cucuk, and M. Tas, "Acute appendicitis together with chylous ascites: is it a coincidence?" *Case Reports in Medicine*, vol. 2010, Article ID 206860, 4 pages, 2010.

[11] M. Yilmaz, S. Akbulut, B. Isik et al., "Chylous ascites after liver transplantation: incidence and risk factors," *Liver Transplantation*, vol. 18, no. 9, pp. 1046–1052, 2012.

[12] R. Kaas, L. D. Rustman, and F. A. Zoetmulder, "Chylous ascites after oncological abdominal surgery: incidence and treatment," *European Journal of Surgical Oncology (EJSO)*, vol. 27, no. 2, pp. 187–189, 2001.

[13] C. Bhatia, U. Pratap, and Z. Slavik, "Octreotide therapy: a new horizon in treatment of iatrogenic chyloperitoneum," *Archives of Disease in Childhood*, vol. 85, no. 3, pp. 234–235, 2001.

[14] P. C. Ward, "Interpretation of ascitic fluid data," *Postgraduate Medicine*, vol. 71, no. 2, pp. 171–178, 1982.

[15] A. Cardenas and S. Chopra, "Chylous ascites," *The American Journal of Gastroenterology*, vol. 97, no. 8, pp. 1896–1900, 2002.

[16] T. Yamamoto, M. Nakahigashi, S. Umegae, T. Kitagawa, and K. Matsumoto, "Impact of long-term enteral nutrition on clinical and endoscopic recurrence after resection for Crohn's disease: a prospective, nonrandomized, parallel, controlled study," *Alimentary Pharmacology & Therapeutics*, vol. 25, no. 1, pp. 67–72, 2007.

[17] Y. Kawaguchi, J.-C. Lin, Y. Kawashima et al., "Relationship between pain and plasma amino acid levels in chronic pancreatitis," *Journal of the Pancreas*, vol. 16, no. 1, pp. 50–52, 2015.

[18] M. Hirota, T. Takada, N. Kitamura et al., "Fundamental and intensive care of acute pancreatitis," *Journal of Hepato-Biliary-Pancreatic Sciences*, vol. 17, no. 1, pp. 45–52, 2010.

26

Idiopathic Nonsurgical Pneumoperitoneum in Healthy Individuals after Endoscopy: Coincidence or Consequence?

Jong Soo Lee[1] **Dong-Hoon Yang,**[2] **Eun Hee Kim,**[1] **Jin Hwa Park,**[2] **Sungwon Park,**[3] **and Hye Won Park**[1]

[1]*Division of Gastroenterology, Health Screening and Promotion Center, Asan Medical Center, University of Ulsan College of Medicine, Seoul, Republic of Korea*
[2]*Department of Gastroenterology, Asan Medical Center, University of Ulsan College of Medicine, Seoul, Republic of Korea*
[3]*Division of Radiology, Health Screening and Promotion Center, Asan Medical Center, University of Ulsan College of Medicine, Seoul, Republic of Korea*

Correspondence should be addressed to Hye Won Park; dexlover93@gmail.com

Academic Editor: Olga I. Giouleme

Idiopathic pneumoperitoneum has an unknown etiology despite exploratory laparotomy. However, it may occur without definite abdominal symptoms; thus, adequate management could be in clinical dilemma. We experienced three cases of idiopathic nonsurgical pneumoperitoneum in healthy individuals during a health check-up. Their cases were not accompanied by any relevant etiology or definite abdominal symptoms. All of the three cases exhibited a benign clinical course. The three patients underwent an abdominal computed tomography (CT) scan as part of a health check-up program, which incidentally revealed free air in the right paracolic gutter without evidence of visceral perforation or inflammation. Among the three cases, two patients underwent colonoscopy before abdominal CT, whereas one patient did not. Two cases were completely asymptomatic and were observed without any treatment in the outpatient clinic. Only the third case with minimal symptoms was treated conservatively for a short time. If a small amount of free air typically located in the right paracolic gutter is detected in the absence of perforation during colonoscopy, close observation without unnecessary treatment would be sufficient.

1. Introduction

Due to increased health concerns and access to medical imaging, computed tomography (CT) scans are occasionally performed after colonoscopy. On postcolonoscopy CT scans, pneumoperitoneum may occur despite the absence of perforation during the procedure. However, pneumoperitoneum does not always correspond to a perforated viscus that requires surgical intervention. Spontaneous or nonsurgical pneumoperitoneum (NSP) may occur due to a variety of intrathoracic, intra-abdominal, gynecologic, and other miscellaneous etiologies [1]. In particular, idiopathic pneumoperitoneum has an unknown etiology despite exploratory laparotomy [1]. Several cases of idiopathic pneumoperitoneum have been reported previously [2–4], but it is rare in patients without any underlying diseases or relevant symptoms. Moreover, only a few clinicians have provided a management for asymptomatic pneumoperitoneum [3–5]. Hence, adequate management could be a clinical dilemma. We share three cases of idiopathic NSP detected incidentally during a health check-up, which were managed conservatively.

2. Case Presentation

2.1. Case 1. A 42-year-old man underwent screening esophagogastroduodenoscopy (EGD) and colonoscopy, which revealed superficial gastritis and normal colonoscopic findings (Figure 1(a)). Room air was used for insufflation. An hour after colonoscopy, he underwent abdominal CT scan as part of a health check-up program, which revealed free air in the right paracolic gutter without any evidence of

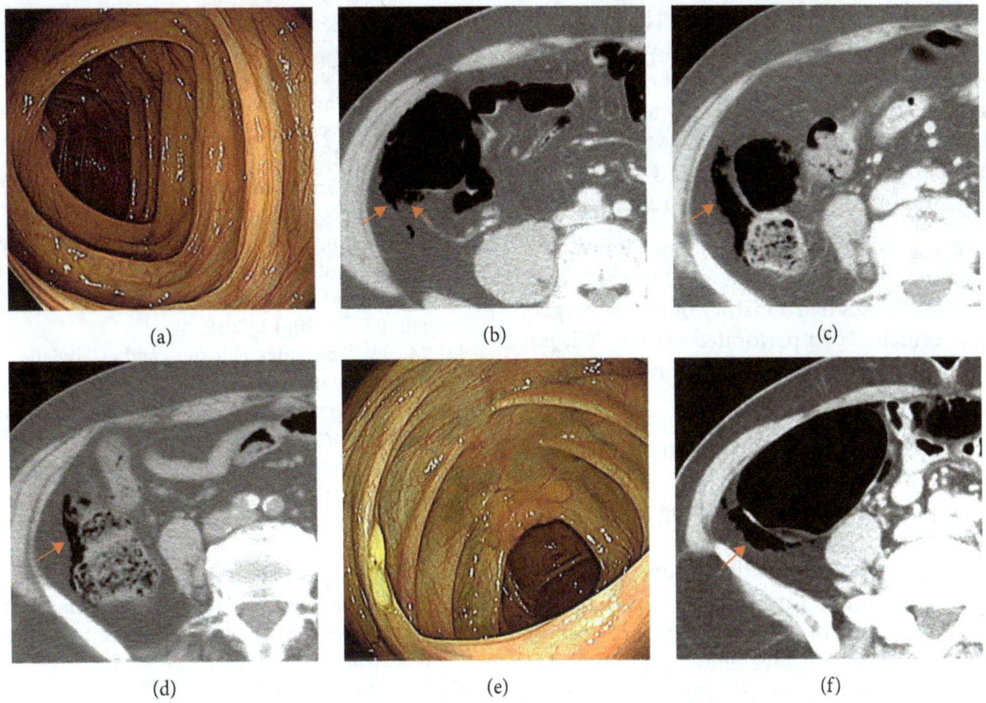

FIGURE 1: (a) Normal colonoscopic findings in case 1. (b) Abdominal computed tomography (CT) shows a small amount of free air in the right paracolic gutter in case 1. (c) Abdominal CT shows a small amount of free air in the right paracolic gutter in case 2. (d) Follow-up CT scan shows a reduced pneumoperitoneum two months after its initial detection in case 2. (e) Normal colonoscopic findings in case 3. (f) Abdominal CT shows a small amount of free air in the right paracolic gutter in case 3.

visceral perforation or inflammation (Figure 1(b)). He did not have any history of abdominal surgery or lung disease. According to the critical value report system in our institution, a radiologist reported the findings to a gastroenterologist and contacted the patient immediately. He was completely asymptomatic postprandial on the day of the test. He was observed without any treatment in the outpatient clinic 10 days later and remained asymptomatic.

2.2. Case 2. A 68-year-old woman underwent screening EGD that revealed atrophic gastritis and had a biopsy at the midbody of stomach. Colonoscopy was not performed. After that, abdominal CT was performed as part of a health check-up program. She had a history of total abdominal hysterectomy decades ago and had no lung disease. We contacted the patient on the third day of the exam since free air was recognized on her CT scan (Figure 1(c)). No immediate evaluation or intervention was considered because she did not demonstrate any symptoms. On the follow-up abdominal CT conducted two months later, pneumoperitoneum was slightly decreased (Figure 1(d)). Colonoscopy was performed four months later and showed normal findings.

2.3. Case 3. A 66-year-old woman without any medical history underwent screening EGD and colonoscopy (Figure 1(e)), which revealed superficial gastritis and normal colonoscopic findings. After that, abdominal CT was performed as part of a health check-up program. Abdominal CT showed free air in the right paracolic gutter (Figure 1(f)). She was admitted due to minimal postprandial abdominal discomfort, although abdominal examination was not suggestive of peritonitis. She was treated with prophylactic intravenous antibiotics and bowel rest for two days. Follow-up abdominal CT scan two days later showed a slight reduction of intraperitoneal free air. She was discharged on the third day of admission. The patient remained asymptomatic in the outpatient clinic two weeks later.

3. Discussion

Pneumoperitoneum usually indicates a perforated viscus, which requires urgent surgical intervention, but the proportion of visceral perforation as the cause of pneumoperitoneum has substantially been reduced [6]. Therefore, clinicians should identify spontaneous pneumoperitoneum or NSP, which can be managed conservatively.

Pneumatosis cystoides intestinalis (PCI) is a frequent cause of NSP [7]. In addition, NSP has been associated with several potential thoracic and gynecological causes and small intestinal diverticulosis [1]. NSP occasionally occurs after colonoscopy. In particular, it has been proposed that microperforation and subsequent air dissection eventually leading to peritoneum via the lymphatic channel are a potential mechanism [1]. In addition, air extravasation through a thinned but intact bowel wall could permit the escape of air without leakage of bowel contents [8]. This can be resolved with conservative management [1, 8]. Finally, idiopathic pneumoperitoneum is a rare clinical entity that has an unclear etiology even after laparotomy [1]. Idiopathic pneumoperitoneum presents with various symptoms including abdominal pain, distension, and elevated inflammatory markers [2]. On the other hand, only a few cases of incidentally detected pneumoperitoneum with thoracic causes, without abdominal symptoms, and with free air, particularly in the subphrenic area, have been reported [3, 4].

In the present cases, we could not identify any clear etiology of pneumoperitoneum radiologically and endoscopically. None of the cases had a history of recent surgery or lung disease or evidence of a perforated viscus, PCI, nor peritonitis. Hence, the present cases were termed as idiopathic NSP.

Previously reported cases of benign pneumoperitoneum after colonoscopy differed from the present ones. In the previous cases, the patients had an underlying condition or definite abdominal symptoms that prompted examination via exploratory laparotomy [5, 9]. In this study, only case 3 exhibited minimal symptoms, for which the patient was subjected to antibiotic treatment and bowel rest for two days. However, it was not clear whether the symptoms were caused by pneumoperitoneum or insufflated air during colonoscopy. Since free air was typically detected in the right paracolic gutter, it could be possible that insufflated air extravasated through the relatively thin right colonic wall. Nevertheless, this mechanism cannot explain case 2, in which the pneumoperitoneum was totally unrelated to colonoscopy. The possibility of ruptured small hidden subserosal PCI cannot be ruled out, considering the frequent location of PCI. Most PCI-associated pneumoperitoneum cases showed typical cystic lesions on colonoscopy or intramural gas of the bowel wall on radiologic exams [10]. These findings were not detected in the present cases. Extraluminal air in NSP usually disappeared within one to two weeks [7]. However, it may last for months as in case 2.

We present three cases of idiopathic NSP with a benign clinical course. In all three cases, CT scans were performed as part of a personalized health check-up program and not to evaluate symptoms after endoscopy. Therefore, this phenomenon is considered as a coincidence rather than a consequence of endoscopy. Once experienced, these conditions would not be difficult to determine. Otherwise, clinical judgement would not be easy. In particular, if a small amount of free air typically located in the right paracolic gutter is detected in the absence of overt perforation during colonoscopy, close observation would be sufficient without unnecessary treatment or bowel rest.

Acknowledgments

The authors would like to thank Jaewon Choe, MD, PhD, Department of Gastroenterology, Asan Medical Center, for providing these cases.

References

[1] R. A. Mularski, J. M. Sippel, and M. L. Osborne, "Pneumoperitoneum: a review of nonsurgical causes," *Critical Care Medicine*, vol. 28, no. 7, pp. 2638–2644, 2000.

[2] G. D. Eslick, V. Chalasani, and A. B. Salama, "Idiopathic pneumoperitoneum," *European Journal of Internal Medicine*, vol. 17, no. 2, pp. 141–143, 2006.

[3] E. Hannan, E. Saad, S. Hoashi, and D. Toomey, "The clinical dilemma of the persistent idiopathic pneumoperitoneum: a case report," *International Journal of Surgery Case Reports*, vol. 63, pp. 10–12, 2019.

[4] M. M. Sidiqi, D. Fletcher, and T. Billah, "The enigma of asymptomatic idiopathic pneumoperitoneum: a dangerous trap for general surgeons," *International Journal of Surgery Case Reports*, vol. 76, pp. 33–36, 2020.

[5] L. A. Joudeh and M. G. Newman, "Nonoperative management of pneumoperitoneum after colonoscopy," *Proceedings (Baylor University. Medical Center)*, vol. 31, no. 4, pp. 465-466, 2018.

[6] A. Kumar, M. T. Muir, S. M. Cohn, M. A. Salhanick, D. B. Lankford, and V. S. Katabathina, "The etiology of pneumoperitoneum in the 21st century," *Journal of Trauma and Acute Care Surgery*, vol. 73, no. 3, pp. 542–548, 2012.

[7] W. Adachi, T. Matsushita, Y. Yashiro, J. Imura, H. Shiozawa, and K. Kishimoto, "Clinical characteristics of pneumoperitoneum with pneumatosis intestinalis detected using computed tomography. A descriptive study," *Medicine*, vol. 99, no. 40, Article ID e22461, 2020.

[8] R. A. Mularski, M. L. Ciccolo, and W. D. Rappaport, "Nonsurgical causes of pneumoperitoneum," *Western Journal of Medicine*, vol. 170, no. 1, pp. 41–46, 1999.

[9] S. Ustek, M. Boran, and K. Kismet, "Benign pneumoperitoneum after colonoscopy," *Case Reports in Medicine*, vol. 2010, Article ID 631036, 3 pages, 2010.

[10] L.-L. Wu, Y.-S. Yang, Y. Dou, and Q.-S. Liu, "A systematic analysis of pneumatosis cystoids intestinalis," *World Journal of Gastroenterology*, vol. 19, no. 30, pp. 4973–4978, 2013.

27

A Rare Granular Cell Tumor with a Center Ulcer of the Rectum

Jeonghun Lee [1] **and Younghye Kim** [2]

[1]*Department of Internal Medicine, Ye Hospital, Anyang, Republic of Korea*
[2]*Green Cross Reference Laboratory, Yongin, Republic of Korea*

Correspondence should be addressed to Jeonghun Lee; tobemd@naver.com

Academic Editor: Hideto Kawaratani

We report a very rare case of granular cell tumor with a center ulcer of the rectum, which was detected in a 47-year-old man during screening colonoscopy. It is difficult to distinguish granular cell tumor from other subepithelial tumors. However, our case had a center ulcer unlike previous cases. We confirmed the diagnosis using histological and immunohistochemical examinations. In addition to our case report, we discuss the morphology, size, layer of invasion, and treatment of rectal granular cell tumors based on a literature review.

1. Introduction

Granular cell tumor (GCT) is a soft tissue neoplasm that arises from Schwann cells. It is usually benign and most commonly found in the skin, subcutaneous tissue, oral cavity, and gastrointestinal tract [1]. About less than 11% of GCTs are incidentally found in the gastrointestinal tract, where they are most commonly found in the esophagus, followed by the duodenum and stomach [2]. Rectal involvement is extremely rare. There are very few reported cases of GCT of the rectum, which usually present a sessile polypoid lesion which is smooth and covered with normal mucosa. We report a very rare case of rectal GCT with a center ulcer in a 47-year-old man and compare our findings with those of previous reports.

2. Case Report

A 47-year-old man presented to our hospital for screening colonoscopy. He had no remarkable medical history or gastrointestinal symptom. A 10 mm reddish pedunculated polypoid lesion with a center ulcer was found in the rectum, 5 cm from the anus (Figure 1). Based on the macroscopic appearance, a tubular adenoma and a carcinoid tumor were included in the differential diagnosis. Although not examined by endoscopic ultrasonography (EUS), the lesion was removed via an endoscopic procedure. Pathologic results showed that the tumor invasion was restricted to the submucosa layer (Figure 2(a)). Tumor cells showed a polygonal or slightly spindle-shaped cytoplasm with mild-to-moderate nuclear atypia and eosinophilic and fine cytoplasmic granules (Figure 2(b)). The cytoplasmic granules had a positive reaction to periodic acid-Schiff staining (Figure 2(c)). Immunohistochemical staining for S-100 protein was also positive (Figure 2(d)). Based on these results, GCT of the rectum was diagnosed. Colonoscopy was performed 3 months later, and no recurrence was observed.

3. Discussion

GCT, also called Abrikossoff tumor or granular cell myoblastoma, was first described by Abrikossoff in 1926 [3]. Colonic involvement is rare, and rectal involvement is extremely rare.

Colorectal GCT occurs predominantly between the ages of 30 and 50 years [4]. It is found incidentally during screening colonoscopy and tends to be asymptomatic. On white-light colonoscopy, it usually presents as a solitary sessile polypoid lesion, measuring less than 2 cm in diameter, which is smooth and covered with normal mucosa. Because finding a "molar-shaped" tumor with a central depression, as seen in esophageal GCT, is rare and the endoscopic

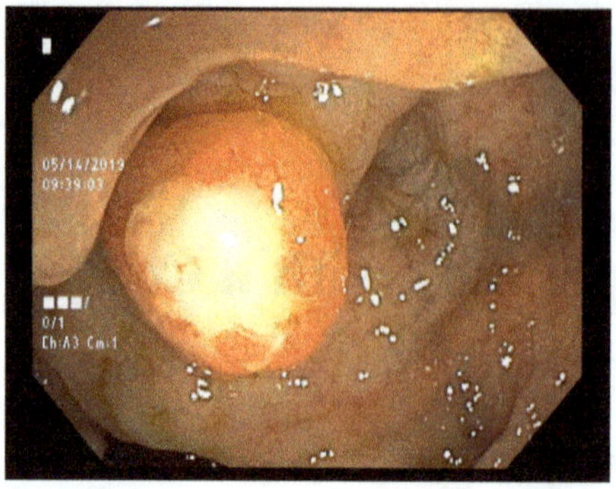

FIGURE 1: A 10 mm pedunculated polyp with a central ulceration was found in the rectum.

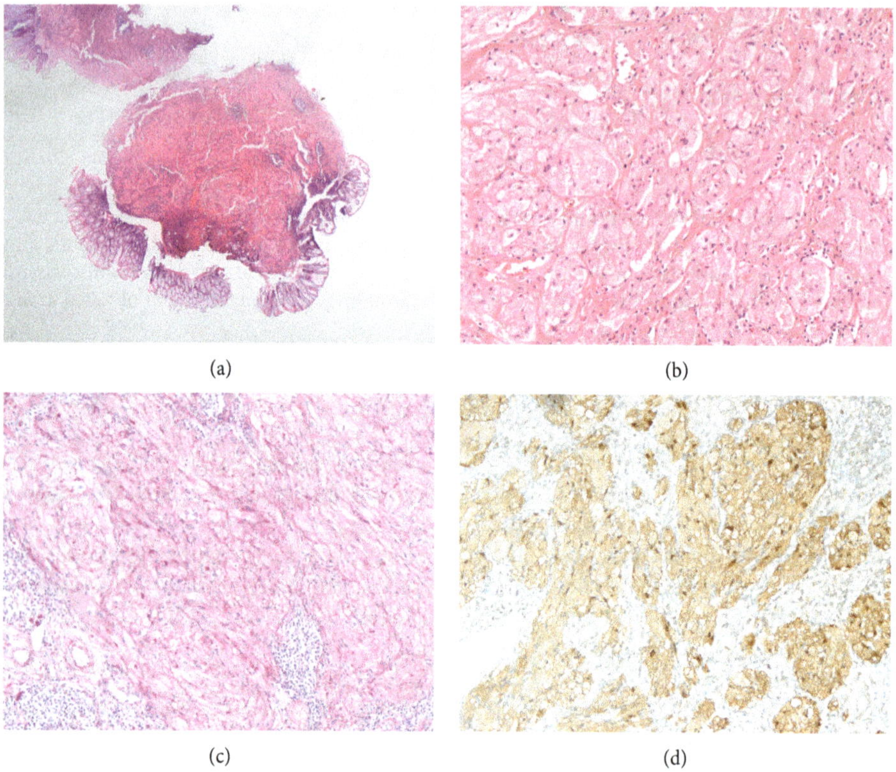

FIGURE 2: Histopathologic features of a rectal granular cell tumor. (a) The tumor was seen in the submucosa (hematoxylin and eosin staining, ×12.5). (b) The tumor cells showed a polygonal or spindle-shaped cytoplasm with mild-to-moderate nuclear atypia and abundant eosinophilic granules (hematoxylin and eosin staining, ×200). (c) Immunohistopathology staining with periodic acid-Schiff was positive (original magnification, ×200). (d) Immunohistopathology staining for S-100 protein was positive (original magnification, ×200).

ultrasonographic findings of GCT are similar to those of other subepithelial tumors (SETs), it is difficult to distinguish GCTs from other SETs, especially carcinoid tumor [5]. The definitive diagnosis of GCT is based on histopathologic findings and positive staining for S-100 protein.

There are only a few studies on GCT of the rectum. We searched on PubMed for cases related to rectal GCT, which were published after the year 2000, using the phrase "granular cell tumor and rectum." We found only six case reports and 13 patients (Table 1) [1, 5–9]. Rectal GCT was more common in men than in women (ratio 12 : 2; including our patient). However, its sex distribution remains unclear because of its rarity [2]. Their average age was 51.7 years. Most affected patients were asymptomatic, and the tumors were identified incidentally. However, in a report from Japan, five of the eight patients had a positive fecal occult blood test. This was probably due to the regular medical check-up system in Japan. Most of the tumors were benign and were removed via endoscopic procedures. Furthermore, most of the rectal GCTs were smooth and covered with normal mucosa, similar to SET. However, our case involved a reddish pedunculated lesion with an ulceration at the top unlike previous cases. This was probably a secondary change due to an inflammatory reaction to the mucosa, and such

Table 1: Patient clinical characteristics from the literature.

Case (no)	Age, years	Sex	Signs and symptoms	Morphology	Size, mm	Layer of invasion	Treatment
1[1]	61	M	None	Normal mucosa, sessile	4	N/A	Endoscopic resection
2[5]	49.9 (mean)	6 M/ 2 F	None: 1, positive FOBT: 5, abdominal discomfort: 2	Yellowish-white: 7; white: 1, all normal mucosa, sessile: 5, pedunculated: 3	<10: 7; 15: 1	Submucosa: most	Endoscopic resection: 5; surgery: 3
3[6]	51	M	None	Yellowish, normal mucosa, sessile	20	Subserosa	Surgery
4[7]	59	M	None	Normal mucosa, sessile	8	Submucosa	Endoscopic resection
5[8]	49	M	N/A	N/A	8	N/A	Endoscopic resection
6[9]	45	M	N/A	N/A	N/A	N/A	N/A
Present case	47	M	None	Reddish, ulcerated, pedunculated	10	Submucosa	Endoscopic resection

M, male; F, female; FOBT, fecal occult blood test; N/A, not available.

lesions are reported in various tumors. Therefore, endoscopists should consider that rectal GCTs may not be similar to SETs, especially carcinoid tumor.

Most GCTs are benign and are fortuitously found. However, less than 2% of them can be malignant [1]. If the tumor size is greater than 4 cm and there is ulceration, cellular necrosis, spindling, pleomorphism, increased nuclear-cytoplasmic ratio, large nucleoli, and increased mitotic activity, the potential for malignancy will be high [7, 10]. Of the factors above, tumor size is the most important factor [11]. Malignant GCTs tend to metastasize, recur, and have a poor prognosis. Therefore, biopsy, EUS, and EUS-guided fine needle aspiration may be valuable for diagnosis. Benign colorectal GCTs that are smaller than 2 cm can be treated via endoscopic resection. Follow-up colonoscopy should be considered valuable as a surveillance modality.

The colonoscopic findings are similar to those of the SETs, but can vary. It is important to analyze the size of the tumor and other features before its treatment because of the possibility of malignancy; most rectal GCTs can be cured via endoscopic resection. Endoscopists should identify the features of GCTs and consider follow-up surveillance via colonoscopy.

Authors' Contributions

J. Lee edited the manuscript. Y. Kim provided the pathology images. J. Lee is the article guarantor.

References

[1] T. Sunkara, S. V. Nagaraj, and V. Gaduputi, "Granular cell tumor of rectum: a very rare entity," *Case Reports in Gastrointestinal Medicine*, vol. 2017, Article ID 3795482, 3 pages, 2017.

[2] Y. Chen, Y. Chen, X. Chen, L. Chen, and W. Liang, "Colonic granular cell tumor: report of 11 cases and management with review of the literature," *Oncology Letters*, vol. 16, pp. 1419–1424, 2018.

[3] A. Abrikossoff, "Über myome," *Virchows Archiv für Pathologische Anatomie und Physiologie und für Klinische Medizin*, vol. 260, no. 1, pp. 215–233, 1926.

[4] P. Guzman Rojas, E. S. Robalino Gonzaga, V. Zayat, and J. Parikh, "Benign granular cell tumor of the cecum," *Cureus*, vol. 11, Article ID e4074, 2019.

[5] T. Nakanome, K. Yokoyama, H. Takeuchi et al., "Rectal granular-cell tumor difficult to distinguish from carcinoid tumor," *Digestive Endoscopy*, vol. 22, no. 4, pp. 325–328, 2010.

[6] S. Y. Yang, B. S. Min, and W. R. Kim, "A granular cell tumor of the rectum: a case report and review of the literature," *Annals of Coloproctology*, vol. 33, no. 6, pp. 245–248, 2017.

[7] S. Sevilla Ribota, J. Perez-Bedmar Delgado, J. J. Dominguez Cancte, A. M. Dotor de Lama, and M. Gomez-Rubio, "Endoscopic resection of rectal granular-cell tumor using elastic band ligation," *Revista espanola de enfermedades digestivas: organo oficial de la Sociedad Espanola de Patologia Digestiva*, vol. 108, pp. 677–680, 2016.

[8] T. Take, Q. Shi, Z. P. Qi et al., "Endoscopic resection of colorectal granular cell tumors," *World Journal of Gastroenterology*, vol. 21, no. 48, pp. 13542–13547, 2015.

[9] J. R. Parfitt, C. A. McLean, M. G. Joseph, C. J. Streutker, S. Al-Haddad, and D. K. Driman, "Granular cell tumours of the gastrointestinal tract: expression of nestin and clinicopathological evaluation of 11 patients," *Histopathology*, vol. 48, no. 4, pp. 424–430, 2006.

[10] J. C. Fanburg-Smith, J. M. Meis-Kindblom, R. Fante, and L.-G. Kindblom, "Malignant granular cell tumor of soft tissue," *The American Journal of Surgical Pathology*, vol. 22, no. 7, pp. 779–794, 1998.

[11] J. M. Cha, J. I. Lee, K. R. Joo et al., "Granular cell tumor of the descending colon treated by endoscopic mucosal resection: a case report and review of the literature," *Journal of Korean Medical Science*, vol. 24, no. 2, pp. 337–341, 2009.

Atypical Manifestation of DRESS Syndrome

Christopher Hakim ,[1] Constantine Melitas,[2] Eric Nguyen,[3] and Kha Ngo[2]

[1]*Department of Internal Medicine, Ascension Providence Hospital, Michigan State University College of Human Medicine, Southfield, USA*
[2]*Department of Gastroenterology, Ascension Providence Hospital, Michigan State University College of Human Medicine, Southfield, USA*
[3]*American University of the Caribbean School of Medicine, Coral Gables, USA*

Correspondence should be addressed to Christopher Hakim; cmhak@msu.edu

Academic Editor: Yoshihiro Moriwaki

The differential for liver transaminases over 1000 units/liter typically includes liver ischemia, acute viral hepatitis, acetaminophen toxicity, and autoimmune hepatitis. Prompt evaluation is imperative as these etiologies can lead to fulminant liver failure. We present a case of transaminases over 1000 units/liter from an atypical etiology. A 52-year-old male, previously treated with allopurinol for an acute gout flare, presented with persistent fevers. Given that he had taken a "high-risk medication" 2–6 weeks before presentation, subsequently presented with fever, rash, renal impairment, elevated liver enzymes in the thousands, and peripheral eosinophilia, DRESS syndrome secondary to allopurinol was diagnosed.

1. Introduction

Elevated liver chemistries (LFTs) include a wide differential diagnosis, and delineating the cause is imperative for treatment. More specifically, LFTs in the thousands include a narrow differential in which assessment for acetaminophen toxicity and testing for acute viral causes, autoimmune hepatitis, ischemic hepatitis/shock liver, and vascular disorders including acute portal vein thrombosis and acute Wilsonian crisis, as well as workup for biliary obstruction, must be performed [1].

We present a case of allopurinol-induced drug reaction with eosinophilia and systemic symptoms (DRESS) syndrome, which presented as a rare cause of liver enzymes in the thousands.

2. Case Report

A 52-year-old African American male presented to the emergency department from his primary care physician's office due to persistent fever. The patient had been discharged from the hospital one week prior after being hospitalized for diarrhea due to *Clostridium difficile* colitis, which was treated with oral vancomycin. During that hospitalization, he was started on allopurinol for an acute gout flare after which he developed a generalized purpuric, morbilliform rash, which started on his chest and spread to his extremities. He was discharged on a prednisone taper for a suspected drug rash, which he completed prior to returning to the hospital.

His past medical history includes hypertension, chronic kidney disease stage 5, osteoarthritis, GERD, and gout. On initial examination, his temperature was 38.3°C with vitals within normal limits. Skin excoriations were noted, but no rash or lymphadenopathy. His cardiopulmonary and abdominal exams were unremarkable. Laboratory data demonstrated a white blood cell count within normal limits, hemoglobin 7.9 gm/dL, platelet count 71K/mcl, creatinine 6.4 mg/dL (baseline 5-6 mg/dL), BUN 60 mg/dL, and elevated LFTs with AST 878 units/L, ALT 1,117 units/L, alkaline phosphatase 169 units/L, and GGT 209 units/L. Of note, the patient had known anemia of chronic disease; however, his thrombocytopenia was a new occurrence. Lactic acid was normal, and urinalysis showed no signs of active urinary tract infection. Chest X-ray demonstrated no acute processes.

During hospitalization, his LFTs continued to increase and thrombocytopenia worsened. The gastroenterology service was consulted on the second day of hospitalization. His temperature of 38.7°C persisted. His LFTs remained elevated with AST 676 units/L, ALT 1,262 units/L, alkaline phosphatase 173 units/L, and total bilirubin 0.6 mg/dl with a normal prothrombin time.

Despite a negative acetaminophen level, *N*-acetylcysteine (NAC) was administered via three consecutive doses given over 21 hours with subsequent decrease in LFTs. Viral serologies (hepatitis A/B/C, EBV, CMV, HSV, and VZV), autoimmune studies (IgG, ANA, smooth muscle antibody, and mitochondrial antibody), and ceruloplasmin were normal as well as serum electrolytes, thyroid function tests, ammonia level, and stool studies. Abdominal ultrasound with doppler demonstrated hepatomegaly without evidence of vascular occlusion or biliary abnormalities.

On the third day, he developed peripheral eosinophilia (13%). Given that he had taken allopurinol two weeks before presentation, subsequently presented with fevers, rash, elevated LFTs, and peripheral eosinophilia, with an extensive workup negative for alternative processes, DRESS syndrome was suspected. LFTs continued to improve significantly. The remainder of testing was negative including infectious workup, alternative autoimmune and genetic etiologies, and toxicology screening leading to discharge on day seven.

3. Discussion

DRESS syndrome is a hypersensitivity drug reaction characterized by rash, hematologic abnormalities, lymphadenopathy, and organ involvement, including liver and kidney with mortality as high as 10% [2, 3]. It has a prevalence of 2.18 per 100,000 patients with specific diagnostic criteria [4, 5]. The pathogenesis is hypothesized to be secondary to an accumulation of toxic drug metabolites due to various enzymatic deficiencies [2].

The presenting symptoms in almost all patients include skin rash, liver involvement, hypereosinophilia, and lymphadenopathy [6]. The first symptoms to present are fever and rash, as were seen in our patient prior to his admission. Skin manifestations occur as a morbilliform eruption, which involves over 50% the body and includes two or more of the following: facial edema, infiltrative lesions, scaling, and/or purpura [6].

The liver is the most common affected organ in DRESS syndrome. Liver involvement is generally mild and infrequently causes liver chemistry elevations in the thousands with rare progression to fulminant hepatic failure [7]. Hematological findings are also commonly seen in DRESS syndrome, with eosinophilia being the most common manifestation, often delayed by 1-2 weeks [6, 8, 9]. Renal dysfunction is also commonly appreciated [8].

Allopurinol has one of the strongest associations with DRESS syndrome [10]. Other high-risk medications include carbamazepine, lamotrigine, phenytoin, and phenobarbital [5].

Diagnosing DRESS syndrome can be challenging but should be suspected in a patient who received a new high-risk medication in the previous 2–6 weeks and presents with characteristic symptoms as outlined above. Bocquet's diagnostic criteria include the presence of three conditions such as drug-induced skin eruption, eosinophilia ≥1500/mm, and at least one of the following systemic abnormalities: lymphadenopathy, hepatitis (LFTs >2 ULN), interstitial nephropathy, interstitial lung disease, or myocardial involvement [5]. The RegisSCAR criteria for diagnosis is another diagnostic tool which classified our patient as "probable" of having DRESS syndrome [11]. Additionally, there is a Japanese diagnostic tool which has been shown to be significantly less accurate [12].

Supportive therapy and prompt withdrawal of the offending agent is the primary treatment. Most patients recover completely in weeks to months after drug withdrawal. Systemic corticosteroids are used by some; however, the literature has not shown a significant benefit [13].

In the setting of significant liver injury, administration of NAC and transfer to a liver transplant center are important considerations. NAC improves overall tissue oxygen delivery to the liver and has been shown to improve mortality. Additionally, studies have demonstrated an increase in transplant-free survival and post-liver transplant survival in several causes of nonacetaminophen acute liver injuries including drug-induced, viral, and autoimmune [14–16].

To avoid complications and death due to DRESS syndrome, prompt diagnosis with removal of the offending agent, supportive care, and administration of NAC in the setting of significant liver injury are imperative.

Disclosure

Prior presentations of this study include the following: (1) Hakim, C., Melitas, C., Nguyen, E., Ngo, K. unDRESSing elevated liver enzymes. Program No. P2547. ACG 2019 Annual Scientific Meeting Abstracts, San Antonio, Texas: American College of Gastroenterology. (2) Hakim, C., Melitas, C., Nguyen, E., Ngo, K. unDRESSing elevated liver enzymes. ACP Michigan Chapter 2019 Annual Meeting, May 3, 2019, Sterling Heights, MI.

References

[1] P. Y. Kwo, S. M. Cohen, and J. K. Lim, "ACG clinical guideline: evaluation of abnormal liver chemistries," *American Journal of Gastroenterology*, vol. 112, no. 1, pp. 18–35, 2017.

[2] S. Choudhary, M. Mcleod, D. Torchia, and P. Romanelli, "Drug reaction with eosinophilia and systemic symptoms (DRESS) syndrome," *The Journal of Clinical and Aesthetic Dermatology*, vol. 6, no. 6, pp. 31–37, 2013.

[3] D. Seth, D. Kamat, and J. Montejo, "DRESS syndrome: a practical approach for primary care practitioners," *Clinical Pediatrics*, vol. 47, no. 9, pp. 947–952, 2008.

[4] A. R. Wolfson, L. Zhou, Y. Li, N. A. Phadke, O. A. Chow, and K. G. Blumenthal, "Drug reaction with eosinophilia and systemic symptoms (DRESS) syndrome identified in the electronic health record allergy module," *The Journal of Allergy and Clinical Immunology: In Practice*, vol. 7, no. 2, pp. 633–640, 2019.
[5] H. Bocquet, M. Bagot, and J. C. Roujeau, "Drug-induced pseudolymphoma and drug hypersensitivity syndrome (drug rash with eosinophilia and systemic symptoms: DRESS)," *Seminars in Cutaneous Medicine and Surgery*, vol. 15, no. 4, pp. 250–257, 1996.
[6] M. Eshki, L. Allanore, P. Musette et al., "Twelve-year analysis of severe cases of drug reaction with eosinophilia and systemic symptoms: a cause of unpredictable multiorga`n failure," *Archives of Dermatology*, vol. 145, no. 1, pp. 67–72, 2009.
[7] S. Tas and T. Simonart, "Drug rash with eosinophilia and systemic symptoms (DRESS syndrome)," *Acta Clinica Belgica*, vol. 54, no. 4, pp. 197–200, 1999.
[8] Y. Kano, T. Ishida, K. Hirahara, and T. Shiohara, "Visceral involvements and long-term sequelae in drug-induced hypersensitivity syndrome," *Medical Clinics of North America*, vol. 94, no. 4, pp. 743–759, 2010.
[9] Z. Husain, B. Y. Reddy, and R. A. Schwartz, "DRESS syndrome part 1. Clinical perspectives," *Journal of the American Academy of Dermatology*, vol. 68, no. 5, p. 693, 2013.
[10] S. Hassan, S. Hassan, R. Wetz, and E. Zouein, "Allopurinol causing drug rash with eosinophilia and systemic symptoms syndrome: a challenging diagnosis," *International Journal of General Medicine*, vol. 4, pp. 789–792, 2011.
[11] A. Pannu and A. Saroch, "Diagnostic criteria for drug rash and eosinophilia with systemic symptoms," *Journal of Family Medicine and Primary Care*, vol. 6, no. 3, pp. 693-694, 2017.
[12] D.-H. Kim and Y.-I. Koh, "Comparison of diagnostic criteria and determination of prognostic factors for drug reaction with eosinophilia and systemic symptoms syndrome," *Allergy, Asthma & Immunology Research*, vol. 6, no. 3, pp. 216–221, 2014.
[13] P. Ichai, A. Laurent-Bellue, F. Saliba et al., "Acute liver failure/injury related to drug reaction with eosinophilia and systemic symptoms: outcomes and prognostic factors," *Transplantation*, vol. 101, no. 8, pp. 1830–1837, 2017.
[14] P. Harrison, J. Wendon, and R. Williams, "Evidence of increased guanylate cyclase activation by acetylcysteine in fulminant hepatic failure," *Hepatology*, vol. 23, no. 5, pp. 1067–1072, 1996.
[15] J. G. Stine and J. H. Lewis, "Current and future directions in the treatment and prevention of drug-induced liver injury: a systematic review," *Expert Review of Gastroenterology & Hepatology*, vol. 10, no. 4, pp. 517–536, 2015.
[16] W. M. Lee, L. S. Hynan, L. Rossaro et al., "Intravenous N-acetylcysteine improves transplant-free survival in early stage non-acetaminophen acute liver failure," *Gastroenterology*, vol. 137, no. 3, pp. 856–864, 2009.

29

EUS-FNA Diagnosis with Core Biopsy of Pancreatic Metastases from Primary Breast Cancer

Samuel Galante Romanini,[1] Juan Pablo Román Serrano,[1] Juliana Silveira Lima de Castro,[1] Isabela Trindade Torres,[1] Alex Ingold,[1] André Lucchiari Borini,[1] Luiz Augusto Sanches Zulske,[1] Maria Bruna Feitosa Matias,[1] Jéssica Said de Marchi,[2] José Andrés Sanchez Pulla,[3] and José Celso Ardengh[1,2,3,4]

[1]*Gastrointestinal Endoscopy, Department of Gastrointestinal Endoscopy, Hospital 9 de Julho, São Paulo, Brazil*
[2]*Department of Radiology, Irmandade da Santa Casa de Misericórdia de São Paulo, São Paulo, Brazil*
[3]*Hospital do Servidor Público Municipal, São Paulo, Brazil*
[4]*Gastrointestinal Endoscopy Service, Department of Gastrointestinal Endoscopy, Hospital das Clinicas, University of São Paulo Riberão Preto, São Paulo, Brazil*

Correspondence should be addressed to Samuel Galante Romanini; samuelromanini@gmail.com

Academic Editor: Yoshihiro Moriwaki

Background. The pancreas as a site of metastasis of other primary tumors is a rare event. Pancreatic metastases may occur years after the start of treatment of a neoplasm of another organ or may be the initial manifestation of an unidentified primary tumor. The most commonly reported primary sites for pancreatic metastases are the kidneys, lungs, breast, bowel, and skin (melanoma). *Case Summary.* The authors report a case of pancreatic metastasis derived from a primary breast cancer that underwent endoscopic ultrasound fine-needle aspiration (EUS-FNA) core biopsy to obtain tissue, which made it possible to perform an immunohistochemical study. *Conclusion.* We emphasize the importance of outpatient follow-up after the treatment of a neoplasia and the completion of control exams. In addition, we should always be aware of the finding of a secondary lesion in patients who have already been diagnosed with cancer, even if it is located in unusual organs, as in this case, where two metastases of a breast carcinoma to the pancreas were detected.

1. Introduction

The pancreas as a site of metastasis of other primary tumors is uncommon and may be difficult to differentiate from a neoplasm derived from the exocrine and/or endocrine pancreas itself, due to the overlap of its clinical presentation, imaging, and cytological features [1].

Pancreatic metastases may occur years after the start of treatment for a neoplasm from another site or may be the initial manifestation of an unidentified primary tumor. The most commonly reported primary sites for pancreatic metastases are the kidneys, lungs, breast, bowel, and skin (melanoma) [1]. Diagnosis before therapy should be the cornerstone of the decision to be made. Pancreatic tissue biopsies accurately detect this type of disease and thus establish the best form of treatment.

The authors report a case of pancreatic metastasis derived from a primary breast cancer that underwent needle puncture to obtain tissue, the result of which allowed the immunohistochemical study.

2. Case Presentation

A 72-year-old, asymptomatic, postmenopausal woman sought medical attention for routine exams with a personal history of systemic arterial hypertension, dyslipidemia, and previous appendectomy. She reported a right breast quadrantectomy in June 2016 by ductal breast adenocarcinoma

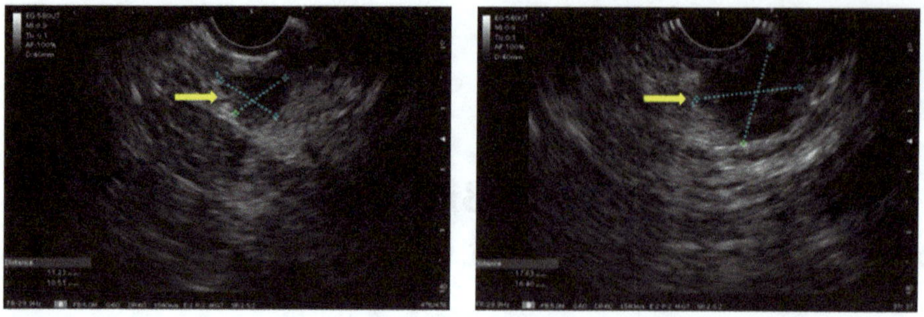

(a) (b)

Figure 1: Sectorial scanning of uncinate process and tail of pancreas. (a) Hypoechoic lesion, homogeneous and well-delimited in the uncinate process and (b) another lesion with the same characteristics but larger in the pancreas tail.

(stage IIA) followed by radiotherapy. She had no family history of breast cancer and denied smoking or alcoholism. Her physical examination showed only a scar from previous surgery on her right breast. Abdominal ultrasonography on February 2019 detected a well-defined nodular lesion on the tail of the pancreas, approximately 2 cm in diameter and without compromising adjacent structures. Other imaging tests were not performed due to a significant allergy to radiological contrast. She underwent endoscopic ultrasound (EUS) which confirmed the finding of abdominal US but detected two more hypoechoic, homogeneous, round areas, with well-defined limits, of soft consistency to elastography, two located in the uncinate process and one in the pancreatic tail, measuring 7 × 8 mm, 11 × 10 mm, and 19 × 12 mm, respectively (Figures 1 and 2). They did not invade or compress the main pancreatic duct or vascular structures. EUS-FNA core biopsy was performed on all lesions with a ProCore 20G needle (Cook Medical) (Figure 3). An additional finding of the exam was the presence of gallbladder stones.

The histological results of the punctures revealed that the lesion located on the tail of the pancreas and the largest in the uncinate process were secondary microduct or small cell-associated epithelial neoplasia isolated (metastatic ductal carcinoma). The smallest located in the uncinate process was negative for neoplasia. The immunohistochemistry of the material was positive for the GATA3 marker, which concluded that it was an invasive carcinoma of mammary origin in the form of triple negative discesa cells (estrogen negative, progesterone negative, and HER2 negative receptors) (Figure 4). The patient was diagnosed with late metastases of breast cancer to the pancreas and resumed follow-up with the oncology team.

3. Final Diagnosis

Metastases of breast cancer to the pancreas.

4. Outcome and Follow-Up

The patient whose case was reported in this article resumed the follow-up with a specialized oncology team for definitive treatment of the diagnosed lesions.

5. Discussion

The pancreas as a site of metastasis is uncommon and difficult to differentiate from ductal adenocarcinoma due to its clinical presentation, imaging findings, and cytological features [1]. Pancreatic metastasis may occur years after the treatment of a primary neoplasm or may be identified even before its diagnosis, and the latter is much rarer than the first [1]. The most frequently identified primary sites for pancreatic metastasis are the kidneys, lungs, breast, bowel, and skin [1].

Few studies in the literature have evaluated the efficacy of EUS-FNA in the diagnosis of this type of lesion [2]. In a study by Fritscher-Ravens A et al. of 207 patients with focal pancreatic mass who underwent EUS-FNA, 116 were diagnosed with malignant neoplasia, of which 32 (27%) were nonmalignant primary pancreatic adenocarcinoma [3]. Recently, the use of harmonic contrast associated with endoscopic ultrasound (CH-EUS) has started to be applied as an adjuvant in the differential diagnosis of pancreatic neoplasms; this is due to the advantage of the method of being able to visualize both the parenchyma and the microvasculature without the artifacts caused by Doppler [4]. The finding of lesions with a pattern of hyperenhancement to the use of contrast, associated, in particular, with a history of hematological or renal neoplasia, are strong predictors for pancreatic metastatic lesion (lymphoma and renal carcinoma metastasis), in some selected cases avoiding, up to even, the EUS-FNA [4].

Pancreatic ductal adenocarcinomas (ADPs) are the most common solid tumors, while others such as neuroendocrine and metastases are the rarest forms [5]. Breast cancer accounts for less than 5% of metastatic pancreatic lesions [6]. Invasive lobular breast carcinoma is the type of breast cancer that most metastasizes to the digestive tract [6]. Ductal carcinoma typically exhibits solitary metastasis and is much rarer in a diffuse pattern in the digestive tract [6].

Immunohistochemistry of the material obtained by puncture is an important tool to confirm the origin of metastatic carcinoma. Mammoglobin (MGB), GCDFP-15, estrogen receptors (ER), and progesterone (PR) act as specific immunohistochemical markers in the evaluation of metastatic breast carcinoma [7]. GATA3 is a member of the

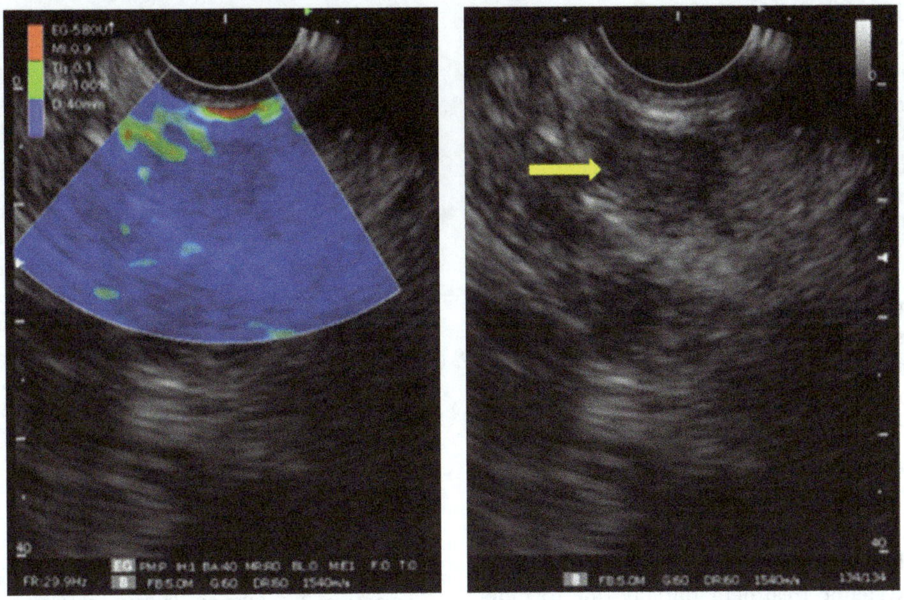

(a) (b)

Figure 2: Elastography performed with a sectorial endoscopic ultrasound device. (a) Elastography of uncinate hardened process lesion (blue image). (b) Yellow arrow indicating hypoechoic lesion of uncinate process.

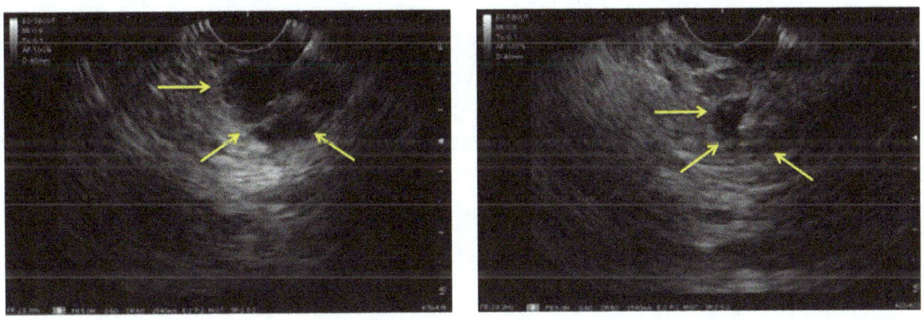

(a) (b)

Figure 3: (a) and (b) EUS-FNA with Procore 20G needle.

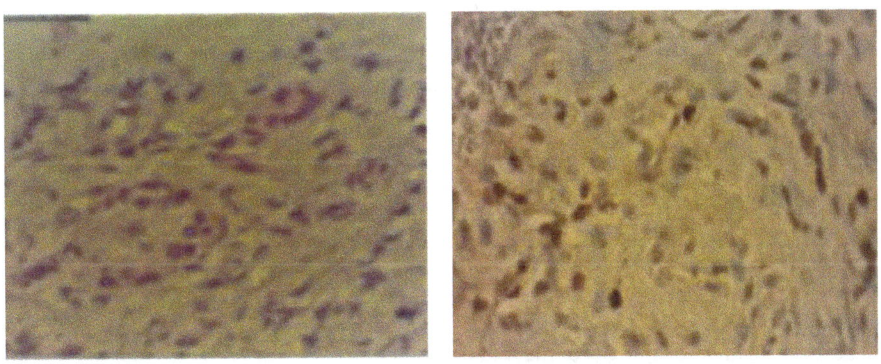

(a) (b)

Figure 4: Material obtained through EUS-FNA and sent for histological and immunohistochemical study. (a) Hematoxylin-eosin revealing atypical microducts and (b) GATA3-labeled immunohistochemistry (+) -secondary breast carcinoma.

zinc-finger transcription factor family [7]. This marker plays an important role in breast development and cell differentiation of the luminal epithelium as well as in the development of other tissues and has been implicated in breast cancer growth, differentiation, progression, and metastasis [7]. GATA3 is widely expressed in estrogen receptor negative luminal breast cancer and is more sensitive than GCDFP-15 and MGB, making it a useful marker for breast carcinoma [7].

The 5-year survival of invasive breast cancer is 90%, but when there are distant metastases, a typical ductal adenocarcinoma becomes incurable and a 5-year survival of approximately 25% [6]. Those with metastasis to the pancreas have a survival range of 1 to 50 months [6].

There is controversy regarding the resection of pancreatic metastases [6]. There are reports that resection of isolated pancreatic lesions may increase the survival and therefore should be the conduct of choice, while other authors advocate systemic treatment initially due to morbidity and mortality associated with duodenopancreatectomy [6].

Among chemotherapeutic drugs, taxanes, docetaxel, and paclitaxel are the drugs of choice in the treatment of metastatic breast cancer [8]. They can be used as single agents or in combination with other chemotherapeutic drugs [8].

6. Conclusion

In conclusion, we emphasize the importance of outpatient follow-up after the treatment of a neoplasm and the completion of control exams. In addition, we should always be aware of the finding of a secondary lesion in patients who have already been diagnosed with cancer, even if it is located in unusual organs, as in this case, where two metastases of a breast carcinoma to the pancreas were detected.

Disclosure

This case report was presented as an e-poster during the ENDO 2020 – 2nd World Congress of GI Endoscopy, March 7–10, 2020.

Authors' Contributions

Romanini S. G. designed the study, drafted the article, and analyzed and interpreted the data; Serrano J. P. R., Castro J. S. L., Torres I. T., Ingold A., Borini A. L., Zulske L. A. S., Matias M. B. F., Marchi J. S., Pulla J. A. S., and Andengh J. C. analyzed the data. Ardengh J. C. approved the final version to be published. All authors read and approved the final manuscript.

References

[1] J. C. Pang and M. H. Roh, "Metastases to the pancreas encountered on endoscopic ultrasound-guided, fine-needle aspiration," *Archives of Pathology & Laboratory Medicine*, vol. 139, no. 10, pp. 1248–1252, 2015.

[2] M. Atiq, M. S. Bhutani, W. A. Ross et al., "Role of endoscopic ultrasonography in evaluation of metastatic lesions to the pancreas," *Pancreas*, vol. 42, no. 3, pp. 516–523, 2013.

[3] A. Fritscher-Ravens, L. Brand, W. T. Knofel et al., "Comparison of endoscopic ultrasound-guided fine needle aspiration for focal pancreatic lesions in patients with normal parenchyma and chronic pancreatitis," *The American Journal of Gastroenterology*, vol. 97, no. 11, pp. 2768–2775, 2002.

[4] P. Fusaroli, M. C. D'Ercole, R. De Giorgio, M. Serrani, and G. Caletti, "Contrast harmonic endoscopic ultrasonography in the characterization of pancreatic metastases (with video)," *Pancreas*, vol. 43, no. 4, pp. 584–587, 2014.

[5] V. Gagovic, B. J. Spier, R. J. DeLee et al., "Endoscopic ultrasound fine-needle aspiration characteristics of primary adenocarcinoma versus other malignant neoplasms of the pancreas," *Canadian Journal of Gastroenterology*, vol. 26, no. 10, pp. 691–696, 2012.

[6] J. Kliiger and M. Gorbaty, "Metastasis to the pancreas and stomach from a breast cancer primary: a case report," *Journal of Community Hospital Internal Medicine Perspectives*, vol. 7, no. 4, pp. 234–237, 2017.

[7] Y. Hou, R. Shen, S. Chaudhary, D. Tonkovich, and Z. Li, "Utility of different immunostains for diagnosis of metastatic breast carcinomas in both surgical and cytological specimens," *Annals of Diagnostic Pathology*, vol. 30, pp. 21–27, 2017.

[8] T. ÇRe, A. Altintas, S. Pasa, Z. Urakçi, and A. Isikdogan, "Breast carcinoma metastasis to the tail of pancreas," *The Journal of Breast Health*, vol. 5, no. 4, pp. 228–230, 2009.

30

Jejunal Ulcer Caused by *Schistosoma japonicum*

Daniela Jaqueline Rivadeneira and Hesheng Luo

Department of Gastroenterology, Renmin Hospital of Wuhan University, Wuhan 430060, China

Correspondence should be addressed to Daniela Jaqueline Rivadeneira; dany_mal3@hotmail.com

Academic Editor: Warwick S. Selby

Intestinal schistosomiasis can be caused by the trematodes *Schistosoma japonicum* that mainly exists in East Asia or the *S. mansoni* in Africa and South America. The adult worms of *S. japonicum* live in the mesenteric veins and excrete eggs that circulate to the liver and colon; the eggs migrate through the intestinal wall and pass out with the stool. Here, we report a case of jejunal ulcer caused by the infection of *Schistosoma japonicum*. A 63-year-old woman from Wuhan, China, was admitted with left quadrant abdominal pain and weight loss for more than 6 months. The patient's computerized tomography reported cirrhotic liver changes, jejunal wall edema, and narrowed lumen; the upper enteroscopy corroborated these findings with the presence of several jejunal ulcers and edema. The pathology report showed chronic inflammation with ulcerative changes and *S. japonicum* eggs deposition. Schistosomiasis is one of the neglected tropical diseases that affect the poorest. Although a great improvement has been made to control it, there is a lot of work that remains to be fulfilled.

1. Introduction

Neglected tropical diseases (NTD) are caused by infectious and parasitic agents that primarily affect the poorest and most vulnerable populations in the world [1]. Currently, the NTD are affecting 41.4 million people, causing approximately 35,000 deaths per day worldwide [2]. By 2014, the World Health Organization (WHO) reported that 258 million people worldwide were infected with trematodes of the genus *Schistosoma* and required treatment and preventive regime [3]. These "neglected" diseases are due to underfinancing and low recognition by the pharmaceutical industries [4, 5].

Schistosomiasis is considered the third most devastating tropical disease in Africa, South America, the Caribbean, Middle East, and Asia [6, 7]. The 2015 death estimates due to schistosomiasis need to be reassessed, as they vary between 24,067 and 200,000 globally per year [8]. *S. japonicum* and *S. mekongi* are found in the Eastern Hemisphere [9]. In China, *S. japonicum* is found along the Yangtze River Basin, and according to a Chinese report for the WHO, *S. japonicum* infects 45 species of animals and remains endemic in seven provinces [10]. China is among the target countries to eliminate schistosomiasis according to the Regional Action Plan for Neglected Tropical Diseases in the Western Pacific (2012-2016), and according to the Ministry of Health, by the end of 2015, China aims to reach the criteria of transmission control threshold of <1% in the lake and marshland provinces and reach transmission interruption threshold in hilly provinces of Sichuan and Yunnan [10, 11].

The physiopathology of chronic schistosomiasis results from the eggs lodging, inducing immune response, granuloma formation, fibrotic changes, and damaging the organs and tissues of the human host. *S. japonicum* and *S. mansoni* adult worms reside in the mesenteric veins and excrete eggs that primarily circulate to the liver and intestines; the eggs migrate through the intestinal submucosa and mucosa, turn into the lumen, and pass out with the feces [12]. In the liver, the chronic progression causes periportal fibrosis, and it will lead to portal hypertension with all the cirrhosis complications if left untreated [12, 13]. Chronic schistosomiasis could be present from months to years after primary exposure; some do not have a clear history of acute phase or just mild and unspecific symptoms. *S. japonicum* or *S. mansoni* causes intestinal manifestations with fatigue, abdominal pain, cramping, anorexia, diarrhea, and dysentery [14]. If the infestation is heavy, the symptoms will be severe and may lead to intestinal ulceration, bleeding, anemia, intestinal polyps, dysplasia, and even bowel strictures [15].

The methods that are being used for schistosomiasis diagnosis depend on the target population and the *Schistosoma* species, but among people living in endemic areas, the approach should be through egg and antigen detection [16]. Another test is the real-time PCR; in stool samples, it can be 94% sensitive and 99.9% specific and may offer added value in diagnosing imported schistosomiasis [17]. The genus-specific PCR methods can detect and perform very well with feces and urine, but not with serum [18].

The treatment for schistosomiasis has important objectives such as reversing acute or early chronic disease and preventing complications. The drug of choice has always been praziquantel with a cure rate up to 90% after one regimen [19].

Prevention strategies to control schistosomiasis in endemic areas include water sanitation, minimizing contact with fresh water, community health-education, eradication of snail species, domestic animals care and treatment, proper work equipment to people at risk of exposition, and mass treatment [10, 19]. We present a case of chronic schistosomiasis with an unusual manifestation of *S. japonicum* in the small intestine.

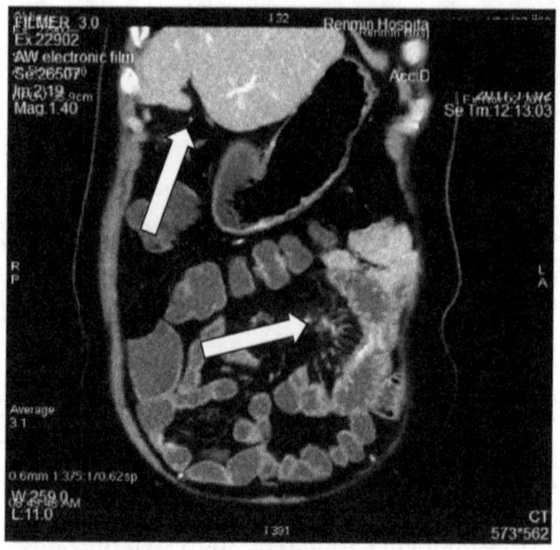

FIGURE 1: CT scan showing atrophy of the right liver lobe with hypertrophy of the left and caudate lobes, mesenteric edema.

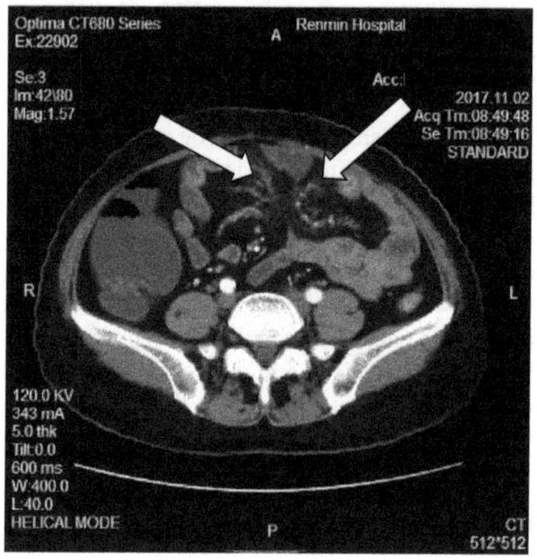

FIGURE 2: CT scan showing mesenteric edema, mesenteric fat blurred.

2. Case Report

A 63-year-old Chinese woman from Wuhan was admitted to the First Affiliated Hospital of Wuhan University in October 2017 with left quadrant abdominal pain and weight loss for more than 6 months. The pain exacerbated after eating and was accompanied with abdominal distension, belching, and reduced flatus. The patient referred was taking traditional Chinese medicine that temporarily relieved the symptoms. She had previous history of hypertension with a poor control. She underwent colonoscopy examination in a local hospital and verbally reported no pathologic findings. The positive findings at the physical examination were the mesogastric tenderness and an enlarged spleen.

The blood laboratory examination reported only mild hypokalemia; the urinary and stool reports were normal. The enhanced computerized tomography showed splenomegaly, the jejunal wall with edema and a narrowed lumen, enlarged lymph nodes, mesenteric edema; the liver cleft was widened with atrophy of the right liver lobe and hypertrophy of the left and caudate lobes; calcification and periportal fibrosis signs were compatible with hepatic schistosomiasis (Figures 1–6).

At the moment of the double balloon enteroscopy, the patient's blood pressure was not stable and we could not reexamine the colon. The upper enteroscopy showed at 150 cm distal to the Treitz ligament a 3.0 x 2.0 cm size ulcer with bottom white coating, peripheral mucosal hyperemia, and edema occupying 2/3 of the lumen so that the endoscope could not pass through. Four biopsies were taken from the ulcer (Figures 7–10). And 20 cm proximal from the ulcer, there were many scattered irregular ulcers from where two biopsies were taken.

The histopathological examination reported chronic jejunal inflammation with ulcerative changes and old *S. japonicum* eggs deposition (Figures 11 and 12).

During hospitalization, the patient received symptomatic treatment with intravenous fluids, electrolytes, antispasmodic medication, and proton-pump inhibitors. Unfortunately, the patient requested for a voluntary discharge from the hospital and decided to continue her treatment and follow-up at a local hospital.

3. Discussion

The importance of this case is the rare finding of jejunal ulcers due to *S. japonicum* infection, causing intestinal symptoms like abdominal pain and weight loss. The patient's CT scan corroborated chronic liver changes due to schistosomiasis; the upper enteroscopy and histopathological exam reported the unusual affection of the jejunal mucosa and diagnosed chronic infection with *S. japonicum*. The patient had abdominal pain for six months; she went to another hospital before arriving to ours and she did not get a correct diagnosis. This

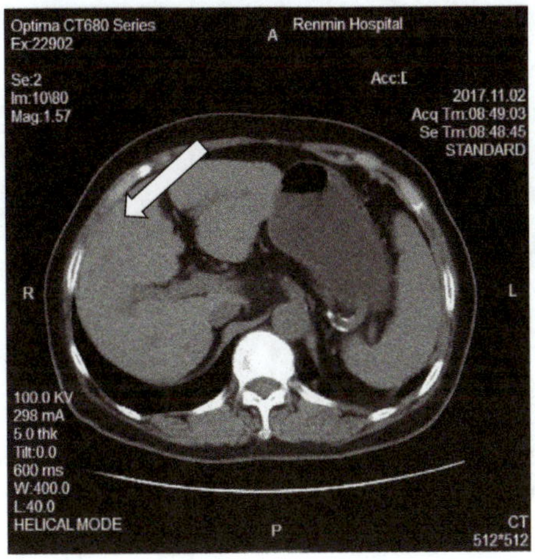

FIGURE 3: CT scan showing a linear calcification consistent with liver fibrosis due to *S. japonicum*.

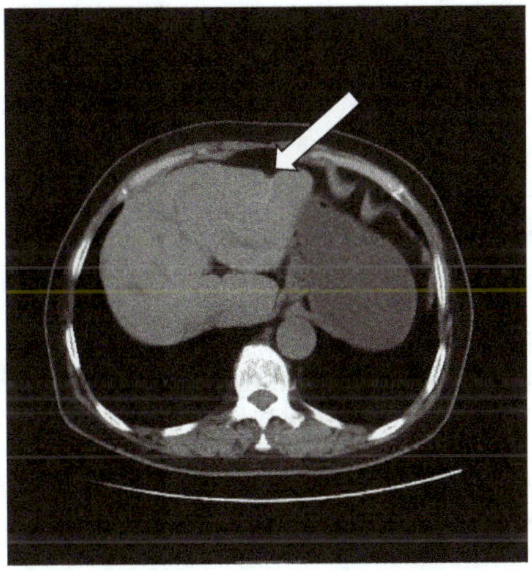

FIGURE 4: CT scan showing a linear calcification consistent with liver fibrosis due to *S. japonicum*.

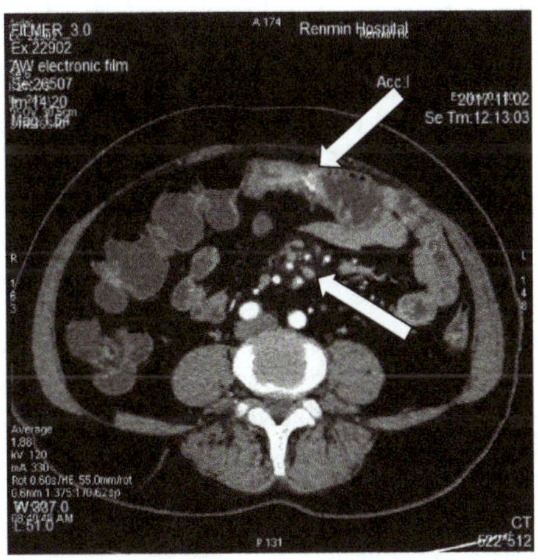

FIGURE 5: CT scan showing thickened intestinal wall, enlarged lymph nodes.

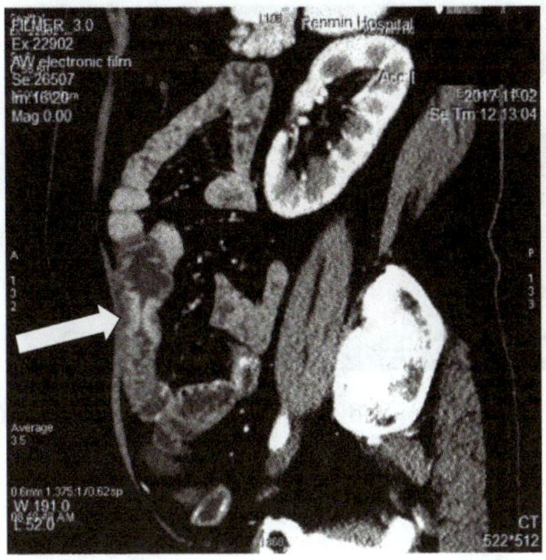

FIGURE 6: CT scan showing thickened intestinal wall and calcification.

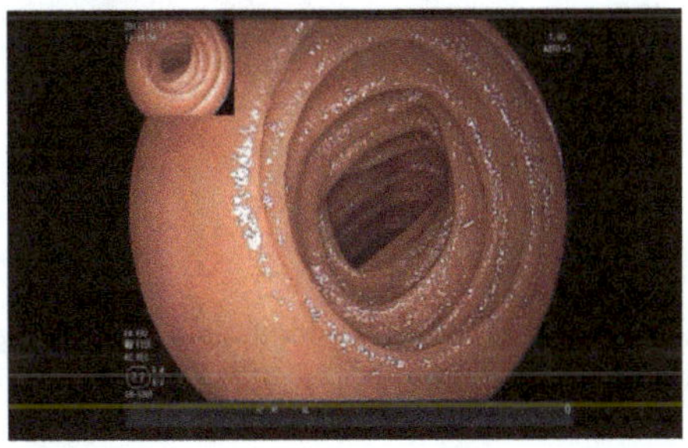

FIGURE 7: Enteroscopy showing normal jejunal mucosa.

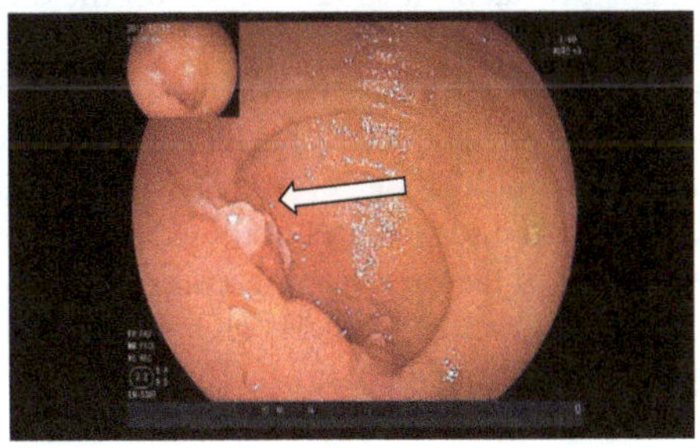

FIGURE 8: Enteroscopy showing a 3.0 x 2.0 cm size jejunal ulcer.

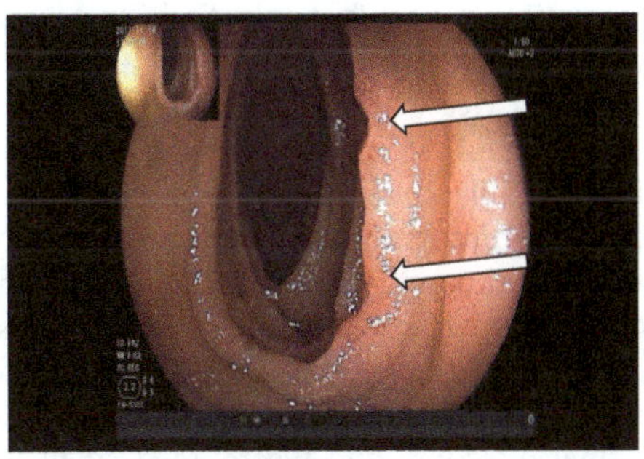

FIGURE 9: Enteroscopy showing several jejunal ulcers.

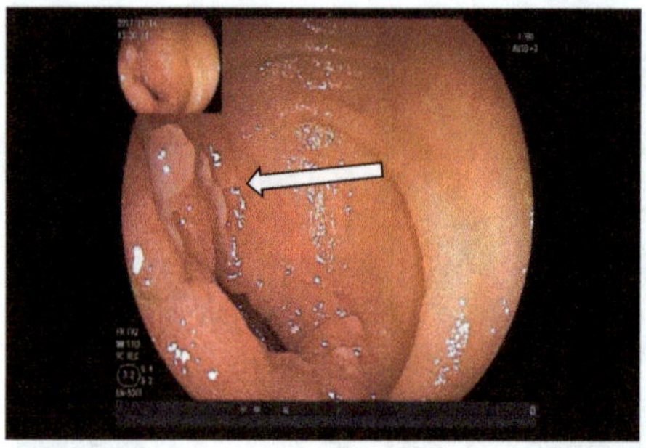

FIGURE 10: Enteroscopy showing a close view of the 3.0 x 2.0 cm size jejunal ulcer.

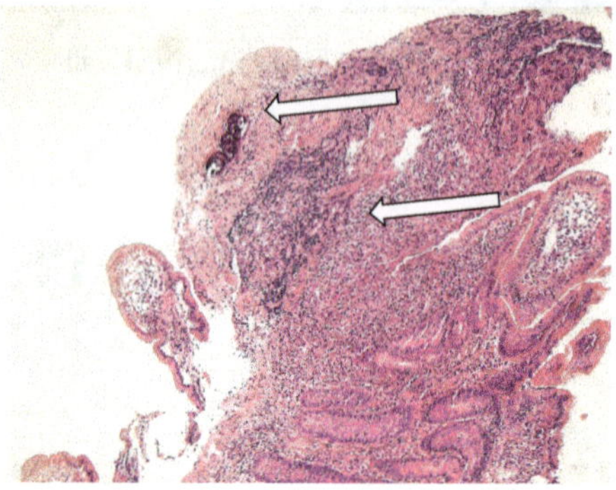

FIGURE 11: 100x histopathology of jejunal mucosa showing chronic inflammation, ulcerative changes, *S. japonicum* eggs deposition.

case teaches us that chronic abdominal pain has a broad range of differential diagnosis and that a well-done anamnesis is very important. In endemic areas like China where schistosomiasis remains prevalent, it should be within the differential diagnosis, and when a patient like ours shows abdominal symptoms, intestinal schistosomiasis should not be forgotten. When medical physicians are considering intestinal schistosomiasis, they should look for small and large intestine infection, and when endoscopists find intestinal ulcers, they should keep in mind this neglected tropical disease.

Despite the governmental and WHO efforts, more attention and support should be paid to this endemic disease, ensuring that the affected population not only receives suitable treatment, but also the education and preventive measures that will not expose them to suffer from this parasitic disease. More support should be given to control the transmission, prevent resistance to praziquantel, and develop a vaccine accessible to people at risk of schistosomiasis.

We encourage the education to endemic areas' population to seek medical advice when gastrointestinal manifestations occur, to medical physicians to consider intestinal schistosomiasis as a differential diagnosis when encountering gastrointestinal symptoms, to keep in mind that *S. japonicum* can also affect the small intestine and that if there are indications for enteroscopy examination, the patients should do it. Small intestine schistosomiasis is a rare manifestation of this tropical disease, but if there exist epidemiological risk, gastrointestinal affection, and ulcers, then small intestinal schistosomiasis should be considered as a possible diagnosis.

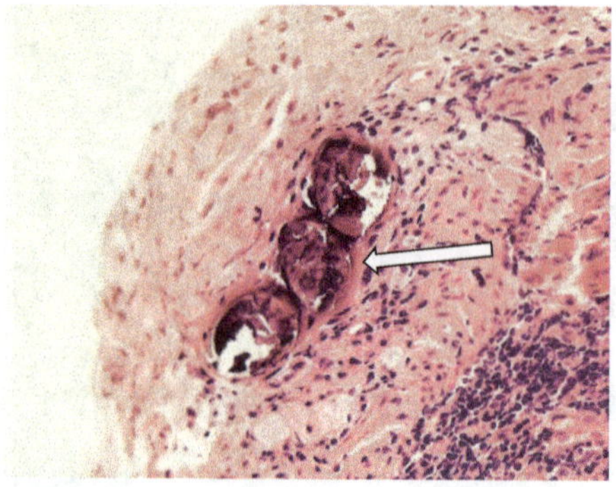

FIGURE 12: 400x histopathology showing old *S. japonicum* eggs deposition.

References

[1] V. K. Sah, L. Wang, X. Min et al., "Human schistosomiasis: a diagnostic imaging focused review of a neglected disease," *Radiology of Infectious Diseases*, vol. 2, no. 3, pp. 150–157, 2015.

[2] J. P. Cohen, G. Sturgeon, and A. Cohen, "Measuring progress in neglected disease drug development," *Clinical Therapeutics*, vol. 36, no. 7, pp. 1037–1042, 2014.

[3] M. Merrifield, P. J. Hotez, C. M. Beaumier et al., "Advancing a vaccine to prevent human schistosomiasis," *Vaccine*, vol. 34, no. 26, pp. 2988–2991, 2016.

[4] L. da Siqueira, D. A. Fontes, C. S. Aguilera et al., "Schistosomiasis: drugs used and treatment strategies," *Acta Tropica*, vol. 176, pp. 179–187, 2017.

[5] J. Clerinx and P. Soentjens, "Epidemiology, pathogenesis, and clinical manifestations of schistosomiasis," *Uptodate database*, 2017.

[6] D. U. Olveda, R. M. Olveda, D. P. McManus et al., "The chronic enteropathogenic disease schistosomiasis," *International Journal of Infectious Diseases*, vol. 28, pp. e193–e203, 2014.

[7] J. J. Xiang, B. J. Cheng, F. Tian, M. Li, X. F. Jiang, and X. M. Hu, "Perforation of small bowel caused by *Schistosoma japonicum*: a case report," *World Journal of Gastroenterology*, vol. 21, no. 9, pp. 2862–2864, 2015.

[8] "Global health estimates 2015: deaths by cause, age, sex, by country and by region, 2000-2015," World Health Organization, Geneva, 2019, http://www.who.int/healthinfo/global_burden_disease/estimates/en/index1.html.

[9] D. G. Colley, A. L. Bustinduy, W. E. Secor, and C. H. King, "Human schistosomiasis," *The Lancet*, vol. 383, pp. 2253-2254, 2014.

[10] J. Balen, Z. Y. Zhao, G. M. Williams et al., "Prevalence, intensity and associated morbidity of Schistosoma japonicum infection

in the Dongting Lake region, China," *Bulletin of the World Health Organization*, vol. 85, no. 7, pp. 519–526, 2007.

[11] World Health Organization, "Schistosomiasis in China. WHO Western PacificRegion," 2015, http://www.wpro.who.int/china/mediacentre/factsheets/schistosomiasis/en/.

[12] K. Gu, Y. Li, P. Rodriguez, X. Zeng, H. Sun et al., "Clinical diagnostic value of viable *Schistosomajaponicum* eggs detected in host tissues," *BMC Infectious Diseases*, vol. 17, no. 244, 2017.

[13] M. J. Lamyman, D. J. Noble, S. Narang, and N. Dehalvi, "Small bowel obstruction secondary to intestinal schistosomiasis," *Transactions of the Royal Society of Tropical Medicine and Hygiene*, vol. 100, no. 9, pp. 885–887, 2016.

[14] A. G. P. Ross, P. B. Bartley, A. C. Sleigh et al., "Schistosomiasis," *The New England Journal of Medicine*, vol. 346, no. 16, pp. 1212–1219, 2002.

[15] A. Mu, I. Fernandes, and D. Phillips, "A 57-year-old woman with a cecal mass," *Clinical Infectious Diseases*, vol. 63, no. 5, pp. 703–705, 2016.

[16] D. G. Colley, T. S. Andros, and C. H. Campbell, "Schistosomiasis is more prevalent than previously thought: what does it mean for public health goals, policies, strategies, guidelines and intervention programs?" *Infectious Diseases of Poverty*, vol. 6, no. 63, 2017.

[17] T. Lier, G. S. Simonsen, H. Haaheim, S. O. Hjelmevoll, B. J. Vennervald, and M. V. Johansen, "Novel real-time PCR for detection of *Schistosomajaponicum* in stool," *Southeast Asian Journal of Tropical Medicine and Public Health*, vol. 37, no. 2, pp. 257–264, 2006.

[18] L. Cnops, E. Tannich, K. Polman, J. Clerinx, and M. Van Esbroeck, "*Schistosoma* real time PCR as diagnostic tool for international travelers and migrants," *Tropical Medicine and International Health*, vol. 17, no. 10, pp. 1208–1216, 2012.

[19] A. Fenwick, D. Rollinson, and V. Southgate, "Implementation of human schistosomiasis control: challenges and prospects," *Advances in Parasitology*, vol. 61, pp. 567–622, 2006.

31

Intentional Foreign Body Ingestion: A Complex Case of Pica

D. Guinan,[1] T. Drvar,[2] D. Brubaker,[3] M. Ang-Rabanes,[4] J. Kupec,[5] and P. Marshalek[6]

[1] *West Virginia University Department of Behavioral Medicine and Psychiatry, General Psychiatry Resident PGY-2, USA*
[2] *West Virginia University, USA*
[3] *West Virginia University School of Medicine, MS-4, USA*
[4] *West Virginia University Department of Behavioral Medicine and Psychiatry, Assistant Professor, USA*
[5] *West Virginia University Department of Medicine Section of Digestive Diseases, Assistant Professor, USA*
[6] *West Virginia University Department of Behavioral Medicine and Psychiatry, Medical Director, USA*

Correspondence should be addressed to D. Guinan; dg0051@hsc.wvu.edu

Academic Editor: Yoshihiro Moriwaki

Intentional ingestion of foreign objects, a form of self-injurious behavior, is rarely discussed in the medical literature but often requires extensive evaluation, management, and resources. It can be especially problematic for gastroenterologists, who are often consulted for removal of the foreign body. Pica is the psychiatric diagnosis for intentional ingestion of nonnutritive objects and is most commonly seen in prison inmates and those diagnosed with intellectual disability or psychiatric illness. This case report presents a challenging case of pica, highlighting the complexity involved in diagnosis and the need for early psychiatric intervention. It also aims to provide a general review of the literature and practical recommendations to assist with managing this form of self-injurious behavior in the inpatient setting. Collaborative efforts among specialties in addition to primary prevention are vital to successful management of these patients.

1. Introduction

Intentional foreign body ingestion is often challenging and frustrating to treat, demanding a considerable amount of time and resources. In many cases, foreign body ingestion occurs repeatedly in a small population of patients and can consume a large percentage of healthcare-related costs. This was demonstrated in a retrospective case study [1] in which 305 cases of intentional foreign body ingestion were associated with only 33 patients. Psychiatric diagnoses were identified in 79 percent of these patients and total cost for management of the cases totaled over $2 million. Elucidating factors contributing to these behaviors could be beneficial to specialists removing the objects to help prevent recurrence and facilitate more cost-efficient and effective care.

Intentional ingestion of foreign bodies has relatively little representation in the medical literature but is most commonly reported by specialists in emergency medicine, general surgery, and gastroenterology [1–4]. These groups tend to focus on the acute management and technique of foreign body removal, particularly the endoscopic techniques that revolutionized treatment approach. In contrast, reports exploring the psychiatric evaluation of these ingestion behaviors are scant. We present a case of repetitive intentional foreign body ingestion which demonstrates psychiatric complexity as well as diagnostic and treatment challenges associated with this self-injurious behavior.

2. Case Report

A 39-year-old male presented to the emergency department after intentional ingestion of multiple objects including 50 paperclips, 50 screws, eight batteries, and seven razor blades covered in paper (Figure 1.). His past psychiatric history included major depressive disorder, generalized anxiety disorder, posttraumatic stress disorder, borderline personality disorder, and pica with a history of more than twenty admissions for ingestion behaviors often requiring endoscopic retrieval. Abdominal radiograph confirmed the presence of multiple metallic objects in the stomach and small intestine

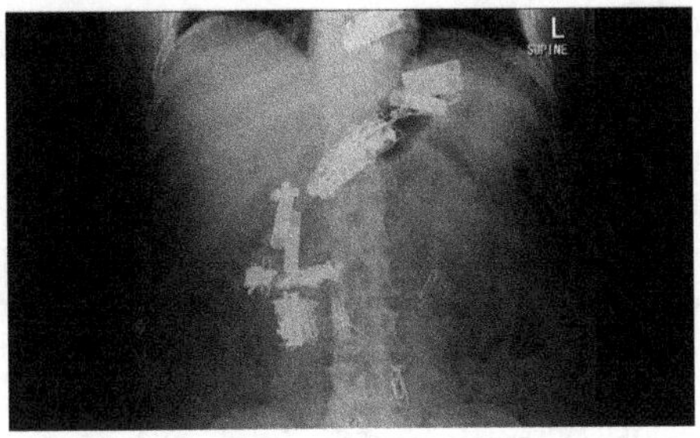

FIGURE 1: Abdominal X-ray showing multiple ingested substances later identified as 50 paperclips, 50 screws, eight batteries, and seven razor blades covered in paper.

which were removed endoscopically by the gastroenterologist. The patient was then admitted to the hospital's adult inpatient psychiatric unit for further care.

The patient cited anxiety and an empty prescription for alprazolam as the primary trigger leading to the ingestions. Multiple psychotropic medications, including antidepressants (sertraline, citalopram, escitalopram, mirtazapine, and bupropion), mood stabilizers (lithium and Depakote), antipsychotics (olanzapine, haloperidol, and aripiprazole), and benzodiazepines (clonazepam and lorazepam), failed to control his ingestion behaviors. His explanations for the ingestions have varied (e.g., coping mechanism for prior sexual trauma, relieving impulses, and getting out of "difficult situations", i.e., jail) but are always nonsuicidal in nature. He denies symptoms of depression but reports multiple symptoms of anxiety including restlessness, feeling tense, and having difficulty with sleep. He denies auditory or visual hallucinations and had no outward signs of paranoid thinking.

During admission, the patient was restarted on alprazolam 2 mg three times daily in conjunction with intensive therapy including Dialectical Behavior Therapy with components of mindfulness, distress tolerance, emotion regulation, and stress management skills. While on the unit, he swallowed a clock battery, screws from the toilet, and a colored pencil. He blamed the ingestion on anxiety and concern that unit staffs were angry with him. He denied the ingestions were a suicide attempt. The patient was subsequently sent back to the emergency department for endoscopy and the objects were successfully removed. He ultimately left against medical advice and no medication changes were made.

The patient was admitted for intentional ingestion four more times that month. During his most recent hospitalization, there was concern for misuse of his alprazolam prescription and he was weaned off and started on venlafaxine 37.5 mg and hydroxyzine 25 mg three times daily as needed for anxiety. He was discharged into a partial hospitalization program for daily psychotherapy groups and medication management. At the time of this writing, he has not been readmitted for pica.

3. Discussion

The Diagnostic Statistical Manual of Mental Disorders 5th Edition defines pica as the persistent eating of nonnutritive, nonfood substances over a period of one month which is inappropriate to the developmental level of the individual and not part of a socially or culturally normative practice. The symptoms must also be severe enough to warrant clinical attention [5]. It is often associated with micronutrient deficiencies (especially iron) and is frequently seen during pregnancy or in those with intellectual disability. Commonly ingested substances include ice, dirt, clay, starch, paper, hair, chalk, and metal artifacts which can occasionally require surgical removal [6]. Treatment of pica involves replacing micronutrients in those with deficiencies or implementing behavioral interventions (e.g., aversive stimuli, overcorrection, and reinforcement) in those with developmental disabilities [7]. In those with comorbid psychiatric illness or in populations where the behavior is used for secondary gain (e.g., prison populations), treatment becomes more challenging due to diagnostic complexity.

Four main diagnostic subgroups of psychiatric diagnoses are associated with intentional foreign body ingestion including malingering, psychosis, pica, and personality disorder [8]. Other psychiatric illnesses including obsessive compulsive disorder and autism spectrum disorder have been implicated in the behavior [9, 10]. Nationwide epidemiologic studies investigating the incidence of intentional foreign body ingestion have yet to be performed; however, one retrospective case series examining ingestions in adults of a lower socioeconomic population found that 92% of the ingestions were intentional and 85% involved patients with psychiatric comorbidities [11]. As highlighted by our case report, a patient may demonstrate several psychiatric comorbidities that accompany their pica.

Treating pica often requires a multidisciplinary approach. Once micronutrient deficiencies have been ruled out, screening for and treating the underlying psychiatric diagnosis may help minimize the intentional ingestion behavior. For the gastroenterologist faced with a patient who intentionally ingests, early involvement of the psychiatric service can facilitate diagnostic clarification. Neuropsychologic testing may assist with identifying mild intellectual disability associated with pica which responds best to behavior modification therapy. Trials of typical and atypical antipsychotics in patients with pica related to an underlying psychotic disorder have been successful in some reports but ineffective in others [12, 13]. Pica related to obsessive compulsive disorder has shown good response to selective serotonin reuptake inhibitor (SSRI) therapy in several cases [14, 15]. In terms of personality disorders, pica is most frequently seen in borderline personality disorder and is proposed to be a form of affect regulation, much like cutting behaviors. Psychiatric admission solely for intentional ingestion related to a personality disorder has not been shown to prevent recurrence of the behavior and may actually lead to escalation of swallowing [16].

Endoscopic retrieval of foreign bodies is costly and, though generally considered a low-risk procedure, can be associated with major complications including bleeding and perforation. Considering repeated ingestions are often seen in patients with comorbid psychiatric illness, prevention of ingestions should be the therapeutic goal of all specialists involved in the care of these individuals. Specific prevention strategies that can be utilized during inpatient admission include the following:

(i) placing patients under constant visual observation status while admitted, whether this be through video monitoring or by having a sitter present at bedside;
(ii) immediately removing potentially ingestible objects from patient's room;
(iii) administering psychotropic medications when indicated;
(iv) utilizing an individualized care plan to prevent reinforcement of behavior and mitigate readmissions and frequent imaging. For example, a specific care plan was implemented by both emergency department and inpatient medical providers in order to improve patient compliance with treatment and promote better outcomes of care. The care plan recommended early involvement of both gastroenterology and psychiatry services and avoidance of intravenous opioids and sedative/hypnotics due to concerns for medication misuse and addiction.

Additionally, a significant amount of frustration and countertransference can arise in healthcare providers when treating patients who repetitively ingest. It is important to remember patients who inflict self-harm, particularly through repetitive foreign body ingestion, have a right to treatment. Continued efforts must be made to best serve patients with pica and comorbid psychiatric diagnoses.

4. Conclusion

Pica is a diagnosis that can be associated with intentional foreign object ingestion and may overlap with multiple other psychiatric conditions. When addressing this behavior, it is important to promote a safe environment while simultaneously screening for and managing any concurrent mental illness. Elucidating and treating specific psychiatric comorbidity can be challenging, and collaborative care from multiple specialists is often required. Early involvement of both gastroenterologists and psychiatrists can prove helpful when determining the best and most comprehensive approach to treatment. Future work is needed to continue to identify successful strategies and specific care plans to meet the needs of these challenging patients.

References

[1] B. L. Huang, H. G. Rich, S. E. Simundson, M. K. Dhingana, C. Harrington, and S. F. Moss, "Intentional swallowing of foreign bodies is a recurrent and costly problem that rarely causes endoscopy complications," *Clinical Gastroenterology and Hepatology*, vol. 8, no. 11, pp. 941–946, 2010.

[2] D. Atluri, C. Veluru, A. Chopra, and K. D. Mullen, "Recurrent intentional foreign body ingestion: an endoscopist's dilemma," *Journal of Gastroenterology and Hepatology*, vol. 8, no. 7, pp. 482–484, 2012.

[3] P. P. Dalal, A. J. Otey, E. A. McGonagle et al., "Intentional foreign object ingestions: need for endoscopy and surgery," *Journal of Surgical Research*, vol. 184, no. 1, pp. 145–149, 2013.

[4] J. Brunner, M. Russel, K. Herr et al., "Nonsuicidal self-injury-related foreign bodies in the emergency department," *Seminars in Ultrasound, CT and MRI*, vol. 36, no. 1, pp. 80–87, 2015.

[5] *Diagnostic and Statistical Manual of Mental Disorders*, American Psychiatric Association, 5th edition, 2013.

[6] R. Mishori and C. McHale, "Pica: An age-old eating disorder that's often missed," *Journal of Family Practice*, vol. 63, no. 7, 2014.

[7] J. L. Matson, M. A. Hattier, B. Belva, and M. L. Matson, "Pica in persons with developmental disabilities: approaches to treatment," *Research in Developmental Disabilities*, vol. 34, no. 9, pp. 2564–2571, 2013.

[8] D. F. Gitlin, J. P. Caplan, M. P. Rogers, O. Avni-Barron, I. Braun, and A. J. Barsky, "Foreign-body ingestion in patients with personality disorders," *Psychosomatics*, vol. 48, no. 2, pp. 162–166, 2007.

[9] B. T. Te Wildt, C. Tettenborn, U. Schneider et al., "Swallowing foreign bodies as an example of impulse control disorder in a patient with intellectual disabilities: a case report," *Psychiatry (Edgmont)*, vol. 7, no. 9, pp. 34–37, 2010.

[10] D. J. Stein, C. Bouwer, and B. Van Heerden, "Pica and the obsessive-compulsive spectrum disorders," *South African Medical Journal*, vol. 86, no. 12, pp. 1586–1592, 1996.

[11] R. Palta, A. Sahota, A. Bemarki, P. Salama, N. Simpson, and L. Laine, "Foreign-body ingestion: characteristics and outcomes in a lower socioeconomic population with predominantly intentional ingestion," *Gastrointestinal Endoscopy*, vol. 69, no. 3, part 1, pp. 426–433, 2009.

[12] S. Kar, R. Kumar, and A. Kamboj, "Pica and psychosis – clinical attributes and correlations: a case report," *Journal of Family Medicine and Primary Care*, vol. 4, no. 10, pp. 149-150, 2015.

[13] N. I. Dumaguing, I. Singh, M. Sethi, and D. P. Devanand, "Pica in the geriatric mentally ill: unrelenting and potentially fatal," *Journal of Geriatric Psychiatry and Neurology*, vol. 16, no. 3, pp. 189–191, 2003.

[14] M. S. Bhatia and R. Gupta, "Pica responding to SSRI: An OCD spectrum disorder?" *The World Journal of Biological Psychiatry*, vol. 10, no. 4, part 3, pp. 936–938, 2009.

[15] D. J. Stein, C. Bouwer, and B. Van Heerden, "Pica and the obsessive-compulsive spectrum disorders," *South African Medical Journal*, vol. 86, no. 12, pp. 1586–1592, 1996.

[16] B. A. Poynter, J. J. Hunter, J. H. Coverdale, and C. A. Kempinsky, "Hard to swallow: A systematic review of deliberate foreign body ingestion," *General Hospital Psychiatry*, vol. 33, no. 5, pp. 518–524, 2011.

From an Incidental Finding to an Emergent Treatment: A Case Report of a Hepatic Adenomatosis and Large Ruptured Hepatic Adenoma

Maria Mironova, [1] **Mohammed K. Mahdi,** [1] **Jyoti Bhatia,** [2] **Rosemarie C. Nielson,** [1] **and Cataldo Doria** [3]

[1] *Department of Medicine, Capital Health Regional Medical Center, 750 Brunswick Ave, Trenton, NJ 08638, USA*
[2] *Department of Gastroenterology, Capital Health Hopewell, One Capital Way, Pennington, NJ 08534, USA*
[3] *Cancer Center, Capital Health Hopewell, Two Capital Way, Pennington, NJ 08534, USA*

Correspondence should be addressed to Maria Mironova; mironova.ma@gmail.com

Academic Editor: Yoshiro Kawahara

Introduction. Hepatic adenoma is an uncommon benign liver tumor presenting as solitary lesions or even rarely as hepatic adenomatosis. Large lesions carry a risk of rupture, hemorrhage, and malignant transformation. This case report aims to increase awareness about risk factors for hepatic adenomas, considering the increasing prevalence of obesity and the widespread use of oral contraceptive pills. *Case Presentation.* A 20-year-old obese female who was taking oral contraceptive pills for seven years presented to the emergency department with vomiting and abdominal pain caused by gastroenteritis. On imaging, multiple hepatic adenomas, including two lesions 6 and 9 cm in diameter, were incidentally found. During the hospitalization, the patient suddenly developed acute anemia and rupture of the largest lesion, which was promptly treated with arterial embolization. *Discussion.* Obesity and exposure to hormones are well-known risk factors for hepatic adenomas. The incidence of hepatic adenomas is steadily increasing because of the prevalence of obesity, especially among females. Lifestyle interventions for weight loss and discontinuation of oral contraceptive pills are considered a conservative treatment of hepatic adenomas. Large lesions possess the risk of malignant transformation and rupture and require surgical excision.

1. Introduction

Hepatocellular or hepatic adenomas (HAs) are benign tumors of presumable epithelial origin that occur in less than 0.004% of the population at risk [1, 2]. Their presentation varies from an asymptomatic solitary lesion, discovered incidentally, to hepatic adenomatosis, characterized by ten or more hepatic adenomas. Lesions bigger than 5 cm occur in less than 20% of cases and have a high potential for malignant transformation, spontaneous hemorrhage, and rupture. Exposure to hormones, including oral contraceptive pills (OCPs), and obesity have been strongly associated with HA occurrence. The risk of HA in women increases with the prolonged use of OCPs [3–5].

We present a case of an obese young female in whom hepatic adenomatosis was found incidentally. Three days after the discovery, the patient developed a rupture of the largest lesion and acute anemia, which led to an emergent, but prompt embolization and partial control of bleeding.

2. Case Presentation

A 20-year-old woman presented to the emergency department for the evaluation of the acute onset of epigastric and chest pain, shortness of breath, and vomiting that started the same day after eating a tuna sandwich. Her medical history was significant for hypothyroidism, depression treated with sertraline, and dysmenorrhea. She was taking OCPs for the

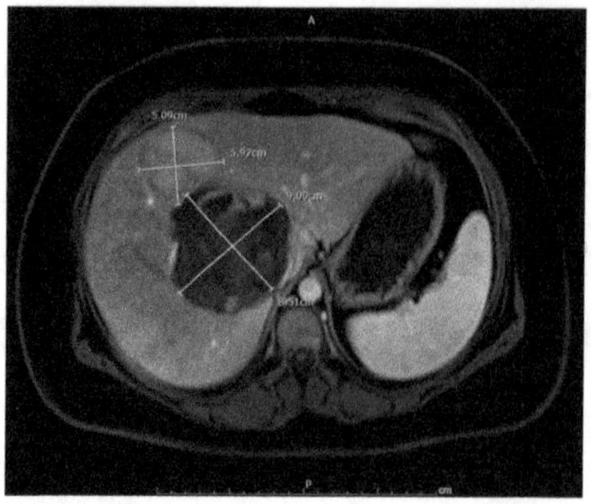

Figure 1: MRI of the liver with contrast showing a sizable hemorrhagic HA measuring 9.0 × 8.5 cm and adjacent nonhemorrhagic HA 5.9 × 5.1 cm (segment 4) and several HAs smaller than 5 cm in diameter.

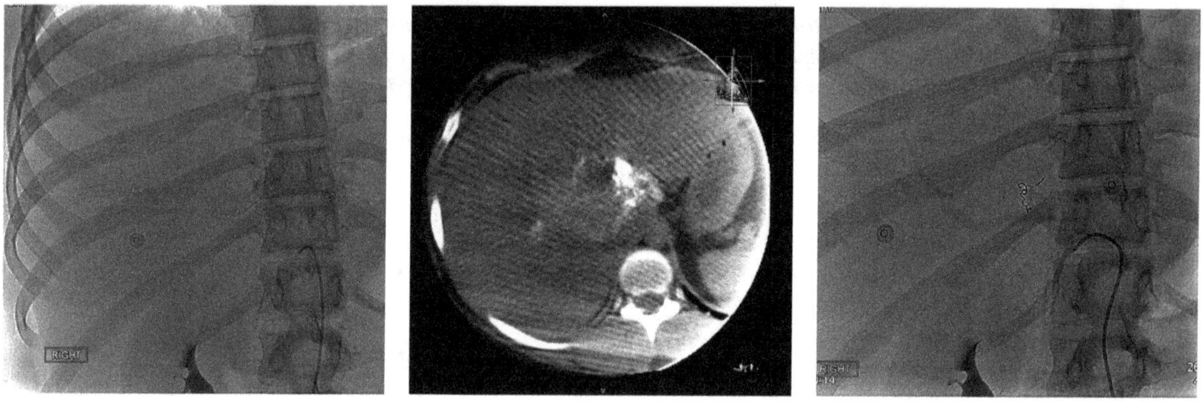

(a) (b) (c)

Figure 2: (a) Subselective catheterization of the hepatic artery, segment 8 branch with arteriography. (b) Cone beam CT demonstrating patency and perfusion of the hepatic adenoma. (c) Coil embolization of segment 8 branch of the hepatic artery.

past seven years. The body mass index was 34, vital signs were prominent for hypertension 164/81 mmHg, and tachycardia 99 bpm. A physical exam revealed palpable hepatomegaly. Laboratory data were remarkable for leukocytosis of 16,000/mm^3 and transaminitis with aspartate transaminase of 267 and alanine transaminase of 333 U/l.

The patient was tested for SARS-CoV-2 infection, considering the ongoing pandemic. The polymerase chain reaction test returned negative. The differential diagnosis also included viral hepatitis, viral or food-borne gastroenteritis, and pulmonary embolism, considering the history of prolonged hormonal treatment. Computerized tomographic (CT) angiography of the chest was negative for pulmonary embolism but noted multiple large hyperenhancing liver masses. The patient was diagnosed with gastroenteritis, and symptomatic treatment was continued. However, the incidental finding of liver masses prompted further investigation. Blood work, including viral hepatitis panel, carcinoembryonic antigen, and cancer antigens 19–9 and 125, were within normal limits. The magnetic resonance imaging (MRI) of the liver was performed to differentiate between possible liver neoplasms, abscesses, hemangiomas, and adenomas. It showed hepatic steatosis and multiple masses involving both lobes. The MRI findings indicated that one of those lesions was an inflammatory hemorrhagic lesion of the hepatic dome, measuring 9.0 × 8.5 cm with severe mass effect and flattening of the intrahepatic inferior vena cava. Another one was a nonhemorrhagic lesion 5.9 × 5.1 cm, inseparable from the dominant mass (Figure 1). There were multiple other nonhemorrhagic HAs smaller than 4.5 cm. The diagnosis of hepatic adenomatosis was postulated as the patient was taking OCPs over a prolonged period. Contraceptives were discontinued, and weight loss was recommended.

After three days at the hospital, the patient developed acute anemia with a drop in the hemoglobin level from 11.5 to 8.7 g/dL. The CT scan of the abdomen showed an increase of the largest adenoma to 9.5 cm in diameter, thus confirming the rupture. The emergent transarterial embolization of the lesion was performed, considering rapid expansion and life-threatening hemorrhage risk (Figure 2). The CT scan completed the next day showed a decrease of adenoma to 8.0 cm × 7.9 cm (Figure 3) along with the increase in hemoglobin levels, confirming the successful embolization.

The patient had a follow-up CT scan of the abdomen two months after embolization. It showed a decrease in the size

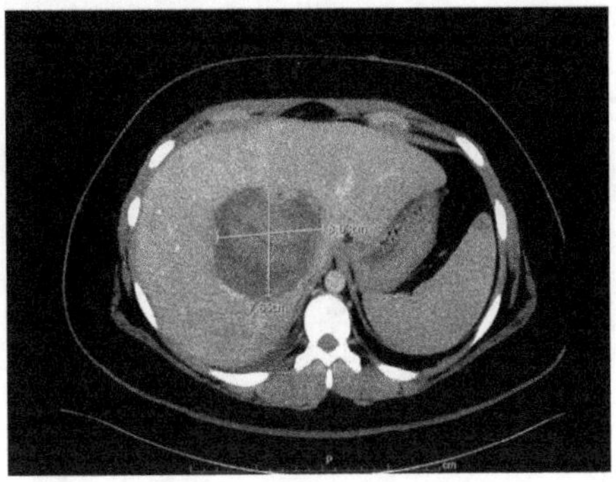

Figure 3: CT scan of the abdomen performed the next day after embolization showing the decrease in the dominant lesion size to 8.0 × 7.9 cm.

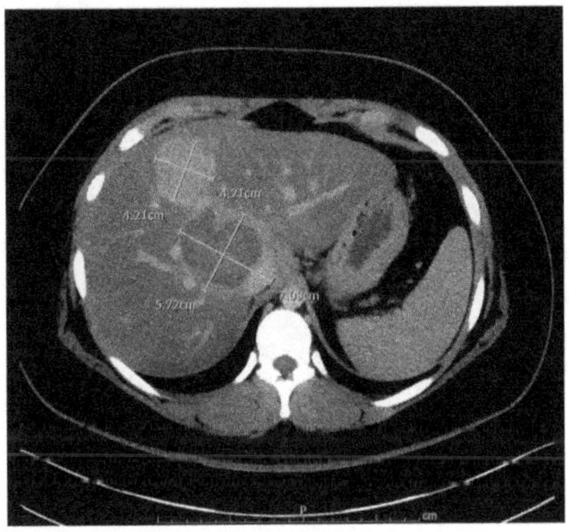

Figure 4: CT scan of the abdomen repeated in two months showing that the dominant HA decreased in size, measuring 7.1 × 5.7 cm, with coils and a resolved hemorrhagic component. The non-hemorrhagic mass in segment four decreased to 4.2 cm in diameter.

of the dominant lesion with a complete resolution of the hemorrhagic component (Figure 4). The option of resection of this lesion was discussed with the patient.

3. Discussion

Exposure to hormones, including OCPs and anabolic steroids, is a known risk factor for HA. It was proven that the use of OCPs for five to seven years carries a 5-fold risk of HA, and after nine years, the risk becomes 25-fold [6]. The injury mechanism is associated with inhibition of bilirubin and bile secretion by estrogens and induction of cholestasis. Discontinuation of hormonal treatment and close monitoring is considered conservative management of HA. Usually, it leads to a regression in tumor size, at least by one-third in 40% of the patients [7, 8].

The modern-generation OCPs are safer and have less impact on the risk of HA. However, the incidence of HA has been steadily growing, driven by the increasing number of overweight and obese female patients [9]. Also, patients with a higher BMI usually develop multiple and inflammatory adenomas, as was seen in this case. Weight loss is strongly encouraged for individuals with HA. Recent studies show that bariatric surgery is associated with tumor regression or even complete resolution [10].

The definite diagnosis of the nature of adenomas is usually made by performing a biopsy of the lesions. In our case, a biopsy was not performed; however, the MRI identified early arterial enhancement without portal washout and a hyperintense signal band on the periphery of the lesion. That finding was strongly suggestive of the inflammatory nature of the adenomas in the patient [11].

HA can result in spontaneous hemorrhage in 20% of the cases and malignant transformation to hepatocellular carcinoma in 5% [1]. The risk of these complications increases with the size of the lesion. Most of the hemorrhages are intratumoral, but in case of massive bleeding, the lesion can rupture, leading to a subcapsular hematoma [12]. Symptomatic lesions or size larger than 5 cm are indications for surgical resection or selective arterial embolization in case of rupture or hemodynamic instability [13]. Radiofrequency ablation can be used in the case of multiple HA, usually requiring several sessions [14, 15].

In conclusion, the combination of hemodynamic compromise and obesity or the history of exposure to hormones in a female should always raise suspicion for the possibility of a ruptured HA and prompt the necessary workup and management.

References

[1] M. G. Thomeer, M. Broker, J. Verheij et al., "Hepatocellular adenoma: when and how to treat? update of current evidence," *Therapeutic Advances in Gastroenterology*, vol. 9, no. 6, pp. 898–912, 2016.

[2] J.-C. Nault, G. Couchy, C. Balabaud et al., "Molecular classification of hepatocellular adenoma associates with risk factors, bleeding, and malignant transformation," *Gastroenterology*, vol. 152, no. 4, pp. 880–894, 2017, e6.

[3] K. Oji, T. Urade, Y. Iwatani et al., "Case of resected multiple hepatocellular adenomas in a young man with severe obesity," *Surgical Case Reports*, vol. 5, no. 1, p. 131, 2019.

[4] A. J. Klompenhouwer, B. V. Rosmalen, M. P. D. Haring et al., "A multicentre retrospective analysis on growth of residual hepatocellular adenoma after resection," *Liver International*, vol. 40, no. 9, pp. 2272–2278, 2020.

[5] C. Bunchorntavakul, R. Bahirwani, D. Drazek et al., "Clinical features and natural history of hepatocellular adenomas: the impact of obesity," *Alimentary Pharmacology and Therapeutics*, vol. 34, no. 6, pp. 664–674, 2011.

[6] M. H. Piper, J. M. Fields, and R. R. Kahl, "Hepatocellular adenoma," 2020, https://emedicine.medscape.com/article/170205-overview Medscape.

[7] M. P. D. Haring, A. S. H. Gouw, R. J. de Haas, F. J. C. Cuperus, K. P. de Jong, and V. E. de Meijer, "The effect of oral contraceptive pill cessation on hepatocellular adenoma diameter: a retrospective cohort study," *Liver International*, vol. 39, no. 5, pp. 905–913, 2019.

[8] A. M. Karkar, L. H. Tang, N. D. Kashikar et al., "Management of hepatocellular adenoma: comparison of resection,

embolization and observation," *HPB*, vol. 15, no. 3, pp. 235–243, 2013.

[9] P. Bioulac-Sage, S. Taouji, L. Possenti, and C. Balabaud, "Hepatocellular adenoma subtypes: the impact of overweight and obesity," *Liver International*, vol. 32, no. 8, pp. 1217–1221, 2012.

[10] T. J. G. Gevers, B. W. Marcel Spanier, P. B. Veendrick, and J. M. Vrolijk, "Regression of hepatocellular adenoma after bariatric surgery in severe obese patients," *Liver International*, vol. 38, no. 12, pp. 2134–2136, 2018.

[11] S. M. van Aalten, M. G. J. Thomeer, T. Terkivatan et al., "Hepatocellular adenomas: correlation of MR imaging findings with pathologic subtype classification," *Radiology*, vol. 261, no. 1, pp. 172–181, 2011.

[12] S. M. van Aalten, R. A. de Man, J. N. M. IJzermans, and T. Terkivatan, "Systematic review of haemorrhage and rupture of hepatocellular adenomas," *British Journal of Surgery*, vol. 99, no. 7, pp. 911–916, 2012.

[13] A. J. Klompenhouwer, R. A. de Man, M. G. Thomeer, and J. N. Ijzermans, "Management and outcome of hepatocellular adenoma with massive bleeding at presentation," *World Journal of Gastroenterology*, vol. 23, no. 25, pp. 4579–4586, 2017.

[14] D. Erdogan, O. M. van Delden, O. R. C. Busch, D. J. Gouma, and T. M. van Gulik, "Selective transcatheter arterial embolization for treatment of bleeding complications or reduction of tumor mass of hepatocellular adenomas," *CardioVascular and Interventional Radiology*, vol. 30, no. 6, pp. 1252–1258, 2007.

[15] O. Mironov, A. Jaberi, R. Beecroft, and J. R. Kachura, "Retrospective single-arm cohort study of patients with hepatocellular adenomas treated with percutaneous thermal ablation," *Cardiovascular and Interventional Radiology*, vol. 41, no. 6, pp. 935–941, 2018.

Somatostatinoma Presented as Double-Duct Sign

Ali Zakaria ,[1] Nour Hammad,[2] Cynthia Vakhariya,[3] and Michael Raphael[1]

[1]*Division of Gastroenterology, Providence-Providence Park Hospital and Medical Center, Michigan State University/College of Human Medicine, Southfield, Michigan, USA*
[2]*Department of Internal Medicine, Providence-Providence Park Hospital and Medical Center, Michigan State University/College of Human Medicine, Southfield, Michigan, USA*
[3]*Division of Hematology & Oncology, Providence-Providence Park Hospital and Medical Center, Michigan State University/College of Human Medicine, Southfield, Michigan, USA*

Correspondence should be addressed to Ali Zakaria; alizakaria86@hotmail.com

Academic Editor: Yoshihiro Moriwaki

Somatostatinoma is a rare neuroendocrine tumor with an incidence rate of 1 in 40 million people. It presents mostly as asymptomatic tumor diagnosed incidentally on imaging or surgery when evaluating or treating possible causes of abdominal pain. It also can present with vague symptoms, or as a clinical triad of glucose intolerance, steatorrhea, and achlorhydria. The majority of somatostatinomas are present in the pancreatic head, followed by the duodenum, the pancreatic tail, and rarely the ampulla of Vater. The prognosis is poor as more than 77% of cases present as advanced disease with local invasion or distant metastasis. Surgical resection is the main treatment for early stage disease. Other treatment options include somatostatin analogue, molecular targeted therapy, and cytotoxic chemotherapy. The scarcity of somatostatinoma cases led to the lack of fully formulated treatment options. Herein, we present a 43-year old male patient who was referred by his primary care physician to our gastroenterology clinic due to elevated liver function test and double-duct sign on CT scan. We performed an ERCP, which revealed 2 cm ampullary lesion with upstream obstruction. Biopsies were taken and histopathology was unrevealing. He underwent a laparoscopic pancreaticoduodenectomy with histopathology revealed stage IIb somatostatinoma. Treating physicians should hold a high index of suspicion and maintain a broad differential diagnosis of elevated liver enzymes.

1. Introduction

Somatostatinoma is a rare neuroendocrine tumor with an incidence rate of 1 in 40 million people. It presents mostly as asymptomatic tumor diagnosed incidentally on imaging or surgery when evaluating or treating possible causes of abdominal pain. It can also present with vague symptoms, or as a clinical triad of glucose intolerance, steatorrhea, and achlorhydria. Somatostatinoma mostly involves the pancreatic head followed by the duodenum.

Due to vague symptomatology it presents in >77% of cases as advanced disease with local invasion or distant metastasis. The rarity of the disease led to lack of fully formulated treatment protocol, with surgical resection, somatostatin analogue, molecular targeted therapy, and cytotoxic chemotherapy being available options. The prognosis is poor in advanced diseases.

2. Case Report

This is a 43-year-old white male patient with past medical history of hypertension and obesity. He was referred to the gastroenterology clinic from his primary care physician due to elevated liver function test found on routine annual physical exam. At the time of evaluation he had no complaint, and he denied any abdominal pain, nausea, vomiting, jaundice, weight changes, skin lesions, or discoloration. He also denied any prior history of illicit drug use, high risk sexual behavior, sexually transmitted diseases, or family history of liver or autoimmune diseases. His physical examination did not reveal any skin lesions suspicious for neurofibromatosis-1.

His initial workup revealed a random glucose level of 85 mg/dl, calcium level 9.5 mg/dl, total bilirubin 1.3 mg/dl, direct bilirubin 0.6 mg/dl, alkaline phosphatase 640 U/L,

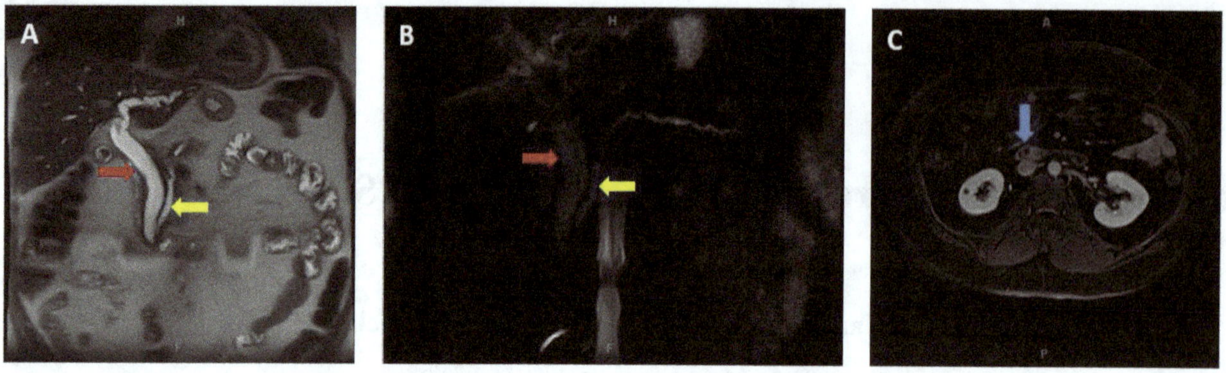

(a) (b) (c)

FIGURE 1: MRI abdomen with and without contrast: (a) T2 image and (b) MRCP image reveal moderate to severe intrahepatic biliary ductal dilation. The common duct measures 1.5 cm in greatest diameter "red arrow". The pancreatic duct is also dilated measuring up to 0.6 cm at the head "yellow arrow". No intraluminal filling defect. (c) T1 image with contrast reveals mild distal common bile duct wall enhancement "blue arrow".

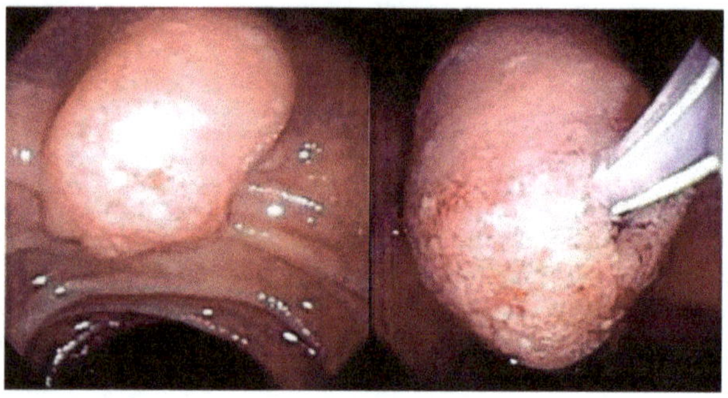

FIGURE 2: Endoscopic (ERCP) images reveal a 2cm ampullary mass.

AST 220 U/L, ALT of 494 U/L, total protein 7.1 g/dl and albumin 4.6 g/dl. Further workup revealed negative viral hepatitis panel, antinuclear antibodies, anti-mitochondrial antibodies and anti-smooth muscle antibodies. Iron studies, ceruloplasmin and alpha-1 antitrypsin were within normal limits.

Abdominal ultrasonography revealed normal liver size and echotexture with no lesions, intrahepatic biliary duct dilatation, common bile duct dilatation 18 mm, contracted gallbladder with no cholelithiasis and no discrete pancreatic mass or ductal dilatation were identified. Magnetic resonance image/magnetic resonance cholangiopancreatography (MRI/MRCP) was performed and revealed moderate to severe intrahepatic and extra hepatic biliary ductal dilatation with mild enhancement of the distal common bile duct without choledocholithiasis or discrete mass, and pancreatic duct dilation with normal pancreas [Figure 1].

An endoscopic retrograde cholangiopancreatography (ERCP) was performed and revealed a large ampullary mass distorting the anatomy, which precluded cannulation of the common bile duct [Figure 2]. During his ongoing evaluation the patient developed pruritus and his repeated liver function test revealed stable levels with numbers around his initial presentation. An advanced endoscopist repeated the ERCP, which revealed 2 cm ampullary lesion with upstream obstruction, pancreatic duct dilatation measuring 4.5 mm, intra- and extra-hepatic biliary dilatation with common bile duct measured 16 mm. A biliary sphincterotomy and balloon sweep was performed, and biopsies were taken of the ampullary tissue. Histopathology revealed congested mixed acute and chronic inflammation with reactive epithelial changes, negative for malignancy. The CA 19-9 level was elevated at 51.4 units/mL.

The patient underwent laparoscopic pancreaticoduodenectomy (Whipple's procedure) with regional lymphadenectomy. Histopathology was consistent with 1.3 cm ampullary neuroendocrine tumor infiltrating the mucosa, submucosa and muscularis propria with angiolymphatic invasion. Immunohistochemical stains were positive for somatostatin, and negative for gastrin, serotonin and pancreatic polypeptide [Figure 3]. There was no local invasion, the specimen margins were negative, and 1/18 lymph nodes were positive. The patient was diagnosed with stage IIb (T2 N1 M0) somatostatinoma.

The post resection surveillance at 3, 6, and 12 months revealed a normal history and physical examination, a fasting somatostatin level of 41, 28, and 19 pg/ml, respectively, and a CT scan abdomen and pelvis with no evidence of recurrence. He is still under yearly surveillance with normal history, physical examination and fasting somatostatin level for the last four years.

3. Discussion

D or delta cells are neuroendocrine cells located in the gastrointestinal (GI) tract and pancreatic islets of Langerhans that secret somatostatin [1]. Somatostatin is a cyclic tetradecapeptide with major inhibitory action on the GI tract hormonal secretion, namely, gastric acid, pepsin and enterochromaffin-like (ECL) cell histamine. Neurotransmitters including acetylcholine and GI peptides are furthermore inhibited by somatostatin. Moreover, somatostatin enhances early gastric emptying and distal intestinal motility and delays late phase gastric emptying and gastroduodenal motility. It

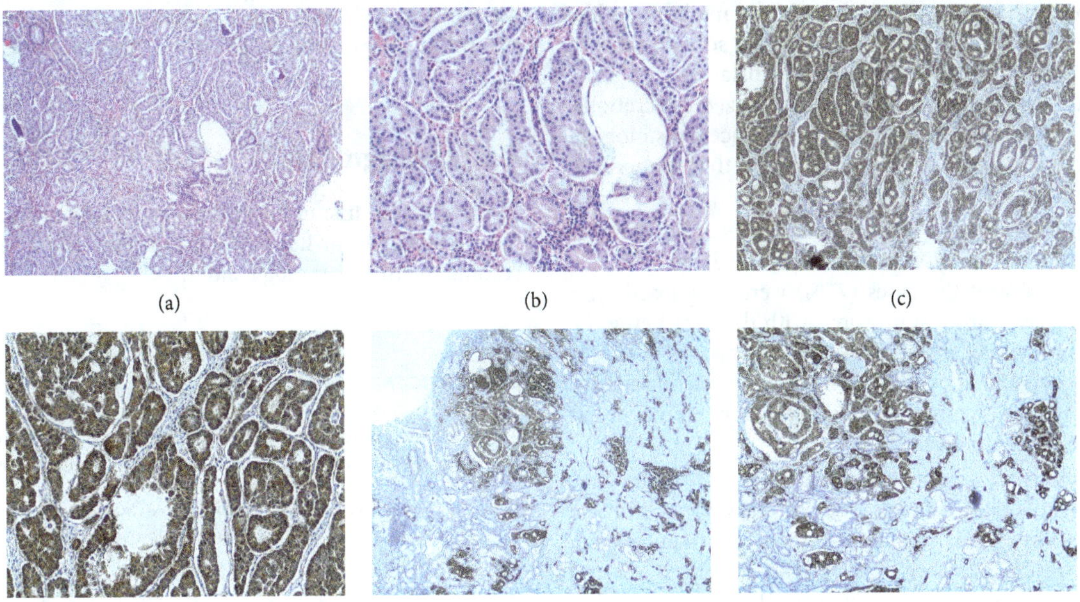

FIGURE 3: Histopathology images H&E [4x (a) and 0x (b)] reveal ampullary neuroendocrine tumor infiltrating the mucosa, submucosa, and muscularis propria with angiolymphatic invasion. Immunohistochemical stain images are positive for somatostatin [4x (c) and 10x (d)], and synaptophysin [2x (e) and 4x (f)].

also hinders intestinal nutrient absorption and splanchnic blood flow [1].

Somatostatin was initially analyzed from the hypothalamus of sheep in 1973 and was later found to be present in the pancreas, lung, adrenal and thymic tissue [1, 2]. Somatostatinoma is a rare tumor with an incidence rate of 1 in 40 million people and an average age of incidence of 50 in men and 52 years in women [2, 3]. Somatostatinoma occurs in association with multiple neuroendocrine syndrome type 1 (MEN-1) in 45% of cases, it is considered one of the least common functioning enteropancreatic neuroendocrine tumors occurring in <1% of MEN-1 cases [4]. It develops also in 10% of patients with neurofibromatosis type 1 [5]. Patients diagnosed with somatostatinoma should be screened for other components of MEN-1 by either serum calcium level (parathyroid hormone and ionized calcium level can be added to enhance sensitivity and specificity) or DNA-based genetic testing. A thorough skin exam looking for signs of NF-1 should also be considered. Larson L et al. initially described somatostatinoma in 1977. They found the tumor incidentally in the pancreas during cholecystectomy. They later performed a retrospective analysis of tumor records and documented another case of pancreatic D cell tumor. They associated the classic triad of glucose intolerance, steatorrhea, and achlorhydria in both patients with somatostatinoma in accordance with somatostatin physiologic effects [6]. It was noted that the somatostatinoma syndrome triad was mostly seen in pancreatic tumors while obstructive symptoms were associated with duodenal masses [7].

The size and location of the tumor has a major influence on the severity and nature of symptoms [8]. The majority of somatostatinomas are present in the pancreatic head (45%), followed by the duodenum (19%), the pancreatic tail (13%) and later the ampulla of Vater (6%) [2]. If symptomatic, somatostatinoma patient's most common complaints are weight loss and abdominal pain [2]. Duodenal somatostatinomas were associated with jaundice and cholestasis in addition to the abdominal pain and weight loss. Many of the somatostatinomas are silent or present with vague symptoms making the diagnosis of such tumors an enigma. Many reported tumors were found incidentally on imaging or surgery when evaluating or treating possible causes of abdominal pain and diagnosis was confirmed by histopathology after resection [7]. When suspected due to presence of somatostatinoma triad, a fasting plasma somatostatin level of more than 30 pg/ml is diagnostic. Other modalities that may aid in diagnosis include computed tomography (CT), magnetic resonance imaging (MRI), endoscopic ultrasound (EUS), somatostatin receptor scintigraphy (OctreoScan) and function positron emission tomography (PET). OctreoScan uses radiolabeled octreotide ([111-In] pentetreotide); it has the advantage of instantaneous whole body scanning, which allows extra-abdominal metastasis detection. Guidelines have different recommendations on when to obtain this study, but experts suggested using this technique as adjunct for tumor staging if finding would change patient management [2]. The functional PET technique uses different tracers (e.g., 68-Ga-DOTATOC, or the newly FDA approved 68-Ga-DOTATATE). It provides higher resolutions, which improves sensitivity for small lesions detections.

Somatostatinoma D cells are located in the submucosa and therefore the yield of the endoscopic biopsies is low. Only 60 to 83% of the biopsies have a positive yield for diagnosis [9]. Histopathological presentation of D cell is marked by the presence of large secretory granules of medium to low intensity. Pathologists use immuno-reactive somatostatin to confirm the presence of the targeted somatostatin in the granules. The spherical, laminated, and mineralized concretions, known as psammoma bodies, are pronounced histological findings that are seen in duodenal rather than pancreatic somatostatinomas [10].

Due to the ambiguity of symptoms at presentation of the somatostatinoma, many of the tumors are diagnosed late. The vast majority of the cases (77%) were diagnosed after distant metastases or local invasion, with the liver being the most common site of invasion (42%). Other areas of tumor invasion are accounted by the lymph nodes (39%), duodenum (13%), spleen (6%), common bile duct, colon, stomach, left kidney, bone and pancreas [2].

The scarcity of somatostatinoma cases led to the lack of fully formulated treatment options. Surgery is still the preferred treatment for smaller tumors of less than 2x2 cm; however, 70-92% of cases present with advanced disease for which surgery is not an option [11]. Larger tumors, locally infiltrative, or tumors with lymph node metastases will mandate pancreaticoduodenectomy. Tumors with extensive distant metastases that are challenging to resect will require other treatment options: Debulking, somatostatin analogue (e.g., octreotide, lanreotide), molecular targeted therapy (e.g., everolimus, sunitinib), and cytotoxic chemotherapy [12, 13]. 5-Flourouracil and streptozocin are chemotherapy agents that were incorporated in the treatment of previous somatostatinoma patients with limited benefit [2]. In patients with extensive liver metastasis other treatment modalities that can be used include hepatic artery embolization, chemoembolization and if small lesions (<3cm) radiofrequency ablation and cryoablation [14]. Liver transplantation is still an investigational approach with no enough data to provide any recommendation for this modality as a cure. Resection of localized somatostatinoma is definitive; however, the prognosis of patient diagnosed with metastatic disease is poor in general with reported survival period of one to two years [8, 15]. Due to limited data regarding somatostatinoma, the survival rate estimate can be roughly reflected from the five- and ten-year survival of the patient who underwent resection of pancreatic neuroendocrine tumors, which was estimated to be 64-75%, and 45-71% in stage I-II disease, compared to 19-60%, and 8-33% in stage III-IV disease, respectively [16]. The National Comprehensive Cancer Network recommendation regarding post-treatment surveillance of somatostatinoma consists of (a) History and physical examination, fasting somatostatin level and imaging studies with CT scan or MRI after 3-12 months; (b) History and physical exam, fasting somatostatin level (every 6-12 months) and imaging studies as clinically indicated after 12 months up until 10 years [17].

4. Conclusion

Somatostatinoma is a very rare neuroendocrine tumor. We reported this case to emphasize the importance of holding a high index of suspicion and maintaining a broad differential diagnosis of elevated liver enzymes. Unfortunately, there is no standardized treatment regimen so far, and the overall survival is poor due to the advanced stage on presentation.

Acknowledgments

Authors would like to express their deepest appreciation to Dr. Hema Govil for her valuable expertise in providing and reading the histopathology slides.

References

[1] T. Debas Haile, *Gastrointestinal surgery: pathophysiology and management*, Springer Science & Business Media, 2004.

[2] G. J. Harris, F. Tio, and A. B. Cruz, "Somatostatinoma: a case report and review of the literature," *Journal of Surgical Oncology*, vol. 36, no. 1, pp. 8–16, 1987.

[3] R. T. Jensen and J. A. Norton, "Endocrine tumors of the pancreas," in *Sleisenger & Fordtran's Gastrointestinal and Liver Disease: Pathophysiology/Diagnosis/Management*, M. Feldman, B. F. Scharschmidt, and M. H. Sleisenger, Eds., p. 988, WB Saunders, Philadelphia, Pa, USA, 7th edition, 2002.

[4] N. Garbrecht, M. Anlauf, A. Schmitt et al., "Somatostatin-producing neuroendocrine tumors of the duodenum and pancreas: incidence, types, biological behavior, association with inherited syndromes, and functional activity," *Endocrine-Related Cancer*, vol. 15, no. 1, pp. 229–241, 2008.

[5] C. Mao, A. Shah, D. J. Hanson, and J. M. Howard, "Von recklinghausen's disease associated with duodenal somatostatinoma: Contrast of duodenal versus pancreatic somatostatinomas," *Journal of Surgical Oncology*, vol. 59, no. 1, pp. 67–73, 1995.

[6] L.-I. Larsson, J. J. Holst, C. Kühl et al., "Pancreatic somatostatinoma: clinical features and physiological implications," *The Lancet*, vol. 309, no. 8013, pp. 666–668, 1977.

[7] G. Nesi, T. Marcucci, C. A. Rubio, M. L. Brandi, and F. Tonelli, "Somatostatinoma: clinico-pathological features of three cases and literature reviewed," *Journal of Gastroenterology and Hepatology*, vol. 23, no. 4, pp. 521–526, 2008.

[8] T. D. O'Brien, G. Chejfec, and R. A. Prinz, "Clinical features of duodenal somatostatinomas," *Surgery*, vol. 114, no. 6, pp. 1144–1147, 1993.

[9] C. Mao, A. Shah, D. J. Hanson, and J. M. Howard, "Von recklinghausen's disease associated with duodenal somatostatinoma: contrast of duodenal versus pancreatic somatostatinomas," *Journal of Surgical Oncology*, vol. 59, no. 1, pp. 67–73, 1995.

[10] Y. Dayal, W. G. Doos, M. J. O'Brien, G. Nunnemacher, R. A. DeLellis, and H. J. Wolfe, "Psammomatous somatostatinomas of the duodenum," *The American Journal of Surgical Pathology*, vol. 7, no. 7, pp. 653–665, 1983.

[11] M. G. House, C. J. Yeo, and R. D. Schulick, "Periampullary pancreatic somatostatinoma," *Annals of Surgical Oncology*, vol. 9, no. 9, pp. 869–874, 2002.

[12] M. E. Caplin, M. Pavel, J. B. Ćwikła et al., "Lanreotide in metastatic enteropancreatic neuroendocrine tumors," *The New England Journal of Medicine*, vol. 371, no. 3, pp. 224–233, 2014.

[13] A. Rinke, M. Wittenberg, C. Schade-Brittinger et al., "Placebo controlled, double blind, prospective, randomized study on the effect of octreotide lar in the control of tumor growth in patients with metastatic neuroendocrine midgut tumors (PROMID): results on long term survival," *Neuroendocrinology*, vol. 104, no. 1, pp. 26–32, 2017.

[14] S. J. Moug, E. Leen, P. G. Morgan, and C. W. Imrie, "Radiofrequency ablation has a valuable therapeutic role in metastatic VIPoma," *Pancreatology*, vol. 6, no. 1-2, pp. 155–159, 2006.

[15] R. Delcore and S. R. Friesen, "Gastrointestinal neuroendocrine tumors," *Journal of the American College of Surgeons*, vol. 178, no. 2, pp. 187–211, 1994.

[16] K. Y. Bilimoria, D. J. Bentrem, R. P. Merkow et al., "Application of the pancreatic adenocarcinoma staging system to pancreatic neuroendocrine tumors," *Journal of the American College of Surgeons*, vol. 205, no. 4, pp. 558–563, 2007.

[17] National Comprehensive Cancer Network (NCCN), "NCCN Clinical practice guidelines in oncology," https://www.nccn.org/professionals/physician_gls/pdf/neuroendocrine.pdf.

34

Simultaneous Massive Esophageal Mucosal Candidiasis and Profound Cytomegaloviral Esophageal Ulcers with Recurrence of Both Infections 12 Years Later in a Patient with Long-Standing AIDS: Endoscopic, Radiologic, and Pathologic Findings

Inayat Gill,[1] Ahmed Edhi,[1] Mitual Amin,[2,3] and Mitchell S. Cappell[4]

[1]*Division of Gastroenterology, Department of Internal Medicine, William Beaumont Hospital at Royal Oak, 3535 W. Thirteen Mile Rd, Royal Oak, MI 48073, USA*
[2]*Department of Pathology, William Beaumont Hospital at Royal Oak, 3600 W. Thirteen Mile Rd, Royal Oak, MI 48073, USA*
[3]*Department of Pathology, Oakland University William Beaumont School of Medicine, 3600 W. Thirteen Mile Rd, Royal Oak, MI 48073, USA*
[4]*Division of Gastroenterology, Department of Medicine, Building 1, Room 3210, Aleda E. Lutz VA Medical Center, 1500 Weiss St, Saginaw, MI 48602, USA*

Correspondence should be addressed to Mitchell S. Cappell; mitchell.cappell@beaumont.edu

Academic Editor: Yoshifumi Nakayama

Immunocompromised patients with acquired immunodeficiency syndrome (AIDS) can develop opportunistic esophageal candidial and cytomegaloviral infections. A case is reported which extends the clinico-endoscopic severity of these infections. A 32-year-old bisexual man with AIDS since 1997, and intermittently compliant with antiretroviral therapy, presented (2007) with dysphagia and 32 kg-weight loss. EGD revealed a massive, cheesy, esophageal mucosal exudate from *Candida albicans*. Cytomegalovirus was isolated by viral culture. The patient improved after fluconazole/ganciclovir therapy. The patient re-presented (2019) with hematemesis and dysphagia. EGD revealed cheesy esophageal exudate and profound "punched out" esophageal ulcers mimicking pseudo-diverticula. Histopathology confirmed candidiasis. Viral cultures revealed cytomegalovirus. Barium esophagram revealed deep esophageal ulcers/pseudo-diverticula. Repeat EGD 8 weeks later after ganciclovir/micafungin therapy revealed mostly healed lesions. This demonstrates that AIDS patients may have massive mucosal esophageal candidiasis; that both infections can recur years after apparent eradication; and that cytomegaloviral esophageal ulcers may be profound and mimic pseudo-diverticula. A comprehensive literature review revealed only one abstract of esophageal pseudo-diverticula associated with cytomegalovirus. Simultaneous esophageal candidial and CMV infections have also been rarely reported in immunocompromised patients without AIDS.

1. Introduction

Immunocompromised patients with acquired immunodeficiency syndrome (AIDS) can develop opportunistic esophageal candidial and cytomegaloviral (CMV) infections. A case is reported which extends the spectrum of clinical, endoscopic, radiologic, and pathologic severity of these infections associated with AIDS by reporting (1)-simultaneous massive esophageal mucosal candidiasis and CMV; (2)-recurrence of both infections 12 years later; and (3)-occurrence of CMV "punched out" ulcers so deep that they mimicked esophageal "pseudo-diverticula" at esophagogastroduodenoscopy (EGD) and barium esophagram. These phenomena are attributed to the patient's poor adherence to antiretroviral therapy.

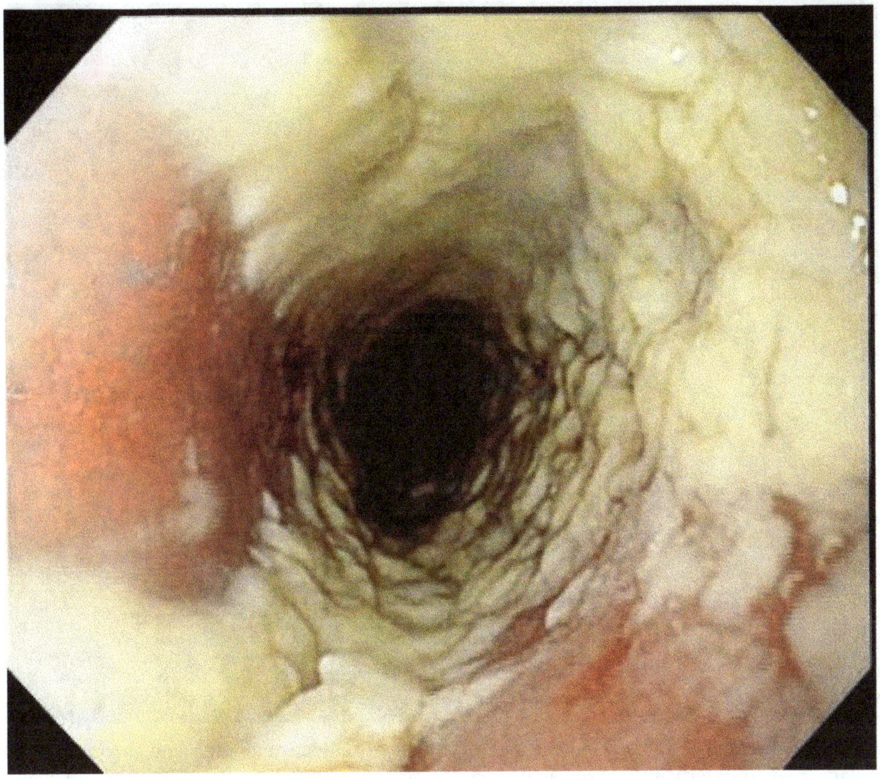

FIGURE 1: Esophagogastroduodenoscopy (EGD) performed in 2007 in a patient with acquired immunodeficiency syndrome (AIDS), carried out for the indications of severe odynophagia, dysphagia, and weight loss revealed massive, cheesy, tightly adherent, esophageal mucosal exudate/esophagitis from candidiasis (see Figure 2). Even though the esophageal candidiasis was massive in 2007, it was very superficial with superficial mucosal ulcers, as opposed to the deep "punched out" ulcers reported in 2019 (Figure 5), attributed to esophageal cytomegaloviral infection.

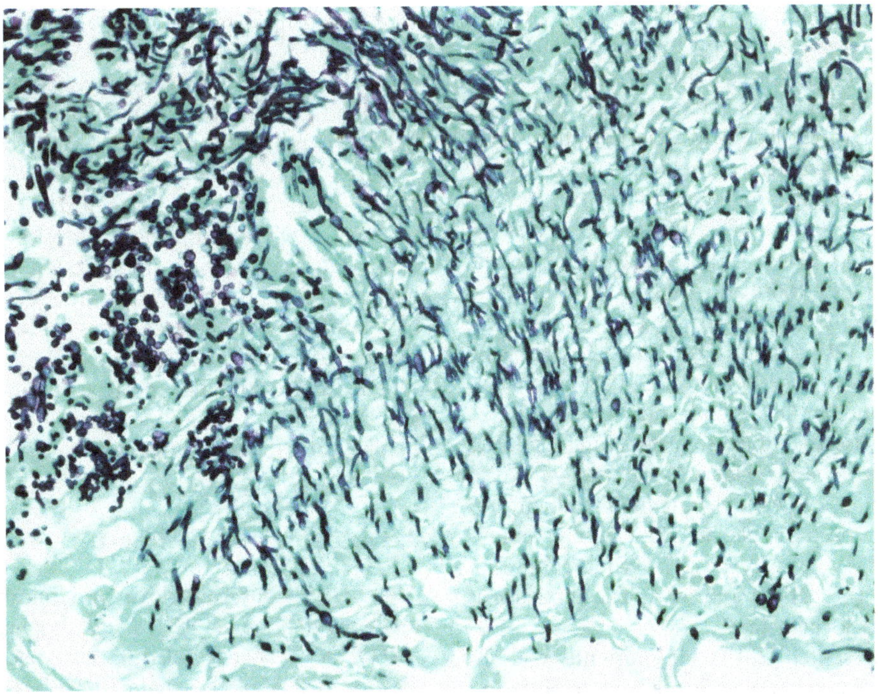

FIGURE 2: Gomori methenamine silver (GMS) stain of endoscopic biopsies of cheesy esophageal exudate demonstrates black spherical yeast forms (upper left) and elongated hyphae (throughout photomicrograph), with the characteristic morphology of *Candida*.

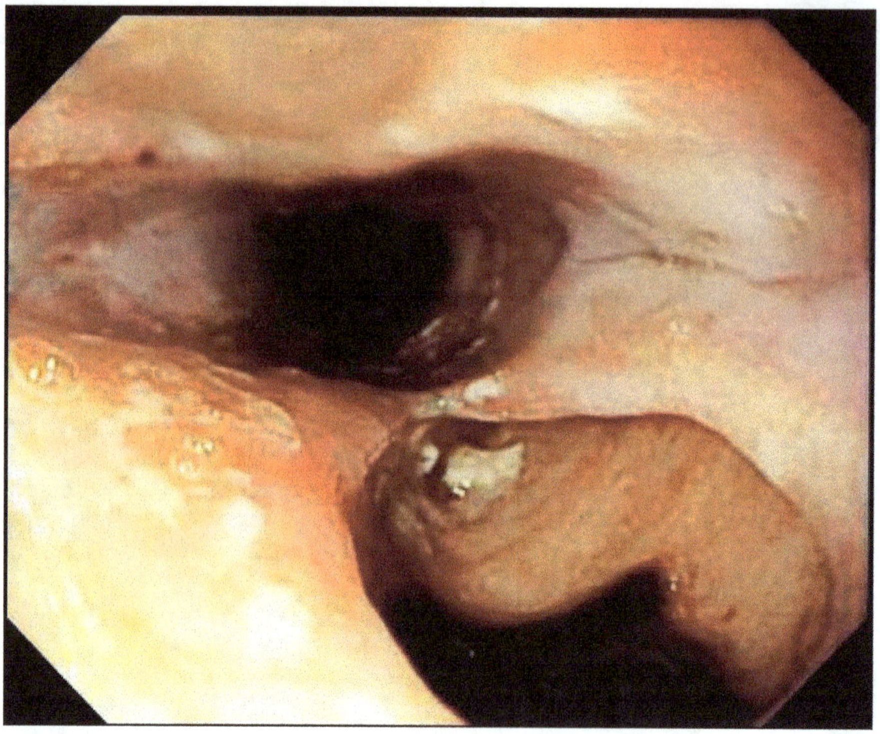

FIGURE 3: Esophagogastroduodenoscopy performed in 2019 for indications of acute hematemesis and chronic odynophagia and dysphagia reveals profound, irregular, "pseudo-diverticular" esophageal ulcers with a maximal diameter of 12 mm and a depth of 15 mm that are located posteriorly to the normal esophageal lumen: Cytomegalovirus was isolated from viral cultures of endoscopic biopsies taken from these esophageal ulcers.

2. Case Presentation

A 32-year-old Black American bisexual man with AIDS since 1997, prior *Pneumocystis carinii* pneumonia, and intermittent compliance with antiretroviral therapy, presented (2007) with chronic odynophagia, dysphagia, and 32 kg-involuntary-weight loss, without prior administration of esophagotoxic medications, corticosteroids, illicit drugs, alcoholism, diabetes mellitus, or gastroesophageal reflux. The patient was relatively indigent with only intermittent employment. Physical examination revealed a temperature of 38.1°C, temporal and intercostal muscle wasting, thrush, and a nontender abdomen. Hemoglobin was 10.1 g/dL (normal: 13.5–17 g/dL), leukocytes were 4.8 bil/L (normal: 3.5–10.1 bil/L), and CD4 cells were 68 mil/L (normal: 433–1722 mil/L). EGD revealed massive, cheesy, adherent, and esophageal mucosal exudate/esophagitis (Kodsi endoscopic candida classification grade 4 [1], Figure 1). *Candida albicans* was isolated from esophageal fungal cultures and demonstrated histologically (Figure 2). Hematoxylin-eosin stain of esophageal biopsies (without immunohistochemistry) revealed insufficiently deep samples to histologically demonstrate CMV, but CMV was isolated by viral culture of esophageal biopsies. The patient improved after intravenous fluconazole and ganciclovir therapy.

The patient re-presented (2019), intermittently compliant with antiretroviral therapy, with acute hematemesis and chronic odynophagia and dysphagia. Physical examination revealed a temperature of 37.9°C, blood pressure of 150/90 mmHg, pulse of 99 beats/minute, orthostasis, BMI = 15.8 kg/m^2, temporal and intercostal muscle wasting, thrush, and nontender abdomen. Hemoglobin was 6.5 g/dL, leukocytes were 4.4 bil/L, and CD4 cells were 4 mil/L.

After transfusing 2 units of packed erythrocytes and administering intravenous pantoprazole, EGD was performed, which demonstrated cheesy esophageal exudate and profound esophageal "punched out" ulcers (maximal depth = 15 mm) that mimicked pseudo-diverticula (Figure 3). Ulcers were not treated endoscopically because high-risk stigmata of recent hemorrhage (SRH) were absent. Histopathology of esophageal biopsies confirmed candidiasis (Kodsi endoscopic candida classification grade 3). Polymerase chain reaction and viral culture of esophageal biopsies (taken from ulcer edges and sides) revealed cytomegalovirus (no Herpes simplex). Barium esophagram revealed deep, irregular, posterior, nonperforating, esophageal ulcers, resembling pseudo-diverticula, without esophageal strictures (Figure 4).

3. Outcome and Follow-Up

After intravenous ganciclovir and micafungin therapy, hemoglobin stabilized at 8.3 g/dl and dysphagia resolved. Repeat EGD 8 weeks later revealed mostly healed esophageal candidiasis and CMV ulcers (Figure 5). He has returned three times to the hospital with recurrent dysphagia during the subsequent 6 months from esophageal candidiasis, each time after self-discontinuing the micafungin therapy.

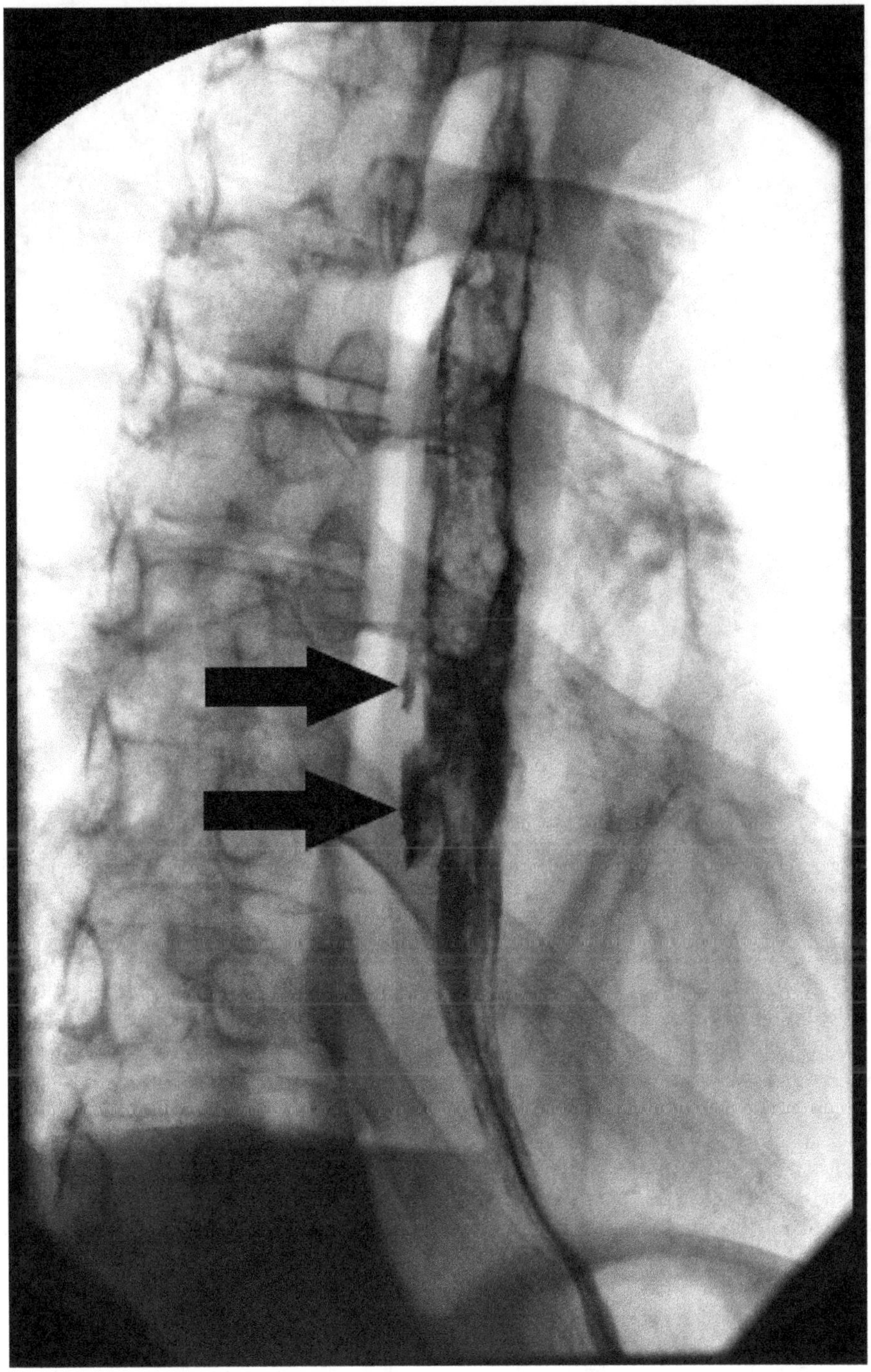

FIGURE 4: Barium esophagram reveals irregular, posterior, nonperforating, deep esophageal ulcers (arrows) that mimic esophageal pseudo-diverticula in extending posteriorly beyond the normal esophageal wall.

4. Discussion

AIDS patients can develop deep esophageal CMV ulcers [2] and widespread candidiasis [3] from immunocompromise. This work demonstrates that, in immunosuppressed patients, esophageal candidiasis may be massive; that both infections can recur 12 years after apparent eradication; and that CMV esophageal infection may cause so profoundly "punched out" ulcers so as to resemble esophageal pseudo-diverticula.

A comprehensive literature review revealed one prior report of esophageal deep ulcers that resembled esophageal pseudo-diverticula associated with CMV [4]. A 52-year-old male, HIV-seropositive patient with <200 CD4 cells/mm^3 presented with dysphagia. EGD revealed esophageal pseudo-diverticula/ulcers. Symptoms improved after unspecified treatment. However, this case was only reported as an abstract, and the ulcer biopsies were reported as "consistent," but not diagnostic, of CMV.

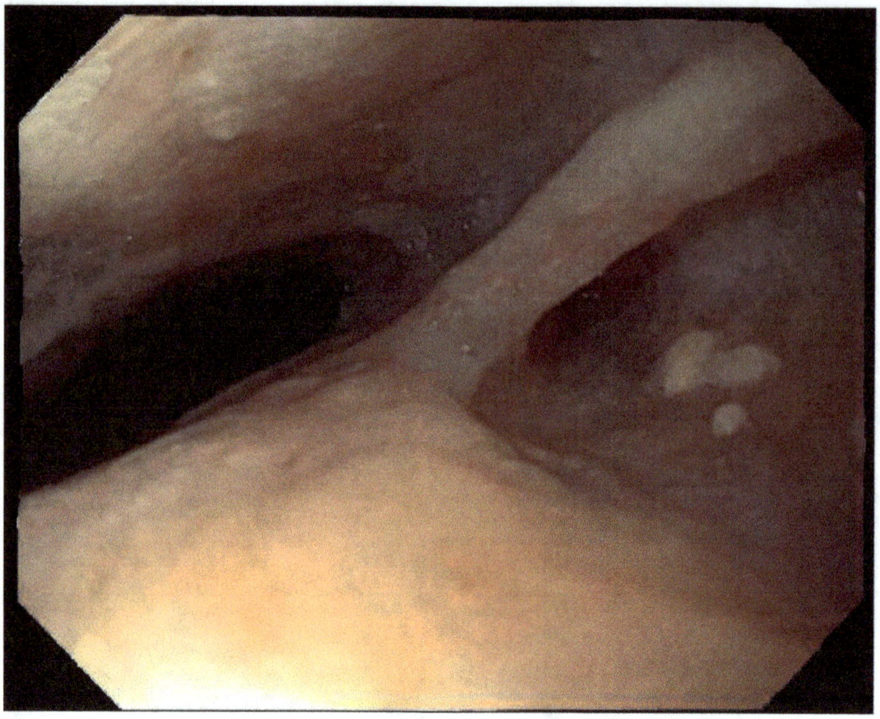

FIGURE 5: Repeat esophagogastroduodenoscopy (EGD) in 2019, 8 weeks after initiating therapy with ganciclovir and micafungin, for profound esophageal pseudo-diverticular ulcers and severe esophageal candidiasis, revealed mostly healed esophageal cytomegaloviral ulcers and esophageal candidiasis.

Oropharyngeal or esophageal candidiasis frequently occurs in patients with AIDS, especially with advanced disease. Esophageal mucosal candidiasis and CMV esophageal ulcers can also occur in other immunocompromised patients without AIDS [5–7]. Esophageal mucosal candidiasis occurs in patients undergoing chemotherapy or having hematologic malignancies, including lymphoma and leukemia [5, 6]. CMV is present in immunocompromised patients with solid organ or bone marrow transplants [7]. Simultaneous presentation of candidial and CMV esophageal infections from other causes of immunosuppression, without HIV infection, is rare [8–12]. One patient with immunosuppression secondary to prednisolone and cyclophosphamide therapy for severe interstitial pneumonia developed simultaneous candida and CMV esophageal infections [8]. Also, a kidney transplant recipient receiving methylprednisolone therapy had recurrent aphthous stomatitis secondary to candida and CMV [9]. Two patients with kidney transplants receiving tacrolimus therapy had simultaneous occurrence of oral mucosal ulcers from candida and CMV [10]. A patient with Hodgkin's lymphoma receiving intravenous immunoglobulin had concurrent candidial and CMV infections [11]. A review of the literature revealed that simultaneous candida and CMV infections can also rarely occur in other organs, such as the cornea [12].

Extreme symptoms (dysphagia and profound weight loss), signs (cachexia evidenced by extreme weight loss, very low BMI, and temporal and intercostal muscle wasting), endoscopic findings (massive cheesy esophageal mucosal exudate), radiologic findings (deep ulcers mimicking pseudo-diverticula), pathologic findings, and recurrence of both infections after 12 years are all attributed to profound immunocompromise (last CD4 cell count = 4 mil/L) from poor adherence to antiretroviral therapy. Study limitations include that it is retrospective, consists of one case, and presents only qualitatively new findings representing a severe spectrum of findings for esophageal candidiasis and CMV. This work illustrates the importance of antiretroviral therapy in AIDS patients to prevent opportunistic infections and the inclusion of esophageal CMV in the differential of esophageal pseudo-diverticula in severely immunocompromised patients. *Candida* unlikely played a significant pathophysiologic role in causing the profound "punched out" esophageal ulcers (Figure 5) that resembled esophageal pseudo-diverticula on barium swallow (Figure 4) reported in 2019, and these profound ulcers are most likely attributable to esophageal CMV infection [3].

CMV is diagnosed by immunohistochemical staining with anti-CMV DNA, in situ hybridization with CMV DNA, or isolation of CMV by viral cultures of esophageal biopsies. In the currently reported patient, CMV infection was confirmed by viral culture as well as by polymerase chain reaction.

Severe esophageal candidiasis is usually treated with fluconazole from 100 to 400 mg once daily orally or intravenously for 14 to 21 days but may require therapy extended to 28 days in patients with advanced AIDS [13]. From 50 to 60% of patients with AIDS experience ≥1 recurrent esophageal candidial infection per year despite episodic therapy and require repeat therapy [14]. CMV esophagitis is usually treated with ganciclovir or valganciclovir. Typical initial therapy is intravenous ganciclovir at 10–15 mg/kg/day in 2-3 divided doses/day for 3 to 6 weeks. Maintenance therapy with IV ganciclovir is indicated for GI infection recurrence after discontinuing therapy [15].

5. Learning Points

(i) We report a novel case of massive esophageal candidiasis and simultaneous profound CMV esophageal ulcers in a patient with AIDS.

(ii) Both esophageal infections recurred 12 years later.

(iii) After 12 years, the cytomegaloviral ulcers were so profound as to mimic esophageal pseudo-diverticula on barium esophagram. This case is only the second reported case of cytomegalovirus infection mimicking esophageal pseudo-diverticula. However, the prior case was only reported as an abstract and only had pathology consistent, but not diagnostic, of cytomegaloviral esophagitis.

(iv) In AIDS patients presenting with dysphagia, the differential diagnosis includes simultaneous esophageal candida and cytomegalovirus and considers cytomegalovirus in the differential of esophageal pseudodiverticulosis.

(v) Patients with other causes of immunocompromise, from chemotherapy, hematologic malignancies, or receiving immunosuppressive drugs after solid organ or bone marrow transplantation, can also rarely develop simultaneous esophageal candidial and CMV infections.

References

[1] B. E. Kodsi, P. C. Wickremesinghe, P. J. Kozinn, K. Iswara, and P. K. Goldberg, "Candida esophagitis: a prospective study of 27 cases," *Gastroenterology*, vol. 71, no. 5, pp. 715–719, 1976.

[2] L. Li and R. C. Chakinala, *Cytomegalovirus Esophagitis*-StatPearls, Treasure Island (FL), 2020.

[3] A. A. Mohamed, X.-l. Lu, and F. A. Mounmin, "Diagnosis and treatment of esophageal candidiasis: current updates," *Canadian Journal of Gastroenterology and Hepatology*, vol. 2019, Article ID 3585136, 6 pages, 2019.

[4] R. Sabbagh, N. Khoury, and F. Antaki, "A case of pseudo-diverticulosis of the esophagus associated with HIV and CMV," *American Journal of Gastroenterology*, vol. 106, p. S174, 2011.

[5] J. Yakoob, W. Jafri, and S. Abid, "Candidaesophagitis: risk factors in non-HIV population in Pakistan," *World Journal of Gastroenterology*, vol. 9, no. 10, pp. 2328–2331, 2003.

[6] M. Rosołowski and M. Kierzkiewicz, "Etiology, diagnosis and treatment of infectious esophagitis," *Gastroenterology Review*, vol. 6, no. 6, pp. 333–337, 2013.

[7] L. Li and R. C. Chakinala, *Cytomegalovirus Esophagitis*-StatPearls Publishing, Treasure Island, FL, USA, 2020, https://www.ncbi.nlm.nih.gov/books/NBK556110/.

[8] T. Yoshioka, M. Ikeda, and N. Kanda, "Sequential infection by herpes simplex virus, candida species, and cytomegalovirus species in esophagus," *Gastrointestinal Endoscopy*, vol. 90, no. 2, pp. 307-308, 2019.

[9] K. Ito, T. Okuno, A. Sawada et al., "Recurrent aphthous stomatitis caused by cytomegalovirus, Herpes simplex virus, and candida species in a kidney transplant recipient: a case report," *Transplantation Proceedings*, vol. 51, no. 3, pp. 993–997, 2019.

[10] D. Olczak-Kowalczyk, J. Pawłowska, B. Cukrowska et al., "Local presence of cytomegalovirus and Candida species vs oral lesions in liver and kidney transplant recipients," *Annals of Transplantation*, vol. 13, no. 4, pp. 28–33, 2008.

[11] M. Mustafa Ali, A. L. Ruano Mendez, and H. E. Carraway, "Hemophagocytic lymphohistiocytosis in a patient with Hodgkin lymphoma and concurrent EBV, CMV, and *Candida* infections," *Journal of Investigative Medicine High Impact Case Reports*, vol. 5, no. 1, Article ID 2324709616684514, 2017.

[12] P. R. Egbert, R. B. Pollard, J. G. Galagher, and T. C. Merigan, "Cytomegalovirus retinitis in immunosuppressed hosts," *Annals of Internal Medicine*, vol. 93, no. 5, pp. 664–670, 1980.

[13] J. Vazquez, "Optimal management of oropharyngeal and esophageal candidiasis in patients living with HIV infection," *HIV/AIDS (Auckland, NZ)*, vol. 2, pp. 89–101, 2010.

[14] M. Bruatto, V. Vidotto, G. Marinuzzi, R. Raiteri, and A. Sinicco, "Candida albicans biotypes in human immunodeficiency virus type 1-infected patients with oral candidiasis before and after antifungal therapy," *Journal of Clinical Microbiology*, vol. 29, no. 4, pp. 726–730, 1991.

[15] L. Li and R. C. Chakinale, *Cytomegalovirus Esophagitis*, Stat Pearls Publishing, Treasure Island, FL, USA, 2021.

35

Hepatic Squamous Cell Carcinoma Diagnosed by Endoscopic Ultrasound-Guided Fine-Needle Aspiration

Koki Yamada[1] **Susumu Shinoura**[2] **and Kaoru Kikuchi**[3]

[1]*Department of Gastroenterology, Okinawa Chubu Hospital, 271 Miyazato, Uruma 904-2293, Japan*
[2]*School of Psychology and Healthcare Management at Akasaka, Department of Healthcare Management, International University of Health and Welfare, 4-1-26 Akasaka, Minato, Tokyo 107-8402, Japan*
[3]*Division of Gastroenterology, Yaeyama Hospital, 584-1 Maezato, Ishigaki 907-0002, Okinawa, Japan*

Correspondence should be addressed to Koki Yamada; yamadakoki@gmail.com

Academic Editor: Chia-Tung Shun

Primary hepatic squamous cell carcinoma (SCC) is a rare malignancy with aggressive clinical features. This is the first case report of a primary hepatic SCC diagnosed by endoscopic ultrasound-guided fine-needle aspiration (EUS-FNA), which is a reliable and safe procedure for the histopathological diagnosis of liver lesions, even if the percutaneous approach is difficult due to ascites or hypervascularity at the puncture site. A 52-year-old man presented to the emergency department of a tertiary referral hospital with right upper quadrant abdominal pain and abdominal distention. Given the laboratory data, a diagnosis of spontaneous bacterial peritonitis (SBP) was made. Concurrently, an abdominal computed tomography (CT) scan revealed an 8 cm hypodense mass with delayed peripheral enhancement in the left hepatic lobe and paraaortic and perihepatic lymphadenopathy. As persistent ascites precluded percutaneous liver biopsy, we performed EUS-FNA of the liver mass, and the obtained specimen showed SCC. As otorhinolaryngological consultation and whole-body investigations, including chest CT, upper and lower endoscopy, and positron emission tomography CT, were all unremarkable except for the liver lesion and lymph nodes, a diagnosis of primary hepatic SCC with systemic lymph node metastasis was made. After treatment of SBP with antibiotics, we initiated chemotherapy concurrent with radiation therapy, adapted to his liver function. Radiation and three cycles of chemotherapy were not effective as the disease progressed, as seen on the follow-up CT scan, and the patient died of hepatic failure on the 134th day after diagnosis. In conclusion, EUS-FNA was a reliable method for tissue sampling in liver malignancies, particularly in selected patients with contraindications for percutaneous biopsy.

1. Introduction

Histopathologic examination of biopsy specimens obtained from atypical liver masses is known to provide essential diagnostic information, thus significantly improving patient care [1]. Occasionally, percutaneous liver biopsy is limited by ascites or coagulopathy secondary to poor liver function. Meanwhile, endoscopic ultrasound-guided fine-needle aspiration (EUS-FNA) has been a reliable method for diagnosing intraabdominal masses [2]. Multiple articles regarding EUS-FNA of the liver have been published, and according to the studies, EUS-FNA has had equivalent efficacy and safety compared with percutaneous liver biopsy [1]. This is the first case report of a hepatic squamous cell carcinoma (SCC) diagnosed by EUS-FNA in a patient with hepatic cirrhosis.

2. Case Presentation

A 52-year-old Japanese man with compensated liver cirrhosis secondary to hepatitis B presented to the emergency room of a tertiary referral hospital with chief complaints of fever, right upper quadrant abdominal pain, and abdominal distension. The patient had gained 4 kgs over the past 3 months. Before arriving at the emergency room, the patient had an episode of chills. His vital signs were as follows: blood pressure, 90/50 mmHg; pulse rate, 136 beats per minute; and body temperature, 39.4°C. On physical examination, the abdomen was distended with hepatomegaly and was positive for shifting dullness and tenderness in the left upper quadrant. Laboratory data were as follows: white blood cell count, 19800/μL; platelet count, 92,000/μL; alkaline phosphatase, 358 U/L; serum albumin, 2.6 g/dL; prothrombin time, 14.6 s; international normalized ratio, 1.27; alpha-fetoprotein, 19.5 ng/mL; carbohydrate antigen, 19-9, 132 U/ml; and protein induced by vitamin K absence-II of 16%. Ascitic fluid analysis showed a white cell count of 10,800/μL (56% neutrophils). Blood and ascitic fluid cultures were negative. With regard to imaging studies, an abdominal ultrasound showed a hypoechoic, mosaic-patterned mass in the lateral segment of the left lobe of the cirrhotic liver (Figure 1(a)). A computed tomography (CT) scan with intravenous (IV) contrast revealed hypodense hepatic masses with peripheral delayed enhancement. The masses in the left and right hepatic lobes measured 8 cm and 2 cm, respectively. The CT scan also showed moderate ascites and paraaortic and perihepatic lymphadenopathy (Figure 1(b)). Marked hyperintensity of both the left and right hepatic lobe masses was revealed on diffusion-weighted magnetic resonance imaging (MRI), while peripheral arterial enhancement was seen on gadolinium ethoxybenzyl diethylenetriamine pentaacetic acid-enhanced MRI (Figures 2(a)–2(d)). A fluorodeoxyglucose-positron emission tomography (FDG-PET) scan showed significant accumulation in the left lobe and multiple hot spots in the paraaortic region (Figure 3).

Given the above laboratory data and imaging findings, a diagnosis of spontaneous bacterial peritonitis (SBP) and bilateral hepatic lobe lesion with multiple lymph node metastases was made. For SBP, IV antibiotics (ceftriaxone 2 g/day) were started. Based on the imaging findings, the radiologist suspected the formation of mixed type hepatocellular carcinoma or intrahepatic cholangiocarcinoma mass. On transabdominal ultrasound, the hepatic lesion was exposed at the hepatic surface without intervening normal hepatic component and ascites was noted at the hepatic surface. These factors precluded percutaneous liver mass biopsy because of the high risk of bleeding. On the other hand, EUS view from the gastric station showed no significant amount of ascites (Figure 4(a)). EUS-FNA targeting the left lobe mass was performed from the gastric station view without worrisome vasculature or ascites, by using a 22-gauge aspiration needle (EXPECT®, Boston Scientific Co., Natick, MA, USA) with 3 passes (Figure 4(b)). Though rapid on-site evaluation was not performed due to the shortage of a pathology technician, an adequate amount of the specimen was obtained without any complications. The histopathological analysis showed a well-differentiated squamous cell carcinoma with necrosis. Components of neither hepatocellular carcinoma nor adenocarcinoma were found in the specimen. Finally, a pathological diagnosis of SCC was made (Figure 4(c)).

As we initially suspected metastatic SCC of the liver, an extensive workup including chest CT, esophagogastroduodenoscopy, colonoscopy, and otorhinolaryngological examination was performed, all of which showed negative findings. Given the above results, a diagnosis of primary SCC of the liver was made.

After 2 weeks of antibiotic treatment for SBP, the patient's liver function gradually improved to a Child–Pugh's score of 6. The patient was fully informed that the diagnosis was primary SCC of the liver and was in agreement with the adjusted chemoradiation therapy. The patient was started on radiation therapy (50 Gy) for the liver mass and paraaortic lymph nodes, followed by chemotherapy comprising cisplatin (50 mg/m^2) and fluorouracil (500 mg/m^2). Given the patient's comorbidity of cirrhosis, the dose of the chemotherapy was reduced. In total, three cycles of chemotherapy were administered. Radiation with three cycles of chemotherapy was not effective as the disease progressed, as seen on the follow-up CT scan, and the patient died of hepatic failure on the 134th day after diagnosis.

Written informed consent was obtained from the patient's family for the publication of this case report and its accompanying images. This study was also approved by the hospital board committee (approval number OCH-66).

3. Discussion

Primary hepatic SCC is rare. Zhang et al. [3] enlisted 31 cases that have been previously reported in the literature and four other patients encountered in their practice. According to the article [3], the average age of the patients was 54 years (range of 18–83 years) with a male to female ratio of 19 : 16. Zhang et al. [3] discussed that of the above 35 patients, 57% (20/35) had liver cysts, 20% (7/35) had bile duct stones, and 5.7% (2/35) had both with a tendency of worse prognosis in SCC patients with accompanying liver cysts than with bile duct stones. Other possible risk factors for primary SCC of the liver were hepatic teratoma, liver cirrhosis, and Caroli's disease [4]. A possible explanation for the occurrence of primary SCC of the liver is a hypothesis—the lesion may have originated from the tumor transformation of the biliary epithelium under chronic inflammation or metaplasia and subsequent neoplastic transformation of the preexisting cysts of the liver [3]. However, no proven explanation for the mechanism is available thus far. The clinical course of primary hepatic SCC, especially with underlying liver cirrhosis, is very aggressive, and it is difficult to achieve survival of >6 months even with several therapies combined (including surgical resection, chemotherapy, radiotherapy, and transcatheter arterial chemoembolization) [5]. The most frequently used chemotherapy regimen for hepatic SCC as described in the literature comprises cisplatin and fluorouracil [6]. However, due to its rarity, the definite management of hepatic SCC has not been established thus far.

Percutaneous liver biopsy remains an essential tool for the evaluation of focal liver masses [7]. Sensitivity, positive predictive value (PPV), negative predictive value (NPV), and overall accuracy were 90%, 100%, 51.7%, and 91%, respectively [8, 9]. Moreover, a percutaneous approach can target

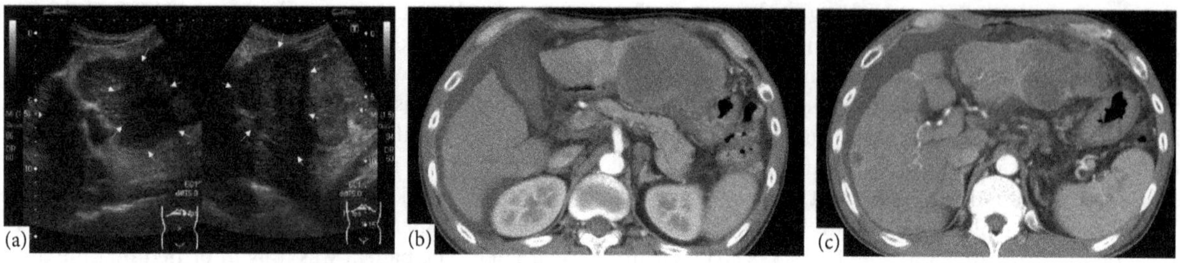

Figure 1: (a) Abdominal ultrasound showing a hypoechoic, mosaic-like, giant mass in the lateral segment of the left hepatic lobe of the cirrhotic liver (arrows). (b), (c) Early arterial phase of a contrast-enhanced computed tomography scan showing an 8 cm hypodense mass in the left hepatic lobe, a hypodense mass with ring-like enhancement in the right lobe, and multiple swollen lymph nodes.

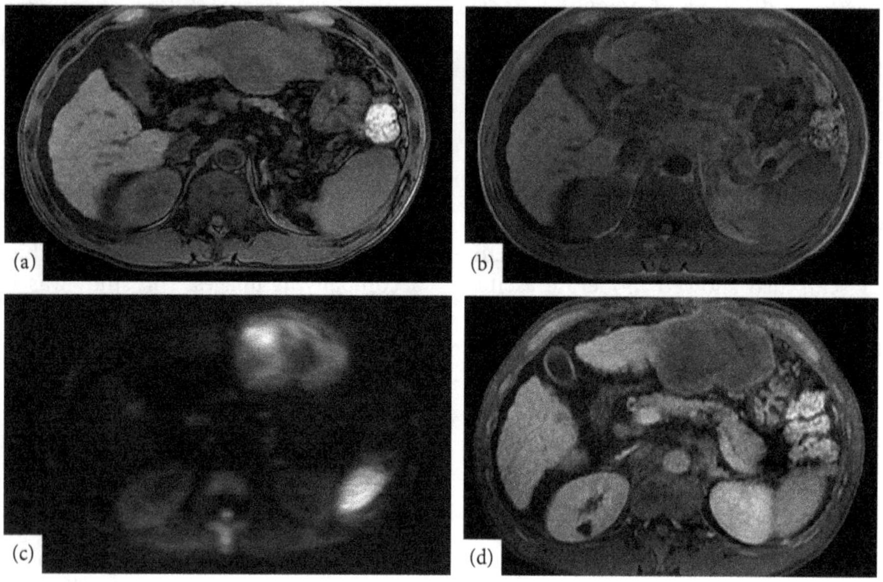

Figure 2: Marked hyperintensity on both the left and right hepatic lobe masses is revealed on diffusion-weighted magnetic resonance imaging (MRI), while peripheral arterial enhancement is seen on gadolinium ethoxybenzyl diethylenetriamine pentaacetic acid-enhanced MRI. (a) T1 in-phase. (b) T1 out-phase. (c) Diffusion-weighted image. (d) Hepatic phase.

multiple parts of the liver including the bilateral and caudate lobes.

The contraindications of percutaneous liver biopsy are thrombocytopenia and coagulopathy [10]. It is suggested that platelet counts of less than 50,000/mm^3 or a PT-INR of above 1.5 should force clinicians to consider suspending the procedure to avoid bleeding [7]. With regard to bleeding complications, the rate is reported to be around 2% [11]. Additionally, a systematic review of 1340 patients evaluated the risk of needle tract seeding following percutaneous liver tumor biopsy, which was reported to be 2.7% overall [12].

In contrast, a prospective study reported the diagnostic accuracy of EUS-FNA in hepatic masses to be between 82% and 100% and the sensitivity, specificity, NPV, and PPV to be 94%, 100%, 78%, and 100%, respectively [13]. Additionally, EUS-FNA can produce specimens at the most comparable to the specimens obtained in percutaneous liver biopsy [13]. One study that directly compared percutaneous liver biopsy (60 patients) and EUS-FNA (30 patients) revealed that EUS-FNA has equivalent feasibility of histological diagnosis (percutaneous liver biopsy = 100% and EUS-FNA = 93%, $p = 0.841$).

If the liver tissue sampling is aimed at a "benign-malignant assessment," a 22-gauge aspiration needle can obtain an adequate specimen for diagnosis [2, 13]. However, to visualize and target the right lobe mass with EUS-FNA is actually difficult [14], and it is suggested that percutaneous biopsy would be a better option for lesions that are located in the right lobe of the liver. When concerned about adverse events, EUS-FNA appears to be a safe and minimally invasive procedure for the normal liver, with an almost equivalent or even less bleeding complication rate as compared with percutaneous tumor biopsy (of less than 2%) [15, 16]. To the best of our knowledge, only one case of needle-track seeding following EUS-FNA of the liver was reported [17].

In the present case, we decided to perform EUS-FNA as the liver masses were mainly located in the left lobe and the visibility from the gastric station on EUS provided us with an excellent view of the liver mass without worrisome vasculature or ascites as compared to the percutaneous view. Based on clinical studies which showed that both 19-gauge and 22-gauge needles attain equivalent feasibility in histological diagnosis [15] and that it is preferable to choose a

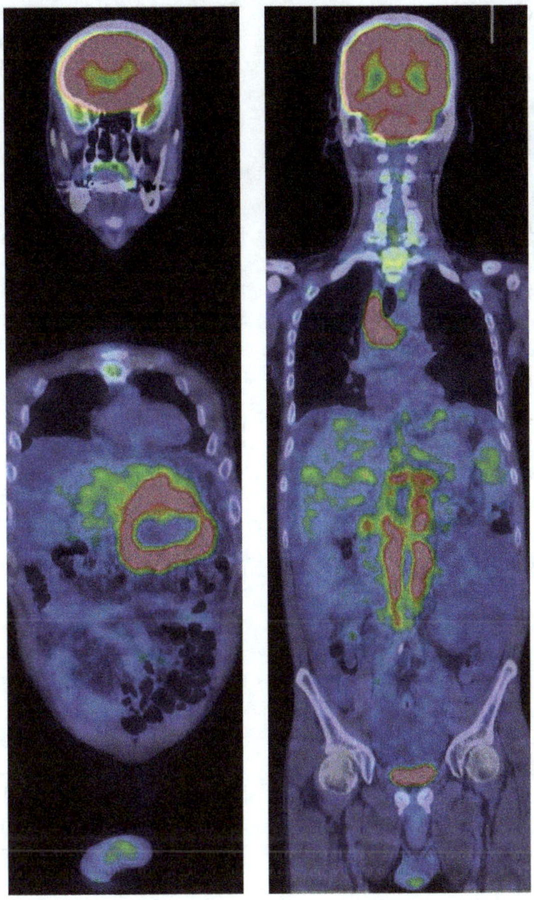

(a) (b)

FIGURE 3: Fluorodeoxyglucose positron emission tomography scan showing significant accumulation in the left lobe and multiple hot spots in the paraaortic region.

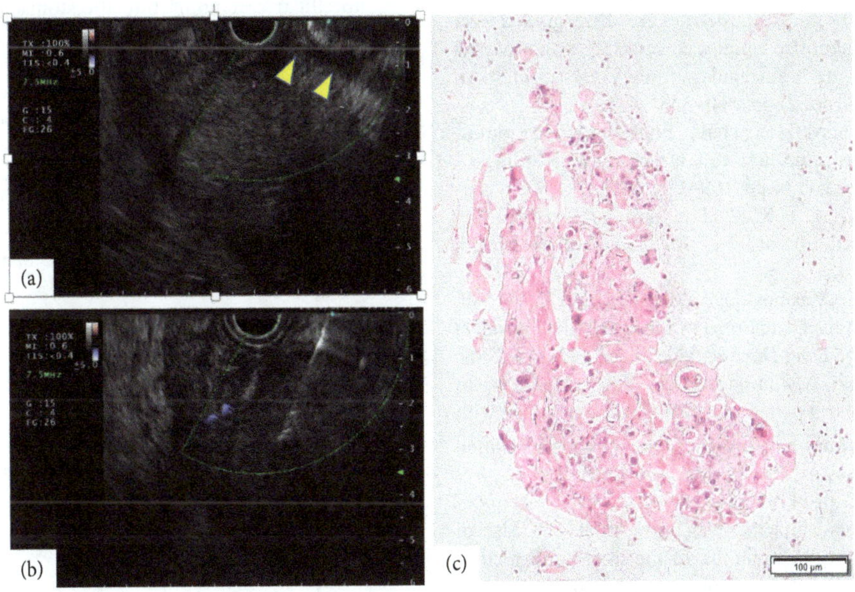

FIGURE 4: (a) Endoscopic ultrasound view from the gastric station showing no significant amount of ascites. Arrowheads correspond to the surface of an exposed hepatic mass. (b) Endoscopic ultrasound-guided fine-needle aspiration of the liver mass performed from the view without worrisome vasculature or ascites. (c) Histopathological view of squamous cell carcinoma with hematoxylin and eosin staining. Components of neither hepatocellular carcinoma nor adenocarcinoma are found.

thinner needle to reduce bleeding complications [18], we chose a 22-gauge needle instead of a 19-gauge to obtain the specimen to minimize the risk of bleeding. An adequate quantity of the specimen was obtained for diagnosing malignancy, and no adverse events were observed after EUS-FNA in this case.

Given the rarity of the primary hepatic SCC, adenosquamous cell carcinoma was a differential diagnosis in the present case; it was less likely from the histopathological evaluation that the specimen was negative for individual cell keratinization, intracellular bridges, glandular differentiation, or intracellular and intraluminal mucin accumulation, which were the characteristic features of adenosquamous cell carcinoma [19].

Primary hepatic SCC is rare and is known for its aggressive clinical course. We concluded that EUS-guided fine-needle biopsy was a reliable method for tissue sampling in liver malignancies, particularly in selected patients with contraindications for percutaneous biopsy.

Authors' Contributions

KY performed conceptualization, formal analysis, and writing; SS performed conceptualization and supervision; and KK performed supervision.

Acknowledgments

The authors thank Editage for English proofreading.

References

[1] J. J. Pineda, D. L. Diehl, C. L. Miao et al., "EUS-guided liver biopsy provides diagnostic samples comparable with those via the percutaneous or transjugular route," *Gastrointestinal Endoscopy*, vol. 83, no. 2, pp. 360–365, 2016.

[2] D. Oh, D. W. Seo, S. M. Hong et al., "Endoscopic ultrasound-guided fine-needle aspiration can target right liver mass," *Endosc Ultrasound*, vol. 6, pp. 109–115, 2017.

[3] X.-F. Zhang, Z.-Q. Du, X.-M. Liu, and Y. Lv, "Primary squamous cell carcinoma of liver," *Medicine*, vol. 94, no. 28, p. e868, 2015.

[4] S. Naik, W. Waris, L. Carmosino, A. Mehrishi, and M. W. Saif, "Primary squamous cell carcinoma of the liver," *The Journal of Gastrointestinal and Liver Diseases*, vol. 18, pp. 487–489, 2009.

[5] T. Yoshida, H. Aoki, A. Kurinaga et al., "An autopsy case of primary squamous cell carcinoma of the liver associated with hepatitis C virus antibody positive liver cirrhosis," *Nihon Shokakibyo Gakkai Zasshi = The Japanese Journal of Gastro-Enterology*, vol. 95, pp. 1141–1146, 1998.

[6] J. Kaneko, M. Matsushita, M. Nagasawa et al., "A case of primary squamous cell carcinoma of the liver confirmed at autopsy," *Kanzo*, vol. 59, no. 2, pp. 125–132, 2018.

[7] C. N. Ghent, "Percutaneous liver biopsy: reflections and refinements," *Canadian Journal of Gastroenterology*, vol. 20, no. 2, pp. 75–79, 2006.

[8] F. Durand, J. M. Regimbeau, J. Belghiti et al., "Assessment of the benefits and risks of percutaneous biopsy before surgical resection of hepatocellular carcinoma," *Journal of Hepatology*, vol. 35, no. 2, pp. 254–258, 2001.

[9] E. Caturelli, L. Solmi, M. Anti et al., "Ultrasound guided fine needle biopsy of early hepatocellular carcinoma complicating liver cirrhosis: a multicentre study," *Gut*, vol. 53, no. 9, pp. 1356–1362, 2004.

[10] G. Menghini, "One-second needle biopsy of the liver," *Gastroenterology*, vol. 35, no. 2, pp. 190–199, 1958.

[11] M. Midia, D. Odedra, O. Devang, A. Shuster, R. Midia, and J. Muir, "Predictors of bleeding complications following percutaneous image-guided liver biopsy: a scoping review," *Diagnostic and Interventional Radiology*, vol. 25, no. 1, pp. 71–80, 2019.

[12] M. A. Silva, B. Hegab, C. Hyde, B. Guo, J. A. C. Buckels, and D. F. Mirza, "Needle track seeding following biopsy of liver lesions in the diagnosis of hepatocellular cancer: a systematic review and meta-analysis," *Gut*, vol. 57, no. 11, pp. 1592–1596, 2008.

[13] E. Akay, D. Atasoy, E. Altınkaya et al., "Endoscopic ultrasound-guided fine needle aspiration using a 22 g needle for hepatic lesions: single-center experience," *Clinical Endoscopy*, vol. 54, no. 3, pp. 404–412, 2021.

[14] J. TenBerge, B. J. Hoffman, R. H. Hawes et al., "EUS-guided fine needle aspiration of the liver: indications, yield, and safety based on an international survey of 167 cases," *Gastrointestinal Endoscopy*, vol. 55, no. 7, pp. 859–862, 2002.

[15] A. H. Ali, S. Panchal, D. S. Rao et al., "The efficacy and safety of endoscopic ultrasound-guided liver biopsy versus percutaneous liver biopsy in patients with chronic liver disease: a retrospective single-center study," *Journal of Ultrasound*, vol. 23, no. 2, pp. 157–167, 2020.

[16] B. J. Hoffman, R. H. Hawes, C. Van Enckevort et al., "EUS-guided fine needle aspiration of the liver: indications, yield, and safety based on an international survey of 167 cases," *Gastrointestinal Endoscopy*, vol. 55, pp. 859–862, 2002.

[17] M. Kasi, S. Rashid, S. A. J. Wallace et al., "Seeding of hepatocellular carcinoma into the stomach wall following endoscopic ultrasound and fine-needle aspiration biopsy," *Oxford Medical Case Reports*, vol. 2018, no. 7, 2018.

[18] D. C. Rockey, S. H. Caldwell, Z. D. Goodman, R. C. Nelson, and A. D. Smith, "Liver biopsy," *Hepatology*, vol. 49, no. 3, pp. 1017–1044, 2009.

[19] S. Gao, D. Chen, L. Huang, L. Wu, R. Dai, and Y. Shan, "Primary adenosquamous carcinoma of the liver: a case report and review of the literature," *International Journal of Clinical and Experimental Pathology*, vol. 8, no. 8, pp. 9687–9692, 2015.

36

Iatrogenic Severe Splenic Injury after Colonoscopy

Ikponmwosa Enofe,[1] Jacob Burch,[1] Julie Yam,[2] and Manoj Rai[1]

[1]*Internal Medicine Resident, Michigan State University, Sparrow Hospital, East Lansing, MI, USA*
[2]*Gastroenterology Fellow, Michigan State University, East Lansing, MI, USA*

Correspondence should be addressed to Jacob Burch; jacob.burch@sparrow.org

Academic Editor: Yoshihiro Moriwaki

Colonoscopy is a low-risk procedure performed for screening and diagnostic purposes. About 15 million colonoscopies were carried out in the United States in 2012 with this number projected to increase. Injury to the spleen as a complication of colonoscopy is still a rather rare occurrence. We report a case of significant splenic injury, American Association of Surgery for Trauma (AAST) grade III with hemoperitoneum, in a patient following diagnostic colonoscopy, managed conservatively without the need for invasive or salvage surgical procedure.

1. Introduction

Colonoscopy is a low-risk procedure for screening, diagnostic, and therapeutic purposes [1]. Bleeding and colonic perforation are the most commonly described complications following colonoscopy [1–3]. Splenic injury is also a complication of colonoscopy, with only about 100 reported cases worldwide, making it a rare complication of colonoscopy [1, 2]. Here, we present a patient who developed significant splenic injury (grade III) [4] with hemoperitoneum as a complication of diagnostic colonoscopy. This case report highlights the importance of a high index of suspicion in patients with vague abdominal symptoms after colonoscopy and the need to increase awareness for splenic injury as a possible complication of colonoscopy, especially among family physicians, emergency room providers, and internists. We also provide an update in the management of this rare but potentially fatal complication of colonoscopy.

2. Case Report

A 72-year-old female presented to the emergency room (ER) with complaints of left upper quadrant (LUQ) abdominal pain and weakness 8 hours after a diagnostic colonoscopy was performed to investigate chronic constipation. Her past medical history was significant for two episodes of unprovoked deep vein thrombosis including one episode with associated pulmonary embolism for which she was on oral anticoagulation with warfarin. The patient was advised to stop warfarin 7 days before her colonoscopy and to use enoxaparin for bridging therapy. Prothrombin time (PT) and the international normalized ratio (INR) measured on the day of the procedure were 19.0 sec and 2.0, respectively. Colonoscopy was performed under monitored anesthesia care (MAC) with propofol. Normal findings were reported with no technical difficulties encountered nor any therapeutic intervention performed or biopsies taken. The duration of the procedure was 16 minutes. At discharge, she remained asymptomatic, and warfarin was resumed.

On return to the ER, examination revealed normal vital signs, a distended abdomen, and left upper quadrant (LUQ) abdominal tenderness. The rest of her physical examination was unremarkable. Laboratory examination showed a hemoglobin concentration of 8.1 g/dl, PT 15.3 s, INR 1.6, and activated partial prothrombin time (aPTT) of 22.3 s. Platelets were 322000 U/L at presentation. The rest of her labs were within normal limits. A computed tomography (CT) scan of the abdomen and pelvis with contrast revealed perisplenic heterogenous and hypodense fluid collection suspicious for hemorrhage or subcapsular hematoma with free fluid extending into the pelvis (Figures 1–3). No pneumoperitoneum was seen. Warfarin was discontinued, and she was managed nonoperatively with serial abdominal exams and hemoglobin measurements. Hemoglobin remained stable during hospitalization, and she did not require any blood transfusions. Warfarin was resumed on day 4. Hemoglobin was monitored for another 48 hours after resuming her on anticoagulation and remained stable at 9.0 g/dl.

The patient was discharged home with follow-up instructions to see her primary care physician for hemoglobin and INR check 48 hours following discharge. On follow-up 48 hours and a month after discharge, her hemoglobin was stable, and she had no abdominal discomfort or pain.

3. Discussion

Splenic injury is a rare complication of colonoscopy [1–3, 5–10]. The symptoms associated with postcolonoscopy splenic injury are nonspecific, and there is significant variability in the timing of onset of symptoms [1]; hence, it poses a diagnostic dilemma for clinicians [4]. Most often, it is diagnosed after it appears on the CT abdomen performed to rule out differentials including colonic perforation or retained gas following colonoscopy [5, 6, 11]. This may lead to a delay in diagnosis and an increased number of critical care admissions, with worse mortality outcomes [6, 12]. Most patients with splenic injury present within 24 hours after procedure [1–12]. However, some patients may present 10 to 14 days after procedure [2, 7, 13, 14] with the longest time reported from procedure to presentation being two weeks [2]. Left upper quadrant abdominal pain is the most commonly reported presenting symptom [6, 7]. Pain radiating to the left shoulders (Kehr's sign) may be present [6, 7] but has been reported to occur in as low as 34.4% of patients [1]. In some cases, patients may be completely asymptomatic [6, 7]. Clinical signs of hypotension, anemia, and elevated white blood cell count may be present [2, 4, 6].

The exact incidence of splenic injury following colonoscopy remains unknown [1, 6, 11] with a reported incidence of 1 per 6,000 to 1 per 100,000 colonoscopies performed [2, 6, 12]. This may be due to underreporting or misdiagnosis, and as such, its real incidence may be much higher [7]. Splenic injury following colonoscopy has a higher occurrence in women and older aged patients with a mean age of about 63 years [1, 7, 8, 11]. Risk factors associated with this complication are frequently a result of excessive manipulation, the presence of a redundant colon, history of previous abdominal surgeries, inflammation from previous intra-abdominal infections, and therapeutic colonoscopies. Splenomegaly, in addition to the use of propofol causing deep sedation, medications that increase bleeding risk (anticoagulants or antiplatelets), and inadequate bowel preparations, has been associated with a higher risk for injury to the spleen during colonoscopies [1, 2, 6–8, 13], although no direct causality has been identified with these risk factors and controversies still exist. In a review of 77 patients by Corcillo et al., anticoagulants and antiplatelets were not associated with an increased risk of injury to the spleen during colonoscopy. In the same review, splenomegaly and technically

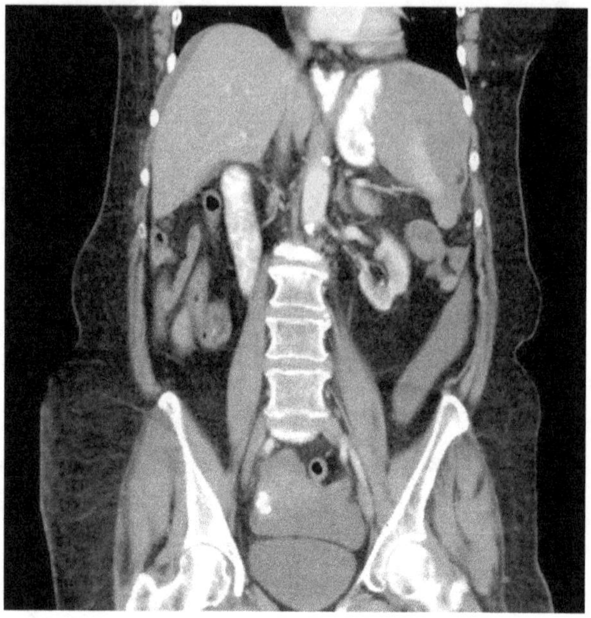

Figure 1: Coronal CT section of the abdomen and pelvis showing a large splenic hematoma.

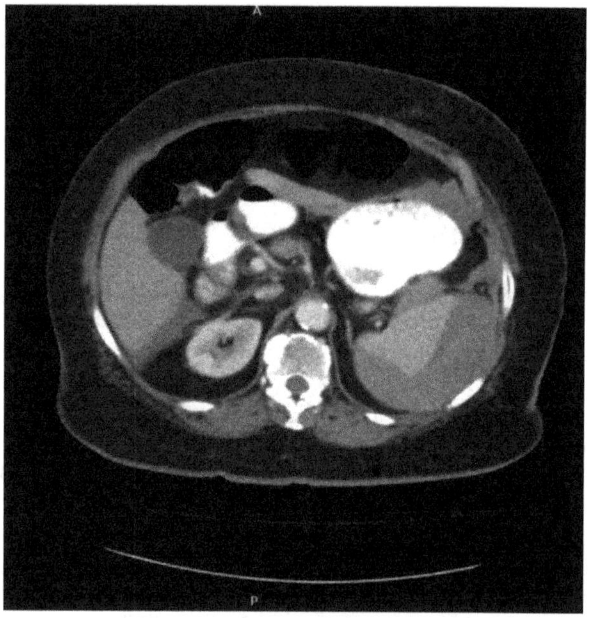

Figure 2: Axial CT scan section showing large subcapsular hematoma of the spleen with hemoperitoneum.

difficult colonoscopies, polypectomies, or biopsies were also not associated with a higher risk for injury to the spleen [8, 13]. Similarly, Singla et al. retrospectively reviewed over 102 cases of splenic injury occurring during colonoscopy reported in the literature over a 30-year period, and no association was observed between risk of splenic injury and the use of antiplatelet or anticoagulants, prior abdominal surgeries, and difficulty during colonoscopy [10].

The exact mechanism by which splenic injury occurs during colonoscopy is unknown. Maneuvers such as the endoscope slide by advancement, alpha maneuver, hooking of

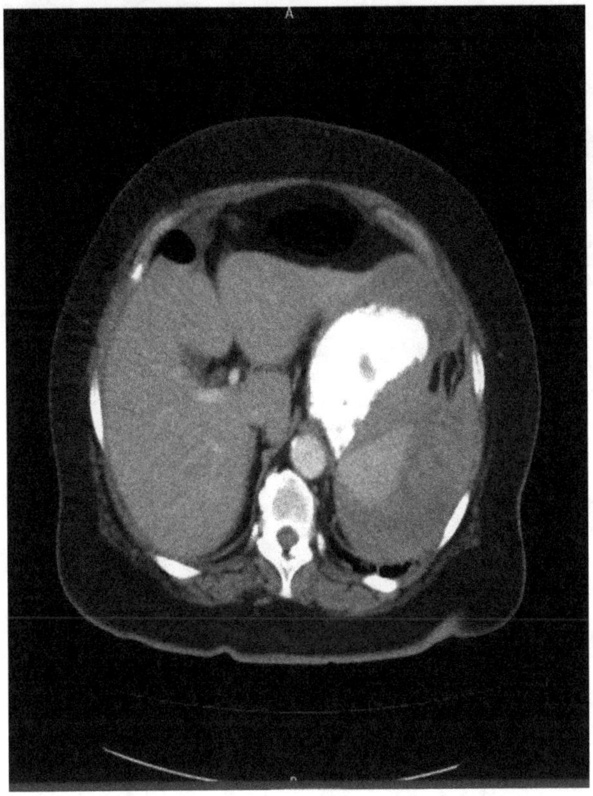

Figure 3: Axial CT scan, cross-section view, showing subcapsular hematoma of the spleen.

the splenic flexure, and straightening of the sigmoid loop may lead to avulsion of the splenocolic ligament resulting in laceration or rupture of the spleen [3, 4, 10–12, 15]. Furthermore, adhesions between the colon and the spleen from previous abdominal surgeries, inflammation, or infections have been suggested to increase traction from decreased mobility of the spleen and colon leading to splenic injury [4, 7, 8]. Precautionary measures such as placing patients in the left lateral position are recommended and are associated with a decreased occurrence in injuries to the spleen [1–6, 13]. This association is best explained by a reduction in the opposing tensions between the colon and the spleen from reduced traction in the splenocolic ligament and adjacent adhesions [1, 3, 7]. Other potential precautionary measures include avoiding looping [3], desufflation, and cautious sedation during the procedure [8]. Furthermore, few cases have reported splenic injury following upper gastrointestinal endoscopy (EGD) and endoscopic retrograde cholangiopancreatography (ERCP) [3, 12, 16, 17]. The exact mechanism of injury is unknown [15, 16] but was attributed to the traction of the greater curvature of the stomach and short gastric vessels [16].

Abdominal CT scan is the most accurate test used for diagnosing splenic injury [3, 5–11, 13, 14], with subscapular hematoma being the most common injury pattern encountered following colonoscopy [7, 13]. A CT scan has 98% specificity and sensitivity in diagnosing splenic injuries [11, 12, 14]. CT scans in hemodynamically stable patients help with grading, provide useful information in management, and exclude other possible differentials. Patients with splenic injury American Association of Surgery for Trauma (AAST) grade III or higher may need surgery [8]. Persistent hemodynamic instability remains the most critical determining factor for surgical versus nonsurgical management which may include radiologic embolization of the splenic artery [7, 11]. Unfortunately, up to 77.4% of patients presenting with splenic injury after colonoscopy may need surgical exploration with as high as 95% of patients needing splenectomy [8, 12]. More recently, the use of proximal splenic artery embolization (PSAE) in patients managed conservatively has been suggested to reduce the need for salvage surgical intervention [8] due to the high failure rates in nonoperative, conservative management compared to patients with injuries from blunt external trauma [4, 8]. There is however no sufficient data to suggest better outcomes and to advocate its use preemptively, as the standard of care in hemodynamically stable patients with grade III or less who are managed conservatively. Fortunately, our patient who had therapeutic INR at the time of colonoscopy and significant (grade III) splenic injury with hemoperitoneum was successfully managed conservatively without the need for invasive or salvage surgical procedure despite high failure rate of conservative management reported in the literature.

Despite several potential risk factors such as female sex, older age, use of propofol (causing deep sedation) during MAC, and use of anticoagulation in our patient, we cannot conclusively say why our patient had injury to the spleen during diagnostic colonoscopy, given there are no clearly identifiable risk factors that predict its occurrence. Due to weak evidence in data concerning risk factors and nonspecific symptoms [4, 13], we advocate more studies to better explain the contribution of each of these identified potential risk factors for developing injury to the spleen during colonoscopy.

4. Conclusion

Splenic injury still is a rare but sometimes fatal complication following colonoscopy. Given the lack of properly identifiable risk factors and variation in its presentation, this rare but potentially fatal complication can present a diagnostic dilemma for clinicians and requires a high index of suspicion in patients with postprocedural pain following colonoscopy. Greater awareness is needed amongst healthcare professionals, including family physicians, emergency room doctors, midlevel staff, and internists about this potentially deadly but rare complication following colonoscopy. Increased awareness may help improve outcomes and decrease mortality.

Disclosure

The abstract of this case was presented at ACG 2019 Annual Scientific Meeting Abstracts San Antonio Texas: American College of Gastroenterology.

References

[1] S. Barbeiro, C. Atalaia-Martins, P. Marcos, J. Nobre, C. Gonçalves, and C. Aniceto, "Splenic rupture as a complication of colonoscopy," *GE-Portuguese Journal of Gastroenterology*, vol. 24, no. 4, pp. 188–192, 2016.

[2] A. Mazulis, A. Lakha, B. Qazi, and A. Shapiro, "Delayed presentation of splenic rupture after endoscopy in a patient with hemophilia A: case report and review of the literature," *ACG Case Reports Journal*, vol. 1, no. 4, pp. 175–177, 2014.

[3] S. Mohammad, A. Ramcharan, and S. Ponnapalli, "Splenic injury after elective colonoscopy," *JSLS*, vol. 13, pp. 616–619, 2009.

[4] D. Thiyagarajan and R. Jeanmonod, "Iatrogenic splenic laceration presenting as syncope," *Case Reports in Emergency Medicine*, vol. 2018, Article ID 7639527, 3 pages, 2018.

[5] M. A. Zappa, A. Aiolfi, I. Antonini, C. D. Musolino, and A. Porta, "Splenic rupture following colonoscopy: case report and literature review," *International Journal of Surgery Case Reports*, vol. 21, pp. 118–120, 2016.

[6] P. F. Lalor and B. D. Mann, "Splenic rupture after colonoscopy," *Journal of the Society of Laparoendoscopic Surgeons*, vol. 11, no. 1, pp. 151–156, 2007.

[7] S. Shankar and S. Rowe, "Splenic injury after colonoscopy: case report and review of literature," *The Ochsner Journal*, vol. 11, no. 3, pp. 276–281, 2011.

[8] A. Corcillo, S. Aellen, T. Zingg, P. Bize, N. Demartines, and A. Denys, "Endovascular treatment of active splenic bleeding after colonoscopy: a systematic review of the literature," *CardioVascular and Interventional Radiology*, vol. 36, no. 5, pp. 1270–1279, 2012.

[9] C. Johnson, M. Mader, D. M. Edwards, and T. Vesy, "Splenic rupture following colonoscopy: two cases with CT findings," *Emergency Radiology*, vol. 13, no. 1, pp. 47–49, 2006.

[10] S. Singla, D. Keller, P. Thirunavukarasu et al., "Splenic injury during colonoscopy-a complication that warrants urgent attention," *Journal of Gastrointestinal Surgery*, vol. 16, no. 6, pp. 1225–1234, 2012.

[11] A. N. Zhang, J. M. Sherigar, D. Guss et al., "A delayed presentation of splenic laceration and hemoperitoneum following an elective colonoscopy: a rare complication with uncertain risk factors," *SAGE Open Medical Case Reports*, vol. 6, 2018.

[12] E. Pavlidis, I. Gkizas, O. Mavromati et al., "Splenic injury following elective colonoscopy: a rare complication," *Journal of Surgical Case Reports*, vol. 2016, no. 12, 2016.

[13] G. Piccolo, M. D. Vita, A. Cavallaro et al., "Presentation and management of splenic injury after colonoscopy," *Surgical Laparoscopy, Endoscopy & Percutaneous Techniques*, vol. 24, no. 2, pp. 95–102, 2014.

[14] P. Ungprasert and V. Jaruvongvanich, "Splenic injury," *Chinese Medical Journal*, vol. 131, no. 3, pp. 372-373, 2018.

[15] D. D. Kingsley, C. R. Schermer, and M. M. Jamal, "Rare complications of endoscopic retrograde cholangiopancreatography: two case reports," *Journal of the Society of Laparoendoscopic Surgeons*, vol. 5, no. 2, pp. 171–173, 2001.

[16] A. Grammatopoulos, M. Moschou, and E. Rigopoulou, "Splenic injury complicating ERCP," *Annals of Gastroenterology*, vol. 27, no. 2, pp. 177-178, 2014.

[17] M. C. Townsend, D. R. Beauchamp, M. B. Evers, and K. L. Mattox, *Chapter 16. Sabiston Textbook of Surgery: The Biological Basis of Modern Surgical Practice*, pp. 407–448, Elsevier Saunders, Philadelphia, PA, USA, 20th edition, 2017.

37

Silica Desiccant Canister: An Unusual Colonic Foreign Body

Rajarajeshwari Ramachandran,[1] **Vikash Kumar**,[2] **Giovannie Isaac-Coss**,[2] **and Denzil Etienne**[1]

[1]*Department of Gastroenterology, Brooklyn Hospital Center, Brooklyn, NY, USA*
[2]*Department of Internal Medicine, Brooklyn Hospital Center, Brooklyn, NY, USA*

Correspondence should be addressed to Rajarajeshwari Ramachandran; rajeeeram@gmail.com

Academic Editor: Matteo Neri

We are reporting a case of incidental identification and removal of two silica desiccant canisters from the cecum in a patient undergoing screening colonoscopy.

1. Introduction

Ingested foreign bodies rarely cause life-threatening manifestations in adults. Once the foreign body moves past the lower esophageal sphincter, which is the narrowest part of the gastrointestinal tract, it usually passes spontaneously [1]. In this case report, we present a 51-year-old man in whom two pill desiccants were identified incidentally during screening colonoscopy.

2. Case Description

A 51-year-old man with a past medical history of vitamin D deficiency presented to the hospital for screening colonoscopy. The patient denied nausea, vomiting, abdominal pain, altered bowel habits, or bloody stools. Colonoscopy revealed two cylindrical foreign bodies labeled as "DO NOT EAT" in the cecum (Figures 1 and 2), and the examination was otherwise unremarkable. Both foreign bodies were removed using a Roth Net (Figure 3). After removal, the foreign bodies were identified as desiccant canisters (Figure 4). In retrospect, our patient indicated that he might have ingested the desiccant canisters mistaking them for the last two vitamin D capsules out of the medication container in the days leading up to the colonoscopy.

3. Discussion

Ingestion of foreign bodies can be accidental or intentional. Accidental ingestion of foreign bodies is common among children and in adults with dementia and visual impairment. Foreign body ingestions are commonly asymptomatic but, in some cases, might lead to complications and, in rare cases, necessitate surgery.

Desiccants are hygroscopic substances that absorb water and are often used in medication containers to maintain dryness inside the package. Desiccants are available as packets or cylinders, and ingredients are either silica gel or calcium oxide. Silica gel is nontoxic, while calcium oxide can react with saliva, reaching a temperature of 100°C within 1 minute, and the product of this reaction is calcium hydroxide and is strongly basic (pH of 12.6) and causes chemical burns of the mucosa as reported by Hagiwara et al. [2].

Pharmaceutical companies have labeled the desiccant packaging as "DO NOT EAT." However, as medications are manufactured in different colors and shapes and consumed by a wide demographic of patients including those with advanced age, lower educational status, language barriers, visual impairment, and memory disturbances, the "DO NOT EAT" labeling alone might not be sufficient to avoid

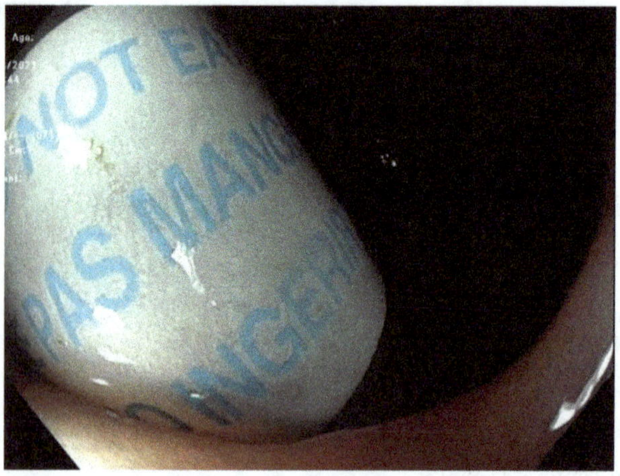

Figure 1: Cylindrical foreign body labeled "DO NOT EAT" in the cecum.

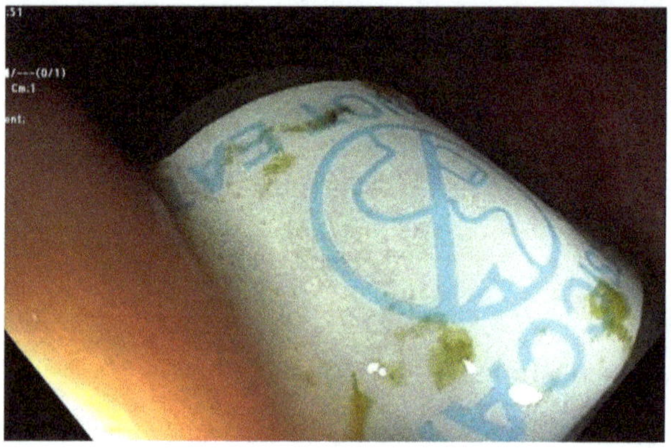

Figure 2: Cylindrical foreign body labeled "DO NOT EAT" in the cecum.

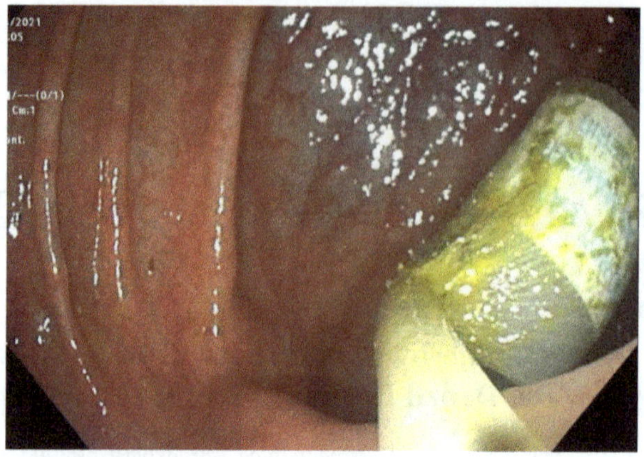

Figure 3: Foreign body removal using Roth Net.

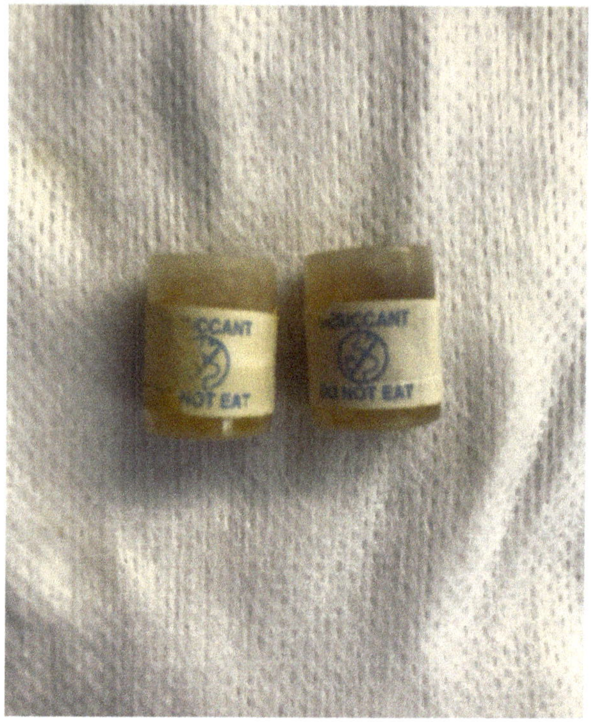

Figure 4: Desiccant canisters after removal.

accidental ingestion. By designing the desiccants in different colors and shapes compared to the medication, anchoring desiccants to the medication bottle, and involving the pharmacists in providing education to the patients regarding the desiccants included in the medication containers, accidental ingestion of desiccants can be reduced significantly [3].

In our literature review, we identified four patients who developed symptoms following accidental ingestion of desiccant canisters. Three elderly patients including a patient with a prior history of esophageal stricture secondary to gastroesophageal reflux disease (GERD) had a desiccant canister lodged in the esophagus causing acute hypoxic respiratory failure and were successfully treated endoscopically [3–5]. Fourth case was reported by Wu et al. in a young woman who developed abdominal pain and unintentional weight loss in the setting of chronic constipation [1]. In this patient, enteroclysis demonstrated a cylindrical foreign body proximal to the terminal ileum. Patient underwent ileocecectomy with removal of the dessicant canister and pathology specimen confirmed the diagnosis of Crohn's disease.

Our case is the first report of accidental ingestion of more than one desiccant canister, and it was identified as an unexpected colonic foreign body. We removed the desiccant canisters due to initial uncertainty regarding the nature of the foreign body and concern for patient safety given the labeling "DO NOT EAT." However, due to the absence of anatomical narrowing in the large intestine in our patient, he would have most likely passed the desiccant canisters spontaneously in his feces.

It is likely that ingestion of desiccant canisters is a more frequent occurrence in the general population but remains largely unrecognized due to lack of symptoms and need for further investigations. The United States Census Bureau estimates patients over age 65 will outnumber children under 18 by 2034 [6]. Due to the increasing aging population and the rising prevalence of GERD which could predispose to esophageal strictures, we anticipate higher rates of symptomatic cases from accidental desiccant ingestions unless additional safety measures are taken by the manufacturers.

Authors' Contributions

R. R. drafted and revised the manuscript for critically important intellectual content. V. K. and G. I. drafted and edited the manuscript. D. E. reviewed the manuscript for critically important intellectual content. All authors approved the final version of the paper.

References

[1] M. L. Wu, W. C. DeVos, and S. L. Flamm, "Desiccant recovered, crohn's disease discovered," *American Journal of Gastroenterology*, vol. 93, no. 12, pp. 2595–2597, 1998.
[2] Y. Hagiwara, K. Seki, and Y. Takahashi, "Oral chemical burn due to accidental ingestion of calcium oxide food desiccant in a patient with dementia," *Journal of International Medical Research*, vol. 48, no. 4, Article ID 030006052092006, 2020.
[3] W. Gerstein and Z. Liu, "Visually impaired elderly patient ingests pill desiccant, leading to acute hypoxic respiratory failure requiring intubation," *BMC Geriatrics*, vol. 17, no. 1, p. 166, 2017.
[4] J. A. Barkin and J. S. Barkin, "Desiccant-induced esophageal obstruction: an emerging patient safety issue," *ACG Case Reports Journal*, vol. 2, no. 1, p. 67, 2015.
[5] N. Lassiter, N. Yang, L. Tiyyagura, and K. S. Whitlow, "A case report highlighting that silica gel products are not always benign," *Clinical Practice and Cases in Emergency Medicine*, vol. 4, no. 4, pp. 576–579, 2020.
[6] J. Vespa, "The U.S joins other countries with large aging populations," 2018, https://www.census.gov/library/stories/2018/03/graying-america.html.

38

Cap-Assisted Endoscopic Mucosal Resection of an Incidental Rectal Traumatic Neuroma

Elias Estifan [1] **Varun Patel** [2] **and Matthew Grossman** [2]

[1] *Department of Internal Medicine, St. Joseph's University Medical Center-New York Medical College, Paterson, NJ 07503, USA*
[2] *Division of Gastroenterology, St. Joseph's University Medical Center-New York Medical College, Paterson, NJ 07503, USA*

Correspondence should be addressed to Elias Estifan; egestifan@gmail.com

Academic Editor: Haruhiko Sugimura

A traumatic neuroma is a well-known complication after acute trauma to a peripheral nerve; the nerve tries to re-establish continuity by an orderly growth of axons from the peripheral to distal stump through the proliferation of Schwann cells. However, this process is not always perfect, and aberrant repair gives rise to a neuroma. We present a 50-year-old female who underwent an initial colonoscopy for change in bowel habits and was found to have a 7 mm submucosal lesion in the proximal rectum. Endoscopic ultrasound was done which showed a hypoechoic lesion in the submucosal plane without muscularis propria invasion. The patient underwent successful cap-assisted endoscopic mucosal resection of the lesion without complication. Pathology of the specimen revealed a traumatic rectal neuroma with immunostaining positive for S100. However, this patient did not have any known risk factors such as previous surgery including polypectomy or hemorrhoidectomy or any previous rectal manipulation. Interestingly, this is the second case of traumatic rectal neuroma reported in the English-language literature.

1. Introduction

A traumatic neuroma develops from a non-neoplastic proliferation of the proximal end of a severed, partially transected, or injured nerve as a result of trauma or surgery. Most commonly, the lesion demonstrates pain whenever palpated or manipulated. The most common location for a traumatic neuroma is the lower extremity after an amputation, followed by the head and the neck area, especially the oral cavity after a tooth extraction [1]. We are presenting a rare case of a traumatic rectal neuroma, which was excised by cap-assisted endoscopic mucosal resection. Only one other case has been reported at this anatomic site in our English literature review [2].

2. Case Presentation

A 50-year-old female with a past medical history of asthmatic bronchitis underwent an initial colonoscopy procedure after complaining of 3 weeks of loose nonbloody bowel movements. The patient denied any rectal pain or prior rectal manipulation. On colonoscopy, an incidental 7 mm submucosal nodule was seen in the proximal rectum at 12 cm from the anal verge (Figure 1). The initial endoscopic biopsies taken from this area, however showed unremarkable rectal mucosa on histology. She then underwent an endoscopic ultrasound (EUS) of the localized submucosal lesion located 12 cm from the anal verge, at the 3 o'clock position (Figure 2). The lesion was homogenously hypoechoic, measuring up to 13 mm in thickness. The lesion was contained within the submucosal plane without muscularis propria invasion. The decision was made to pursue a cap-assisted endoscopic mucosal resection with an adult endoscope. A Carr-locke needle was used to inject approximately 5 ml of a mixture of saline and methylene blue, which provided an adequate lift of the lesion from the muscularis propria layer. An *en bloc* endoscopic mucosal resection with a cap and snare was achieved (Figure 3). Two hemostatic clips were placed to close the mucosal defect (Figure 4). The resected specimen was examined, showing no muscular fibers. Pathology of the specimen revealed a well-circumscribed 4 mm submucosal traumatic neuroma comprised of haphazardly proliferating spindle cells

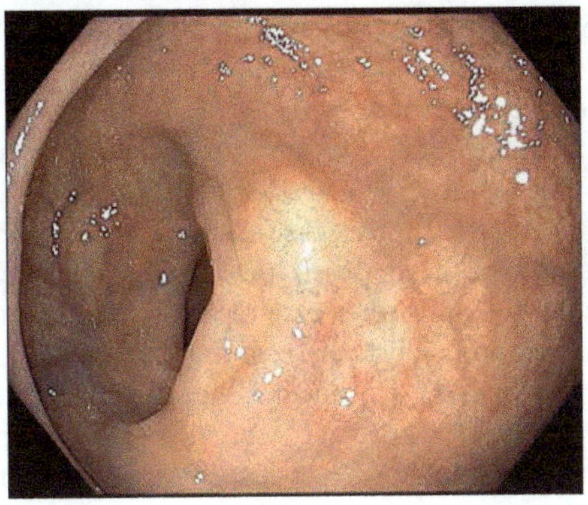

FIGURE 1: Endoscopic image showing a submucosal nodule in the rectum at the 3 o'clock position located 12 cm from the anal verge.

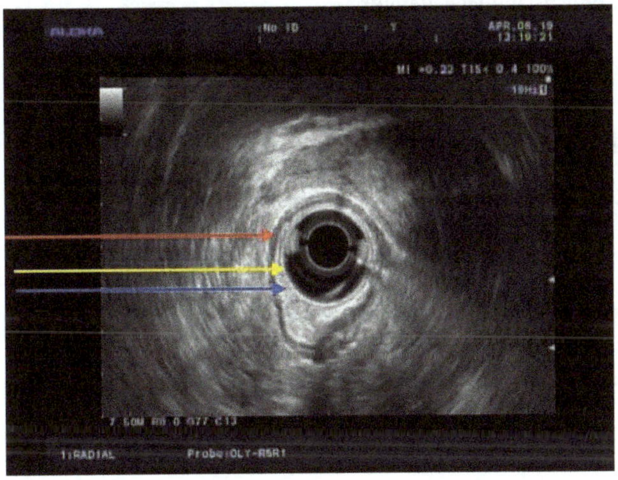

FIGURE 2: Rectal endoscopic ultrasound (EUS) showing a localized hypoechoic submucosal lesion with tiny hyperechoic bands without muscularis propria invasion. Muscularis mucosae (yellow arrow), submucosa (blue arrow), and muscularis propria (red arrow).

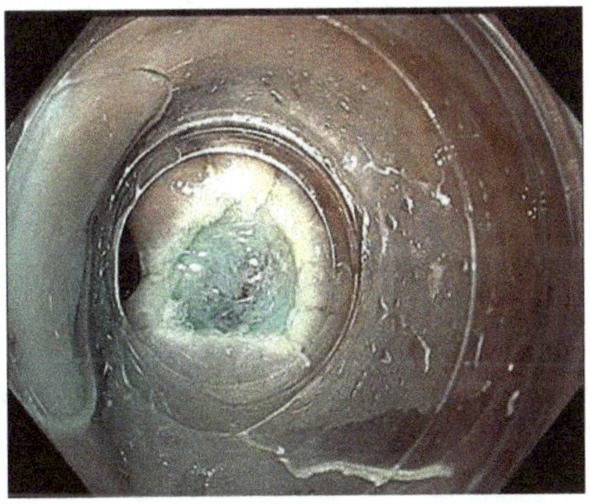

FIGURE 3: Endoscopic image showing *en-bloc* cap-assisted endoscopic mucosal resection of the rectal lesion.

consistent with Schwann cells embedded in a fibrous stroma (Figure 5). Immunostaining was positive for S100 (Figure 6). The patient tolerated the procedure well and had no complications on one-month follow-up.

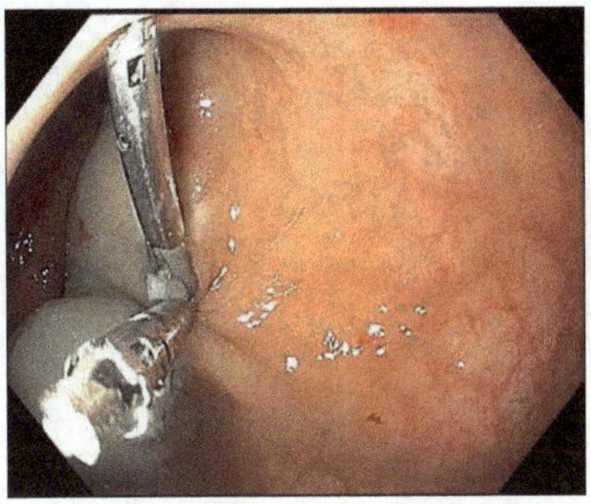

FIGURE 4: Endoscopic image showing successful closure of the rectal mucosal resection with two hemostatic clips.

3. Discussion

Neuromas are benign neural proliferations that occur after nerve injury. A neuroma can occur after a laceration which results in micro-trauma of peripheral nerves from stretching or compression of local tissues and can arise 1–12 months after transection or injury [1, 3, 4]. Transection of the peripheral nerve will cause loss of essential macromolecules and stimulate the distal portion of the nerve to undergo Wallerian degeneration followed by regeneration of the nerve by expression of growth factors at the transection site of Schwann cell. This process, however, is not always perfect, as it can grow aberrantly, forming dense nerve tangles called neuromas. Extending the distance between two injured nerve segments or an absence of a distal segment could result in a haphazard growth [5–8].

Traumatic neuromas are divided into spindle neuroma and terminal neuroma. A spindle neuroma is characterized by an internal, focal, fusiform swelling secondary to constant friction or irritation due to a nondisrupted, injured, but intact nerve trunk [1]. A terminal neuroma is the result of severe trauma with partial avulsion, disruption, or total transection of a nerve [1]. Histologically, it corresponds as a non-neoplastic, nonencapsulated tangled masses of axons, Schwann cells, endoneurial cells, and perineurial cells in a dense collagenous matrix with surrounding fibroblasts [1]. On high-resolution endoscopic ultrasound (EUS), a neuroma appears homogenously hypoechoic, sometimes with small hyperechoic internal bands. Our patient's EUS demonstrated that the lesion was contained to the submucosal layer, giving rise to a differential diagnosis of lipoma, carcinoid, or ectopic pancreas. However, the stains were negative for these pathologies.

In rat models, it has been demonstrated that inhibiting nerve growth factor (NGF) following nerve injury could reduce neuroma formation and neuropathic pain without damaging the cell bodies [5]. Therefore, management of traumatic neuroma in extremities consists of steroid injections, nerve stimulation and/or physical therapy, however half of the patients will ultimately require surgical resection for definitive management [1, 2, 6]. There are no clear established recommendations for treating a traumatic rectal neuroma; however, as shown in our case, using cap-assisted endoscopic mucosal resection (EMR) technique was safe and successful, achieving

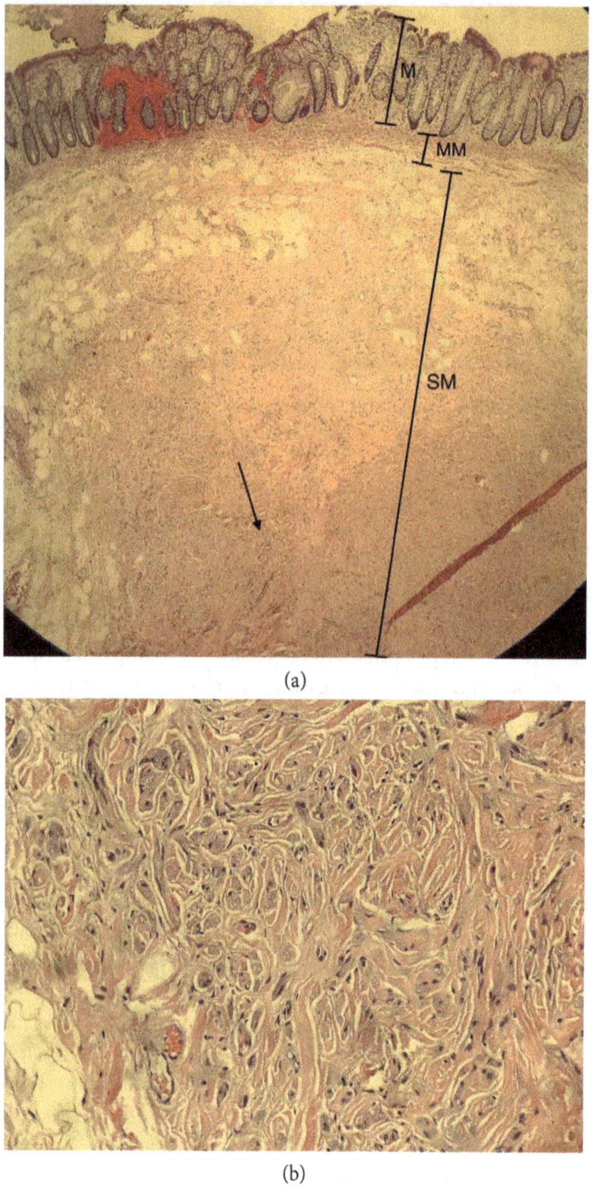

FIGURE 5: Pathology images of the traumatic rectal neuroma. (a) Low-power view. Note the mucosa on the top (M), the muscularis mucosae (MM), and the submucosa (SM). The lesion contained in the submucosal (arrow). (b) High-power view of the neural cells in the submucosa comprised of haphazardly proliferating spindle cells.

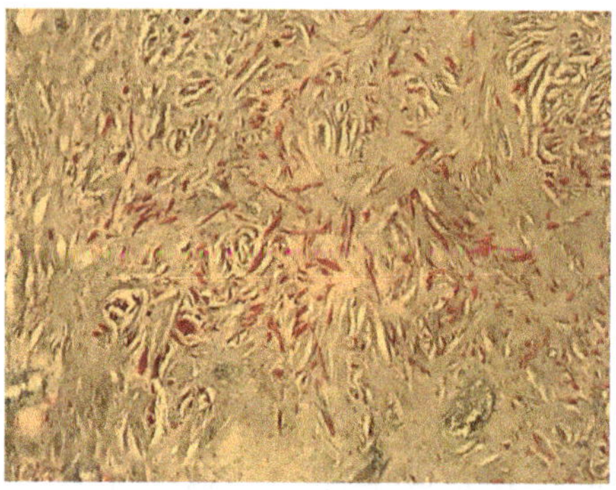

FIGURE 6: Pathology images of Immunostaining for S100, which including spindle and epithelioid neuro cells.

en bloc resection. Nevertheless, the risk of recurrence has been reported to be high, and therefore, surveillance colonoscopy should be recommended.

The usual presentation of a traumatic neuroma is of pain; however, our patient presented asymptomatically. This can possibly be attributed to the lack of somatic innervation within the rectal submucosa as opposed to neuromas located in an extremity. In the only other case report of a traumatic rectal neuroma, the authors hypothesized the lesion likely arose as a result of trauma to the submucosal Meissner's plexus fibers or Auerbach's plexus fibers after a previous polypectomy [2]. Interestingly, our patient never had a previous colonoscopy, rectal trauma/manipulation or anal receptive intercourse, which could have precipitated a neuroma. To our knowledge, this is the second case of a traumatic rectal neuroma, however the first case of incidental traumatic rectal neuroma was reported in the English-language literature.

References

[1] M. D. Murphey, W. S. Smith, S. E. Smith, M. J. Kransdorf, and H. T. Temple, "From the archives of the AFIP. imaging of musculoskeletal neurogenic tumors: radiologic-pathologic correlation," *Radiographics*, vol. 19, no. 5, pp. 1253–1280, 1999.

[2] T. Curran, V. Poylin, R. Kane, A. Harris, J. D. Goldsmith, and D. Nagle, "Case report of a traumatic rectal neuroma," *Gastroenterology Report*, vol. 4, no. 4, pp. 331–333, 2016.

[3] E. Abreu, S. Aubert, G. Wavreille, R. Gheno, C. Canella, and A. Cotten, "Peripheral tumor and tumor-like neurogenic lesions," *European Journal of Radiology*, vol. 82, no. 1, pp. 38–50, 2013.

[4] K. M. C. Oliveira, L. Pindur, Z. Han, M. B. Bhavsar, J. H. Barker, and L. Leppik, "Time course of traumatic neuroma development," *PLoS ONE*, vol. 13, no. 7, Article ID e0200548, 2018.

[5] G. S. Kryger, Z. Kryger, F. Zhang, D. L. Shelton, W. C. Lineaweaver, and H. J. Buncke, "Nerve growth factor inhibition prevents traumatic neuroma formation in the rat," *The Journal of Hand Surgery*, vol. 26, no. 4, pp. 635–644, 2001.

[6] P. D. Wall and M. Gutnick, "Ongoing activity in peripheral nerves: the physiology and pharmacology of impulses originating from a neuroma," *Experimental Neurology*, vol. 43, no. 3, pp. 580–593, 1974.

[7] R. P. Bunge, "The role of the Schwann cell in trophic support and regeneration," *Journal of Neurology*, vol. 242, no. S1, pp. S19–S21, 1994.

[8] A. Faroni, S. A. Mobasseri, P. J. Kingham, and A. J. Reid, "Peripheral nerve regeneration: experimental strategies and future perspectives," *Advanced Drug Delivery Reviews*, vol. 82–83, pp. 160–167, 2015.

39

Recalcitrant Esophageal Stricture Secondary to Mycophenolate Mofetil

Joyce J. Kim,[1] Ramzi H. Mulki,[2] and Kavya M. Sebastian[2]

[1]*Department of Medicine, Emory University School of Medicine, Atlanta, Georgia*
[2]*Department of Medicine, Division of Digestive Diseases, Emory University School of Medicine, Atlanta, Georgia*

Correspondence should be addressed to Joyce J. Kim; joyce.kim@emory.edu

Academic Editor: Yoshifumi Nakayama

Mycophenolate mofetil (MMF) is associated with various gastrointestinal toxicities. However, limited literature studies exist reporting MMF-related gastrointestinal toxicity manifesting as esophageal strictures. We report a case of a 62-year-old male with kidney transplant on MMF, tacrolimus, and prednisone, presenting with progressive dysphagia and odynophagia. Esophagogastroduodenoscopy revealed severe esophageal stricturing with near food bolus impaction, requiring dilations, esophageal stent, and ultimately gastrostomy tube. Biopsies revealed nonspecific inflammation with no evidence of infectious/neoplastic process; thus, our multidisciplinary esophageal group determined that the process was secondary to MMF. This case demonstrates that, though rare, MMF can result in severe esophageal strictures causing significant morbidity.

1. Introduction

Advances in immunosuppressive agents have transformed the field of transplantation, improving graft and patient outcomes [1, 2]. Unfortunately, these medications also commonly lead to gastrointestinal (GI) complications. Specifically, mycophenolate mofetil (MMF) has been associated with increased risk of infectious esophagitis [3], GI malignancies [4], as well as injury to both upper and lower gastrointestinal mucosa manifesting as constellation of symptoms including nausea, vomiting, abdominal discomfort, and diarrhea [5–8]. However, limited literature exists on esophageal stricture as a complication of MMF. Herein, we present a rare case of recalcitrant esophageal stricture caused by MMF.

2. Case Report

We report a case of a 62-year-old male with a history of renal transplant (5 months prior to presentation) on an immunosuppressive regimen consisting of MMF, tacrolimus, and prednisone, who presented with progressive solid and liquid dysphagia and odynophagia for one month, with associated 20-pound weight loss. An EGD was performed, and upon careful inspection, a shallow 1 cm × 1 cm ulcer was seen on the right side of the soft palate (Figure 1). With further advancement, multiple, deeply cratered ulcers, in a circumferential manner, were found starting 23 cm from the incisors to the GE junction (40 cm from the incisors) (Figure 2(a)). Food debris were adherent to the ulcers, causing severe narrowing of the esophageal lumen in a near bolus food impaction, and was only traversable with an ultrathin endoscope (Figure 2(b)). Biopsies were obtained from the center and the edge of the ulcers, which revealed reactive squamous mucosa with fragments of granulation tissue and neuroinflammatory debris (Figure 3). Immunostains for CMV, HSV1/2, and fungal organisms were negative. Otolaryngology obtained a biopsy of the ulcerative lesion found in the soft palate during initial EGD, which revealed nonspecific findings of acute and chronic inflammation and negative for infectious causes.

The patient was discharged on high-dose proton pump inhibitor, liquid diet, and total parenteral nutrition. MMF was suspended given the suspicion of MMF-induced esophageal injury. A repeat EGD 4 weeks later revealed a pin-point esophageal lumen starting from 23 cm from

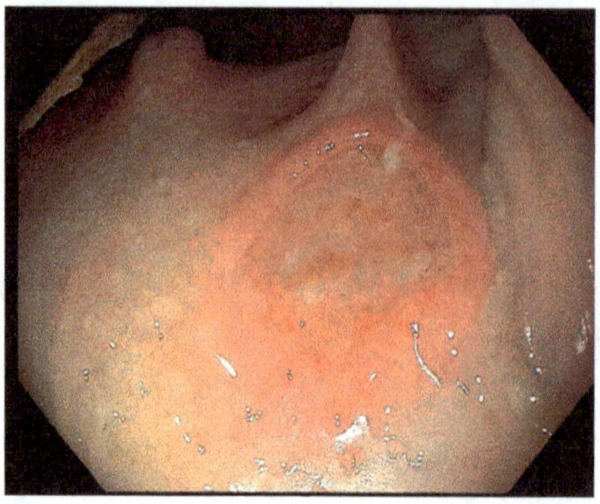

FIGURE 1: Soft palate ulcer in the right oropharynx, which was biopsied and revealed nonspecific findings of acute and chronic inflammation.

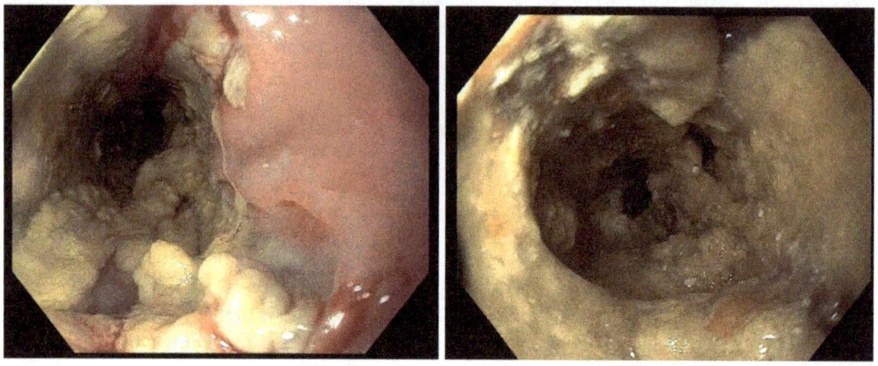

FIGURE 2: Multiple, deeply cratered ulcers, in a circumferential manner with adherent food debris (a), causing severe narrowing of the esophageal lumen, in a near complete food bolus impaction (b).

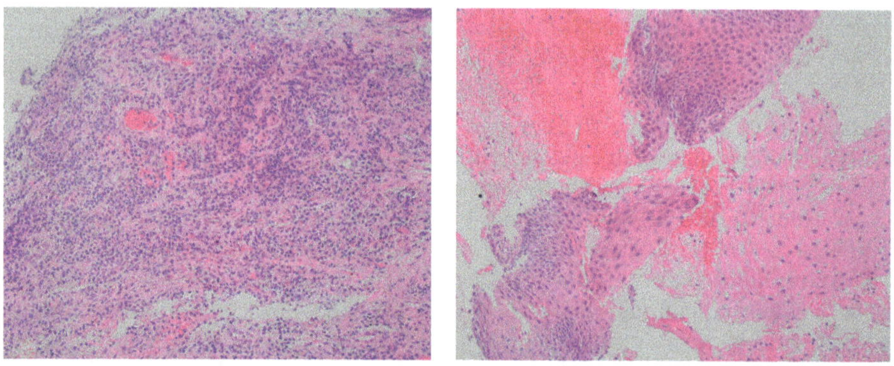

(a) (b)

FIGURE 3: Nonspecific histologic findings included granulation tissue and necroinflammatory debris (a) consistent with endoscopically identified ulcer. Fragments of squamous epithelium showed reactive features (basal cell hyperplasia and balloon cell change) (b).

incisors not traversable with the ultrathin upper endoscope (Figure 4). A barium swallow demonstrated the extent of the narrowing in the mid and distal esophagus with proximal esophageal dilation (Figure 5). The patient was referred for a surgically placed feeding gastrostomy tube, with plans for serial dilation under fluoroscopic guidance. Several attempts at endoscopic dilation were performed using a through-the-scope (TTS) balloon dilator from 6 mm to 10 mm. The esophageal stricture was recalcitrant despite dilation and maximal medical therapy. After discussion in multidisciplinary dysphagia conference, the decision was made to proceed with esophageal stenting. This was performed using a 18 mm × 12.3 cm fully covered stent, which was placed under fluoroscopic guidance (Figure 6). The patient tolerated the procedure initially, but due to chest discomfort, the stent was subsequently removed. Esophagectomy was considered but deferred due to the patient's comorbid conditions; he opted for maximal medical therapy

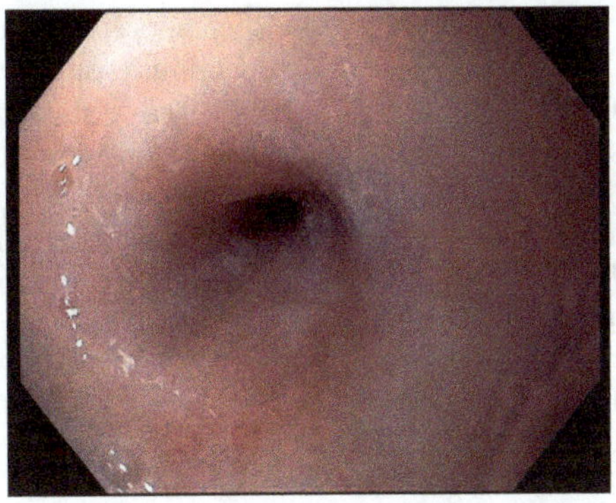

Figure 4: EGD revealing a pin-point esophageal in the midesophagus.

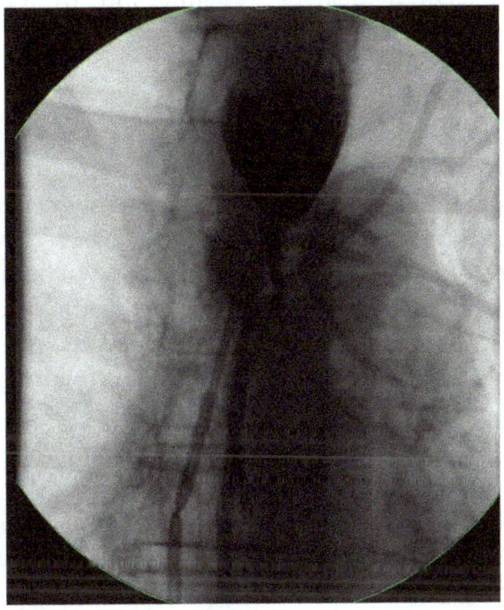

Figure 5: Barium swallow demonstrating a severe narrowing in the mid and distal esophagus with proximal dilation.

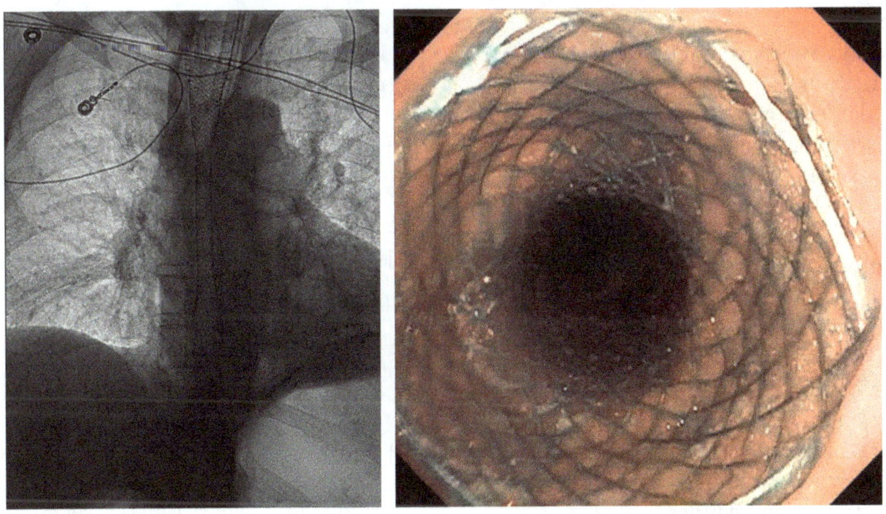

Figure 6: A fully covered esophageal metal stent placement under fluoroscopy.

(fluticasone 2 puffs of 220 mcg/inhalation aerosol twice daily, lansoprazole 30 mg twice daily, and sucralfate 1 g/ 10 mL solution 4 times daily) and serial dilations with intralesional steroid injections. A year and a half after initial presentation, his oral intake is improving with slow weaning off of dependence on feeding tube.

3. Discussion

MMF is an immunosuppressive agent that selectively acts on T and B lymphocytes and is commonly used to prevent graft rejection after transplantation [9]. Unfortunately, MMF has been associated with gastrointestinal toxicities with reported incidence varying from 40% to 85% [10]. Previous studies have suggested that mucosal injuries throughout gastrointestinal tract can occur particularly within the first twelve months of initiating MMF; one study found that, among those with kidney transplants on immunosuppressants, 46% developed ulcers in the first year, with MMF being an independent risk factor [11].

Though not fully understood, MMF-related complications in the GI tract have been attributed to its mechanism of inhibiting lymphocyte proliferation by blocking de novo guanosine nucleotide synthesis, upon which the rapidly replicating enterocytes partially depend, thereby disrupting the gastrointestinal epithelial barrier [12]. In addition, its metabolites including mycophenolic acid acyl-glucuronide (AcMPAG) can trigger the immune system, leading to hypersensitivity and autoimmune-like reactions [5]. Interestingly, the reported pathologic features of MMF-related toxicity of upper and lower GI tract are dissimilar. Most extensively documented are graft-versus-host disease such as changes of the colon and small intestines including mild crypt disarray, crypt loss, and increased epithelial apoptosis (features that are nonspecific on their own) [7, 8, 13], symptomatically manifesting as diarrhea, and a presentation similar to inflammatory bowel disease. In contrast, upper GI toxicities of MMF have been found to be similar to features of nonsteroidal anti-inflammatory drug use with topical irritation and damage, leading to ulcerative esophagitis, reactive gastropathy, and duodenal ulcers [7, 14, 15]. This can symptomatically manifest as nausea/vomiting, dysphagia, and dyspepsia.

However, to our knowledge, manifestation of MMF-related upper GI toxicity as esophageal stricture is not well-reported. This case demonstrated an example of a recalcitrant esophageal stricture causing near food bolus impaction, requiring multiple dilations, esophageal stent placement, and ultimately gastrostomy placement. Given multiple biopsies of nonspecific findings (reactive squamous mucosa) with negative stains for infectious or neoplastic processes, the disease process was attributed to MMF. One of these biopsies included an ulcerative lesion of the oral cavity that was found during the initial EGD; an oropharyngeal examination is often overlooked during a routine EGD but may reveal incidental findings with important implications [16]. The recurring nature of the stricture in this case suggests that there likely was an underlying fibrotic process that occurred in an irreversible manner.

This report contributes to a better understanding of atypical presentation of MMF-induced esophagitis in immunocompromised patients, expanding upon prior reports regarding upper GI manifestation of MMF. Specifically, this report demonstrated a new potential consequence of MMF in the esophagus, namely, strictures. This diagnosis should be considered in a posttransplant patient with dysphagia when more common etiologies (e.g., reflux esophagitis or infectious esophagitis) have been excluded. Furthermore, an improved systematic surveillance may be needed among patients on immunosuppressants, particularly MMF, given that delay in appropriate diagnosis and treatment can result in significant morbidity, as well as possible life-threatening consequences, as in our case.

Disclosure

A preliminary result from this work was presented at the American College of Gastroenterology 2019, but differs significantly from the final findings presented in this report.

Authors' Contributions

JK was involved in data collection and drafting/revising the paper. RM was involved in conception of the paper, interpretation of findings, and drafting/revising the paper. AG provided pathologic images and description and revised the paper. KS was involved in interpreting findings, reviewing, and revising the paper. All authors reviewed the final manuscript.

Acknowledgments

The authors thank Ashley Greer, MD, and the Emory Pathology Department for providing histologic images used in this paper.

References

[1] M. A. Lim, J. Kohli, and R. D. Bloom, "Immunosuppression for kidney transplantation: where are we now and where are we going?" *Transplantation Reviews*, vol. 31, no. 1, pp. 10–17, 2017.

[2] M. N. Scherer, B. Banas, K. Mantouvalou et al., "Current concepts and perspectives of immunosuppression in organ transplantation," *Langenbeck's Archives of Surgery*, vol. 392, no. 5, pp. 511–523, 2007.

[3] J. H. Helderman and S. Goral, "Gastrointestinal complications of transplant immunosuppression," *Journal of the American Society of Nephrology: JASN*, vol. 13, no. 1, pp. 277–287, 2002.

[4] E. B. Haagsma, V. E. Hagens, M. Schaapveld et al., "Increased cancer risk after liver transplantation: a population-based study," *Journal of Hepatology*, vol. 34, no. 1, pp. 84–91, 2001.

[5] N. M. Davies, J. Grinyó, R. Heading, B. Maes, H.-U. Meier-Kriesche, and M. Oellerich, "Gastrointestinal side effects of mycophenolic acid in renal transplant patients: a reappraisal," *Nephrology Dialysis Transplantation*, vol. 22, no. 9, pp. 2440–2448, 2007.

[6] K. Liu and L. Kia, "Mycophenolate mofetil–induced esophagitis," *Clinical Gastroenterology and Hepatology*, vol. 17, no. 12, p. e139, 2019.

[7] J. R. Parfitt, S. Jayakumar, and D. K. Driman, "Mycophenolate mofetil-related gastrointestinal mucosal injury: variable injury patterns, including graft-versus-host disease-like changes," *The American Journal of Surgical Pathology*, vol. 32, no. 9, pp. 1367–1372, 2008.

[8] A. Jehangir, B. Shaikh, J. Hunt, and A. Spiegel, "Severe enteropathy from mycophenolate mofetil," *ACG Case Reports Journal*, vol. 3, no. 2, pp. 101–103, 2016.

[9] M. Behrend, "Adverse gastrointestinal effects of mycophenolate mofetil," *Drug Safety*, vol. 24, no. 9, pp. 645–663, 2001.

[10] W. Arns, "Noninfectious gastrointestinal (GI) complications of mycophenolic acid therapy: a consequence of local GI toxicity?" *Transplantation Proceedings*, vol. 39, no. 1, pp. 88–93, 2007.

[11] G. Telkes, A. Peter, Z. Tulassay, and A. Asderakis, "High frequency of ulcers, not associated with Helicobacter pylori, in the stomach in the first year after kidney transplantation," *Nephrology Dialysis Transplantation*, vol. 26, no. 2, pp. 727–732, 2011.

[12] M. Qasim, H. Rahman, R. Ahmed, M. Oellerich, and A. R. Asif, "Mycophenolic acid mediated disruption of the intestinal epithelial tight junctions," *Experimental Cell Research*, vol. 322, no. 2, pp. 277–289, 2014.

[13] M. K. Selbst, W. A. Ahrens, M. E. Robert, A. Friedman, D. D. Proctor, and D. Jain, "Spectrum of histologic changes in colonic biopsies in patients treated with mycophenolate mofetil," *Modern Pathology*, vol. 22, no. 6, pp. 737–743, 2009.

[14] I. S. Kim, H. Lee, J. C. Park, S. K. Shin, S. K. Lee, and Y. C. Lee, "Increased incidence of endoscopic erosive esophagitis in solid organ transplant recipients," *Gut and Liver*, vol. 6, no. 3, pp. 349–354, 2012.

[15] T. Nguyen, J. Y. Park, J. R. Scudiere, and E. Montgomery, "Mycophenolic acid (cellcept and myofortic) induced injury of the upper GI tract," *The American Journal of Surgical Pathology*, vol. 33, no. 9, pp. 1355–1363, 2009.

[16] H. Fatima, "Oropharyngeal findings at upper endoscopy," *Clinical Gastroenterology and Hepatology*, vol. 17, no. 12, pp. 2423–2428, 2019.

Endoscopic Mucosal Resection of a Proximal Esophageal Pyogenic Granuloma

Elias Estifan,[1] Varun Patel,[2] and Matthew Grossman[2]

[1]*Department of Internal Medicine, St. Joseph's University Medical Center, New York Medical College, USA*
[2]*Division of Gastroenterology, St. Joseph's University Medical Center, New York Medical College, USA*

Correspondence should be addressed to Elias Estifan; egestifan@gmail.com

Academic Editor: Matteo Neri

Pyogenic Granuloma (PG), also known as lobular capillary hemangioma, is usually seen as a polypoid red lesion found on the skin or the mucosal surface of the oral cavity. PG of the gastrointestinal tract is rare, in particular involving the esophagus, only 14 cases have been reported in the English literature. We present an 80-year-old male who underwent endoscopy for evaluation of dysphagia and was found to have a single, red, bilobed 10 mm polyp with adherent white exudate approximately 19 cm from the incisors. Endoscopic ultrasound was performed with a 20 mHz miniprobe which showed the lesion contained to the mucosal layer with no muscularis propria invasion. A decision was made to perform endoscopic mucosal resection (EMR). A mixture of saline and methylene blue was injected into the submucosal plane to raise the lesion with subsequent successful mucosal hot snare resection. The resection defect was then approximated and closed with a hemostatic clip to prevent bleeding. Pathology of the specimen revealed small capillary vessels growing in a lobular architecture with an edematous stroma and a florid inflammatory infiltrate representing a pyogenic granuloma. EMR allows for an en bloc resection of mucosal lesions with tumor-free margins, thereby providing both diagnostic and prognostic information. Comparing EMR with the novel technique of endoscopic submucosal dissection (ESD), the incidence of bleeding and perforation is much lower; making EMR the best and safest resection option for this rare hemangioma. In this case, we demonstrate that EMR is a safe technique in removing a pyogenic granuloma in the esophagus.

1. Introduction

Pyogenic Granuloma (PG) is a polypoid form of a hemangioma that frequently occurs on the skin or in the oral cavity. It is a benign tumor with frequent recurrence, with no cases of malignant transformation having been reported [1]. PG of the gastrointestinal tract is rare, in particular involving the esophagus, only 14 cases have been reported in the English literature. Most PG are managed by snare polypectomy, endoscopic mucosal resection (EMR), laser photocoagulation therapy, endoscopic submucosal dissection (ESD) or regional radiation therapy [2]. In our case, we describe the safety of EMR of a pyogenic granuloma in the esophagus.

2. Case Report

An 80-year-old male with a past medical history of hypertension and diabetes mellitus type II underwent endoscopy for evaluation of dysphagia and was found to have a single, red, bilobed 10 mm polyp with white exudate in the proximal esophagus measuring 19 cm from the incisors (Figure 1). Endoscopic ultrasound was performed with a 20 mHz miniprobe which showed the lesion contained to the mucosal layer with no muscularis propria invasion. A standard gastroscope was introduced and careful examination of the surrounding area and the remaining esophagus was done with no evidence of esophagitis or Barrett's esophagus seen. Thereafter, a mixture of saline and methylene blue was injected into the submucosal plane to raise the lesion. The lesion lifted symmetrically, and a mucosal snare resection was performed successfully with en bloc retrieval of the specimen (Figures 2 and 3). The post-polypectomy site was then carefully examined with no residual tissue or prominent blood vessels seen. The polypectomy defect was then approximated and closed with a hemostatic clip successfully to prevent post-polypectomy bleeding (Figure 4). No bleeding was observed throughout the

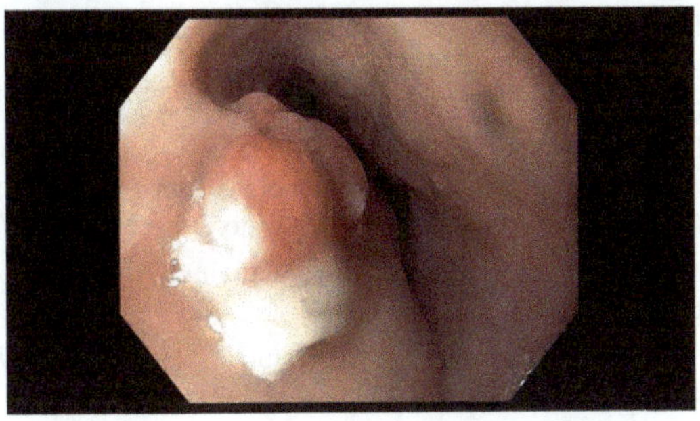

FIGURE 1: Endoscopic image showing a single, red, bilobed 10 mm polyp with whitish exudate in the proximal esophagus.

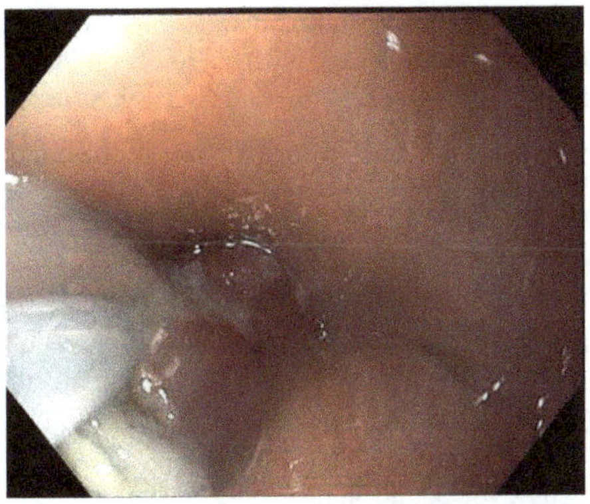

FIGURE 2: Endoscopic image of the mucosal snare resection being performed after saline and methylene blue injection.

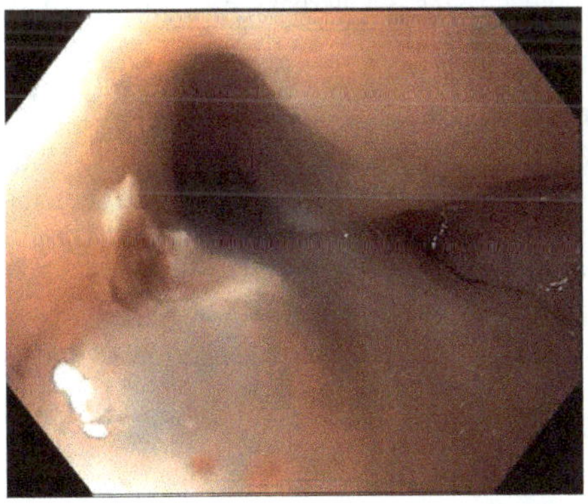

FIGURE 3: Endoscopic image of the post-polypectomy site with no residual tissue remaining and no evidence of bleeding.

procedure. Pathology of the specimen revealed small capillary vessels growing in a lobular architecture with an edematous stroma and a florid inflammatory infiltrate representing a lobular capillary hemangioma or pyogenic granuloma (Figure 5).

3. Discussion

PG or lobular capillary hemangioma is a hemorrhagic, benign, polypoid neoplasm which was first described in 1897, at that time it was called botryomycosis hominis [3–5]. The lesion is most commonly found on the skin and the

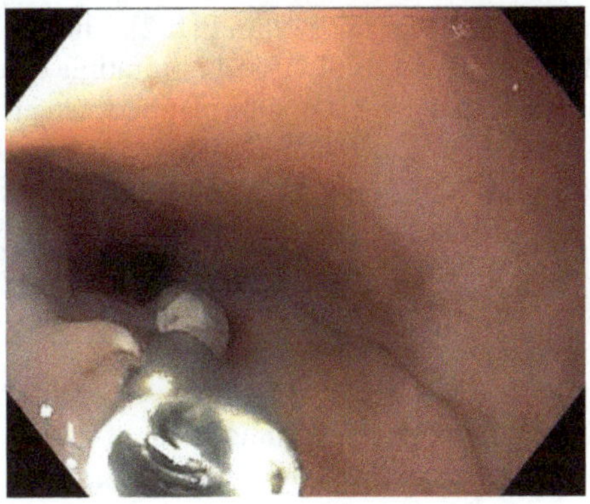

FIGURE 4: Endoscopic image of successful closure of the post-polypectomy site with a hemostatic clip.

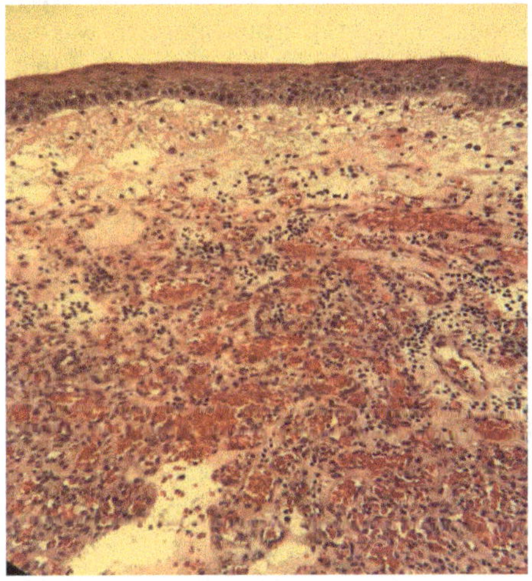

FIGURE 5: Pathology imaging revealed small capillary vessels growing in a lobular architecture with an edematous stroma and a florid inflammatory infiltrate representing a pyogenic granuloma.

mucosal surface of the oral cavity, nasal cavity, and tongue [6, 7]. Only a few cases have been reported in the gastrointestinal tract including the stomach, duodenum, jejunum, ileum, and colon, with the esophagus being the most common [2]. PG is seen in all parts of the esophagus, with the distal segment (57.1%) being most common, followed by the middle segment (35.7%) [2, 6]. On endoscopy, the lesion is usually solitary, appearing in a variety of colors ranging from a bright red/pink to a dark color. Most esophageal PG are confined to the mucosal layer, however submucosal extension has been reported. The size of the lesion can range from several millimeters to a few centimeters. It tends to be friable and hemorrhagic with occasional ulceration and white exudate noted on the surface of the lesion [2, 5, 6, 8, 9].

Most patients who are found to have PG are asymptomatic. However, some symptoms associated with PG are upper gastrointestinal bleeding, epigastric discomfort, chest discomfort, dysphagia, and/or heartburn.

Histological characteristics are proliferation and lobular arrangement of multiple capillaries, inflamed, and edematous stroma, and endothelial cell swelling [1, 2]. The etiology has been a matter of debate as discussed in multiple case reports and its theorized that there is an interplay between mechanical irritation, trauma from foreign body, iatrogenic irritation from biopsy, hormonal factors as in pregnancy, and infections from *Staphylococci*, *Helicobacter pylori*, *Botryomycosis*, *Campylobacter enteritis*, and *Candida* which may affect the morphology of the lesion [5, 10, 11]. Two cases of PG published in the literature were associated with Barrett's esophagus, which illustrates the possibility of PG arising due to chronic gastric acid damage to the esophageal mucosa [1, 7]. In addition, it is important to differentiate the lesion from Kaposi's sarcoma, which typically is encountered in patients with acquired immune deficiency syndrome (AIDS). Kaposi's sarcoma is less well circumscribed, more bluish in color and mostly covered by a moistly glistening intact mucosa. Also, microscopically Kaposi's has slit-like vascular channels lined by atypical endothelial cells which is a feature not found in PG [11]. In our case, there was no identified underlying infection or foreign body irritation that could be linked as an etiologic factor for the formation of a PG.

With the advent of new technology and rapid progression of minimally invasive techniques, endoscopy is becoming integral in providing both diagnostic and therapeutic interventions with virtually no morbidity and mortality [12]. Endoscopy aided with endoscopic ultrasound allows for evaluation of the size, depth, and surface characteristics for early-stage lesions based on Paris classification [13]. EMR, was first described in 1973, is an endoscopic resection technique that provides both diagnostic and prognostic information for mucosal-based lesions [12, 14]. In comparison to cold forceps biopsy, EMR is able to obtain complete tissue resection with a lower recurrence rate [12]. EMR has a high success rate in en bloc resection of mucosal lesions less than 10 mm in size. Lesions that are more extensive up to 20 mm can be resected by EMR; however, ESD has better resection rates with a lower recurrence rates [15]. In one meta-analysis study, the estimate complications of esophageal ESD such as bleeding was 2.1%, whereas the perforation rate was 5.0% [16]. However, in other studies of esophageal EMR, the rate of bleeding post-procedure was between 2.4% and 25% and the perforation rate was equal to ESD of 5.0% [17].

Pyogenic granuloma or lobular capillary hemangioma is a polypoid form of a hemangioma that is usually found as an incidental lesion; however, patients can present with symptoms of dysphagia, bleeding, or pain. Therefore, when discovered on endoscopy, these lesions should be resected to prevent possible complications. EMR provides a lift from the muscularis propria layer to ensure an adequate cushion which minimized the perforation risk, thus entailing a safer resection technique than a polypectomy. We illustrate that EMR, if done appropriately, is the most safe and best treatment modality for such high-risk bleeding lesions.

References

[1] E. R. Hoekstra, P. Fockens, and P. Scholten, "A 15-year-old boy with an esophageal pyogenic granuloma and subsequent Barrett's esophagus (with videos)," *Gastrointestinal Endoscopy*, vol. 65, no. 7, pp. 1086–1088, 2007.

[2] D. A. Suarez-Zamora, P. A. Rodriguez-Urrego, J. Solano-Mariño, F. Sierra-Arango, and M. A. Palau-Lazaro, "Esophageal pyogenic granuloma: a case report and review of the literature," *International Journal of Surgical Pathology*, vol. 26, no. 8, pp. 735–738, 2018.

[3] A. D. L. Poncet, "Botryomycose humaine," *Rev Chir*, vol. 18, pp. 996–1003, 1897.

[4] M. B. Hartzell, "Granuloma pyogenicus," *Journal of Cutaneous Diseases*, vol. 22, pp. 520–523, 1904.

[5] S. N. Bhaskar and J. R. Jacoway, "Pyogenic granuloma–clinical features, incidence, histology, and result of treatment: report of 242 cases," *Journal Oral Surgery*, vol. 24, no. 5, pp. 391–398, 1966.

[6] S.-Y. Park, C.-H. Park, W.-S. Lee, H.-S. Kim, S.-K. Choi, and J.-S. Rew, "Pyogenic granuloma of the duodenum treated successfully by endoscopic mucosal resection," *Gut and Liver*, vol. 3, no. 1, pp. 48–51, 2009.

[7] R. M. Craig, S. Carlson, H. A. Nordbrock, and H. Yokoo, "Pyogenic granuloma in Barrett's esophagus mimicking esophageal carcinoma," *Gastroenterology*, vol. 108, no. 6, pp. 1894–1896, 1995.

[8] H. G. Seoung, G. H. Kim, G. A. Song et al., "Esophageal pyogenic granuloma: endosonographic findings and endoscopic treatments," *Clinical Endoscopy*, vol. 46, no. 1, pp. 81–84, 2013.

[9] N. Okada, T. Matsumoto, K. Kurahara et al., "Pyogenic granuloma of the esophagus treated by endoscopic removal," *Endoscopy*, vol. 35, no. 4, pp. 375–375, 2003.

[10] M. Iwamuro, H. Okada, T. Tanaka et al., "Morphological changes in a pyogenic granuloma of the esophagus observed over three years," *Internal Medicine*, vol. 54, no. 14, pp. 1737–1740, 2015.

[11] S. Van Eeden, G. J. A. Offerhaus, F. H. Morsink, B. P. van Rees, O. R. C. Busch, and C. J. M. Van Noesel, "Pyogenic granuloma: an unrecognized cause of gastrointestinal bleeding," *Virchows Archiv*, vol. 444, no. 6, pp. 590–593, 2004.

[12] Ş. Çolak, B. Gürbulak, E. Çakar, and H. Bektaş, "Resection of mucosal and submucosal gastrointestinal lesions and a double endoscope experience," *Journal of the Society of Laparoendoscopic Surgeons*, vol. 23, no. 1, Article ID e2018.00096, 2019.

[13] Participants in the Paris Workshop, "The paris endoscopic classification of superficial neoplastic lesions: esophagus, stomach, and colon," *Gastrointestinal Endoscopy*, vol. 58, no. 6, pp. S3–S43, 2003.

[14] P. Deyhle, S. Jenny, and I. Fumagalli, "Endoscopic polypectomy in the proximal colon. A diagnostic, therapeutic (and preventive?) intervention," *Deutsche Medizinische Wochenschrift*, vol. 98, no. 5, pp. 219–220, 1973.

[15] T. Yamashita, A. Zeniya, H. Ishii et al., "Endoscopic mucosal resection using a cap-fitted panendoscope and endoscopic submucosal dissection as optimal endoscopic procedures for superficial esophageal carcinoma," *Surgical Endoscopy*, vol. 25, no. 8, pp. 2541–2546, 2011.

[16] J. S. Kim, B.-W. Kim, and I.-S. Shin, "Efficacy and safety of endoscopic submucosal dissection for superficial squamous esophageal neoplasia: a meta-analysis," *Digestive Diseases Sciences*, vol. 59, no. 8, pp. 1862–1869, 2014.

[17] M. di Pietro, M. I. Canto, and R. C. Fitzgerald, "Endoscopic management of early adenocarcinoma and squamous cell carcinoma of the esophagus: screening, diagnosis, and therapy," *Gastroenterology*, vol. 154, no. 2, pp. 421–436, 2018.

41

Endoscopic Ultrasound in Guiding Local Resection and Ampullary Preservation of a High-Risk Periampullary GIST

Andrew Spiel ,[1] Ravi Patel,[1] Rebecca Minter,[2] Amir Ali Rahnemai Azar,[2] Rashmi Agni,[3] Antonio Bosch ,[1] and Deepak Gopal [1]

[1]*Division of Gastroenterology & Hepatology, Department of Medicine, Univeristy of WIsconsin School of Medicine and Public Health, Madison, WI, USA*
[2]*Division of Surgical Oncology, Department of Surgery, University of Wisconsin School of Medicine and Public Health, Madison, WI, USA*
[3]*Department of Pathology & Laboratory Medicine, University of Wisconsin School of Medicine and Public Health, Madison, WI, USA*

Correspondence should be addressed to Andrew Spiel; aspiel@uwhealth.org

Academic Editor: Hideto Kawaratani

Gastrointestinal stromal tumors (GISTs) typically develop in the stomach or small intestine and rarely involve the ampulla of Vater, with only 13 cases reported in the world literature since 2004. Most authors advocate performing pancreaticoduodenectomy for such lesions. However, this operation can carry higher rates of morbidity and mortality compared to local resection. We present a case of a high-risk, invasive periampullary GIST and the multidisciplinary management approach to local resection with the aid of endoscopic ultrasound. In addition, this case shows no local recurrence at 3 months and a favorable clinical outcome at 1 year.

1. Introduction

The ampulla of Vater can be home to a variety of neoplasms including adenomas, adenocarcinomas, choledochocele (type III), and neuroendocrine tumors [1]. Rarely, do these lesions represent gastrointestinal stromal tumors (GISTs). A GIST is generally defined as a spindle-cell tumor of the GI tract originating from the cells of Cajal (an intestinal pacemaker cell) [2]. By definition, they express *KIT* protein (CD117), which is a tyrosine kinase receptor protein [3]. Malignant potential of GIST is defined by size and mitotic index [4]. GISTs typically develop in the stomach or small intestine and rarely involve the ampulla of Vater, with only 13 cases reported in the literature [5]. Most authors advocate performing pancreaticoduodenectomy (PD) for such lesions [6]. Endoscopic ultrasound (EUS) can aid in surgical planning for local resection. We present a case of a high-risk, invasive periampullary GIST and the multidisciplinary management approach to local resection with preservation of the biliary tree and ampullary complex.

2. Case

A 61-year-old male presented to his primary care provider (PCP) for medication management. He had a history of chronic back pain, depression, anxiety, and peptic ulcer disease (PUD). On routine laboratory testing, he was noted to be anemic with a hemoglobin of 8.8 g/dL and, upon further questioning, endorsed 2 weeks of melena. Repeat Hgb was 9.2 g/dL, iron, 17 ug/dL, and ferritin, 6 ng/mL. Upper endoscopy revealed a 2.5 cm submucosal lesion with a central ulceration adjacent to the ampulla of Vater (Figures 1(a) and 1(b)). Standard forceps biopsy was obtained which revealed CD117- and DOG1-positive spindle-cell subtype GIST but was insufficient for risk assessment. CT of abdomen and pelvis was read as 2.6×1.4 cm intraluminal mass involving the proximal duodenum extending to the level of the ampulla (Figure 2). Endoscopic ultrasound (EUS) was performed showing a hypoechoic round mass in the area of the major papilla extending from the mucosa to the muscularis propria and measuring 2.5 cm by 1.6 cm in

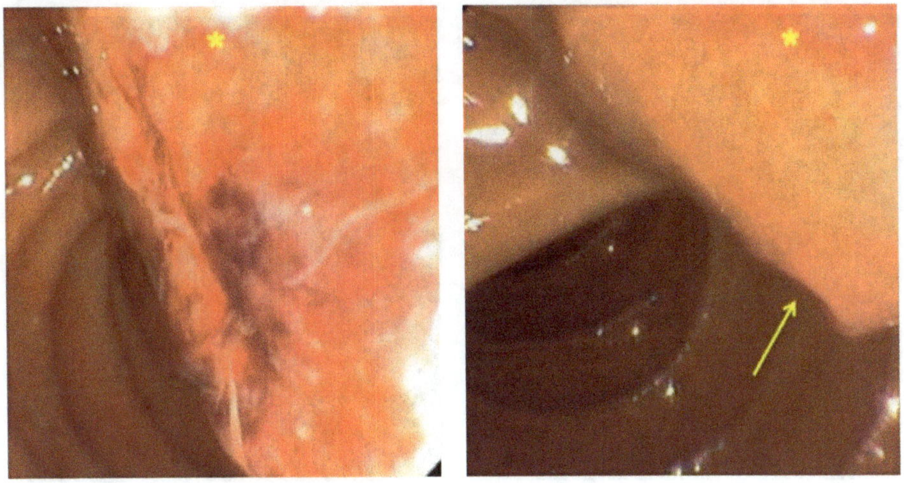

(a) (b)

FIGURE 1: (a, b) Endoscopy. Ulcerated mass (*) adjacent to ampulla of Vater (arrow).

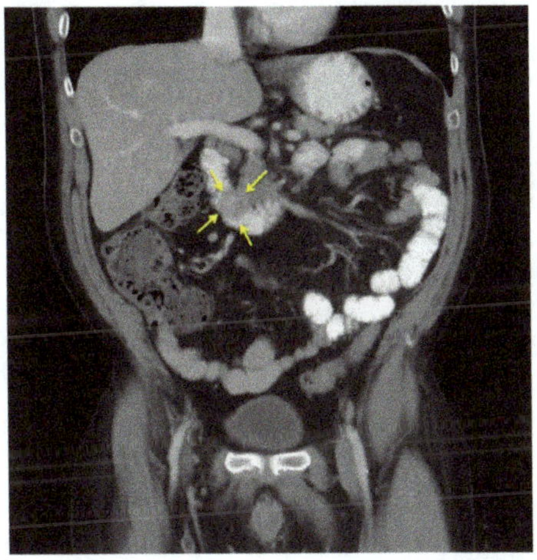

FIGURE 2: CT imaging showing a 2.6 × 1.4 cm intraluminal mass involving the proximal duodenum extending to the level of the ampulla.

maximum cross-sectional dimensions. Biliary and pancreatic ducts were of normal caliber, and the papillary orifice was identified (red arrow) (Figure 3(a)). A core biopsy was obtained with a 22-gauge fine-needle biopsy (SharkCore™, Medtronic) (Figure 3(b)). EUS and side-viewing duodenoscope assisted in demonstrating that there was no involvement of the distal bile duct or head of the pancreas. Liver chemistry evaluation at that time showed total bilirubin of 0.6 mg/dL, AST of 29 U/L, ALT of 22 U/L, and alkaline phosphatase of 103 U/L. Core biopsy histopathology confirmed GIST but again was unable to further risk stratify by mitotic index. EUS images were reviewed with the pancreatobiliary surgeons in order to guide an operative plan. The preoperative distance of the tumor to the major papilla estimated <4 mm (approximated at 3-4 mm on EUS imaging), and the tumor deemed periampullary. The patient was therefore planned for surgery preparing for local excision based on EUS findings and normal liver chemistries, suggesting no invasion by the tumor of the adjacent pancreaticobiliary structures. Laparotomy was performed, and palpation confirmed that the ampullary complex and tumor capsule were thinly separated, on the order of millimeters as suggested by EUS. This allowed for completion of a duodenal excision with complex reconstruction, pyloric exclusion, and Billroth II jejunostomy (Figure 4) instead of a pancreaticoduodenectomy. Tumor capsule remained intact; a small portion of pancreatic head was resected due to extrinsic tumor adherence. Duodenal reconstruction involved 2 layers of suture to bring the cut edges of the duodenum together within the head of the pancreas. Final pathology showed a mixed-subtype, high-risk GIST staining positive for CD117 (Figure 5(a)) and 8 mitotic bodies per 5 mm^2 (Figure 5(b)). Negative margins were obtained. His hospitalization was complicated by gastrojejunal anastomotic ulcer bleed and acute kidney injury. He underwent upper endoscopy with control of bleeding with full recovery. The patient's renal function returned to normal prior to discharge. Imatinib adjuvant chemotherapy was initiated, and he is currently tolerating with a brief treatment break due to lower extremity edema and fatigue in the first month.

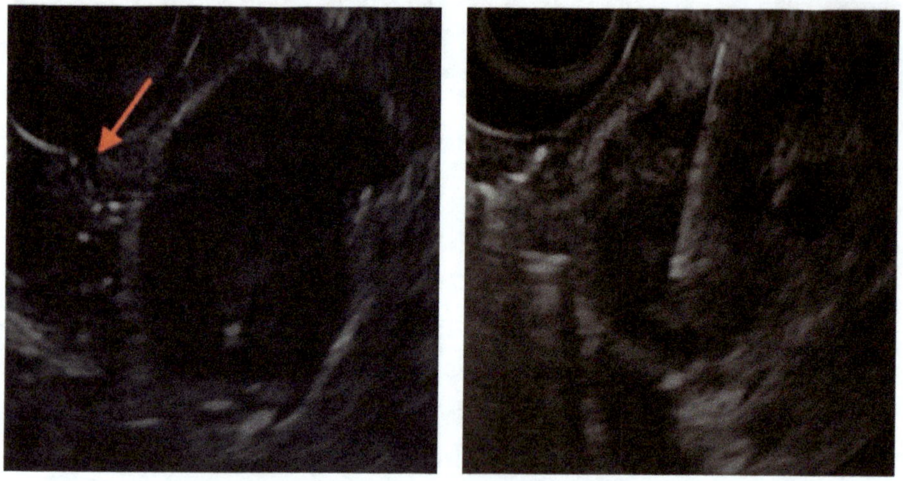

(a) (b)

Figure 3: EUS. (a) Tumor extending from muscularis propria with identification of the papillary orifice (red arrow). Fine-needle biopsy of tumor (b).

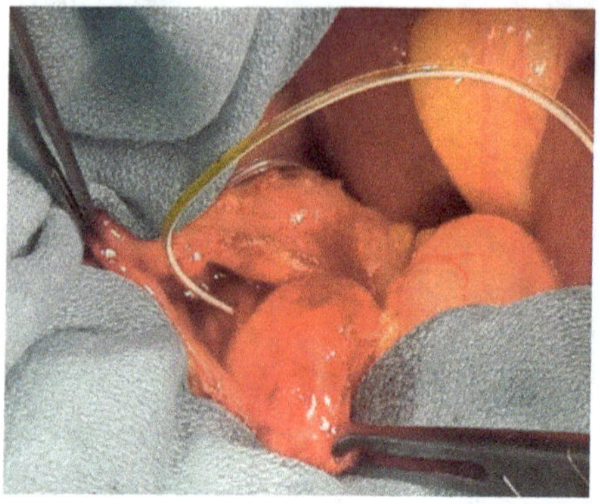

Figure 4: Intraoperative resection. Biliary catheter exiting ampulla.

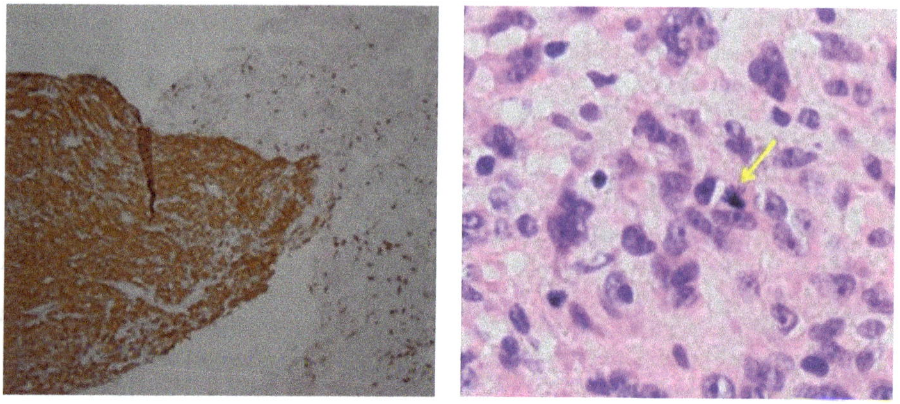

(a) (b)

Figure 5: Pathology results. CD117-positive GIST (a). Mitotic body (arrow) 8 per 5 mm^2 (high risk) (b).

Surveillance imaging 3 months after resection shows no evidence of recurrence. 12 months after resection, he is clinically well and tolerating imatinib therapy.

3. Discussion

An ampullary or periampullary GIST is an extremely rare neoplasm. The majority of GISTs are located in the stomach (60%–70%) and the small intestine (20%–25%), with only 4% occurring in the duodenum [6]. These tumors classically arise from the cells of Cajal, and malignant potential is largely based on mitotic index >5/50 hpf and size [4].

Complete resection with negative margins carries the highest potential for cure of GIST [7]. Universally, surgical resection should be the approach to the treatment of these tumors when feasible. Lymphatic spread remains exceedingly rare, and lymphadenectomy is not routinely warranted. Many authors still advocate for pancreaticoduodenectomy (PD or Whipple Procedure) for treatment of these tumors, which are adjacent to or involve the ampulla of Vater. However, PD carries significant morbidity and mortality [8].

Of the 13 cases of ampullary GIST available for comparison in the literature, 3 were locally resected [5, 9, 10]. Surgical decision-making and feasibility of resection were aided by use of endoscopic ultrasound in 2 of these cases. This is the third case where local resection of a periampullary GIST is aided by use of EUS preoperatively.

Additionally, the utility of EUS with fine-needle aspiration or core biopsy to make a preliminary diagnosis is instrumental in surgical planning. Neuroendocrine tumors (NETs) and GISTs can appear similarly on endoscopy and imaging. Differentiation is critical with regard to surgical approach, as there is typical indication for lymphadenectomy in the case of NET [11]. The yield of standard forceps biopsy of subepithelial lesions is typically <10% and as low as 4% in one study [12].

A 2008 study by Goh et al. suggests similar disease-specific survival with local resection compared to PD for duodenal GIST's [13]. Of the total 7 patients who underwent local resection in this study, the median disease-specific survival was 144 months. Given the EUS findings of preserved ductal anatomy, our patient was referred and underwent successful local resection of the GIST with sparing of the ampullary complex.

Ultimately, this case demonstrates how local resection can be achieved with a multidisciplinary approach and use of EUS. This approach can lead to preservation of the ampullary and biliary complex while achieving negative margins in a high-risk periampullary GIST. Prior to referral for PD of a high-risk periampullary GIST, the authors would advocate for the use of EUS in confirming the diagnosis and consideration of local resection.

Disclosure

This work was presented at the ACG Annual Scientific Meeting on Monday, October 8, 2018, titled "Endosonography in Guiding Local Resection and Ampullary Preservation of a High-Risk Peri-Ampullary GIST-A Novel Approach."

Authors' Contributions

Andrew Spiel, MD, was responsible for drafting the manuscript, data collection, and interpretation. He was also the guarantor. Ravi Patel, MD, Rebecca Minter, MD, Amir Ali Rahnemai Azar, MD, Rashmi Agni, MD, Antonio Bosch, MD, collected the data. Deepak Gopal, MD, FRCP(C), FACG, was involved in organization, data collection and interpretation, and manuscript editing.

References

[1] J. L. Buck and A. M. Elsayed, "Ampullary tumors: radiologic-pathologic correlation," *Radiographics*, vol. 13, no. 1, pp. 193–212, 1993.

[2] L. G. Kindblom, H. E. Remotti, F. Aldenborg, and J. M Meis-Kindblom, "Gastrointestinal pacemaker cell tumor (GIPACT): gastrointestinal stromal tumors show phenotypic characteristics of the interstitial cells of Cajal," *The American Journal of Pathology*, vol. 152, no. 152, pp. 1259–1269, 1998.

[3] C. D. M. Fletcher, J. J. Berman, C. Corless et al., "Diagnosis of gastrointestinal stromal tumors: a consensus approach," *Human Pathology*, vol. 33, no. 5, pp. 459–465, 2002.

[4] A. L. Faulx, S. Kothari, R. D. Acosta et al., "The role of endoscopy in subepithelial lesions of the GI tract," *Gastrointestinal Endoscopy*, vol. 85, pp. 1117–1132, 2017.

[5] K. Leung, M. Worni, J. Galeotti, and D. Blazer, "A novel approach: local resection for ampullary GIST case report and review of literature," *Journal of Gastrointestinal Cancer*, vol. 48, no. 4, pp. 376–378, 2017.

[6] M. Kobayashi, N. Hirata, S. Nakaji et al., "Gastrointestinal stromal tumor of the ampulla of vater: a case report," *World Journal of Gastroenterology*, vol. 20, no. 16, pp. 4817–4821, 2014.

[7] R. P. DeMatteo, J. J. Lewis, D. Leung, S. S. Mudan, J. M. Woodruff, and M. F. Brennan, "Two hundred gastrointestinal stromal tumors," *Annals of Surgery*, vol. 231, no. 1, pp. 51–58, 2000.

[8] F. Panzeri, S. Crippa, P. Castelli et al., "Management of ampullary neoplasms: a tailored approach between endoscopy and surgery," *World Journal of Gastroenterology*, vol. 21, no. 26, pp. 7970–7987, 2015.

[9] D. K. Filippou, N. Pashalidis, P. Skandalakis et al., "Malignant gastrointestinal stromal tumor of the ampulla of Vater presenting with obstructive jaundice," *Journal of Postgraduate Medicine*, vol. 52, no. 3, pp. 204–206, 2006.

[10] D. Singhal, M. Kumar, R. Sud et al., "Image of the month-quiz case," *Archives of Surgery*, vol. 142, no. 9, pp. 899-900, 2007.

[11] Y. Futo, S. Saito, H. Miyato et al., "Duodenal gastrointestinal stromal tumors appear similar to pancreatic neuroendocrine

tumors: a case report," *International Journal of Surgery Case Reports*, vol. 53, pp. 358–361, 2018.

[12] M. J. Cantor, R. E. Davila, and D. O. Faigel, "Yield of tissue sampling for subepithelial lesions evaluated by EUS: a comparison between forceps biopsies and endoscopic submucosal resection," *Gastrointestinal Endoscopy*, vol. 64, no. 1, pp. 29–34, 2006.

[13] B. K. P. Goh, P. K. H. Chow, S. Kesavan, W.-M. Yap, and W.-K. Wong, "Outcome after surgical treatment of suspected gastrointestinal stromal tumors involving the duodenum: is limited resection appropriate?" *Journal of Surgical Oncology*, vol. 97, no. 5, pp. 388–391, 2008.

Unusual Presentation of Recurrent Gallstone Ileus: A Case Report and Literature Review

Osayande Osagiede,[1] **Paula Pacurari**,[2] **Dorin Colibaseanu**,[1] **and Nezar Jrebi**[3]

[1] *Mayo Clinic, Department of Surgery, Jacksonville, FL, USA*
[2] *West Virginia University School of Medicine, Morgantown, WV, USA*
[3] *West Virginia University, Department of Surgery, Morgantown, WV, USA*

Correspondence should be addressed to Nezar Jrebi; nejrebi@hsc.wvu.edu

Academic Editor: Yoshifumi Nakayama

Background. Gallstone ileus (GSI) is a rare form of small bowel obstruction (SBO) in patients with cholelithiasis, which is often poorly managed. Enhanced abdominal computed tomography (CT) with contrast is considered the most helpful diagnostic tool, as it is highly sensitive, specific, and accurate. We report an interesting case of recurrent GSI that was not detected by CT but diagnosed intraoperatively. *Case Presentation.* A 49-year-old female with a previous history of choledocholithiasis and ERCP presented to the emergency department following episodes of sudden cramping, epigastric pain, and nausea. An abdominal CT revealed evidence of SBO with clear evidence of GSI and a cholecystoduodenal fistula. Laparoscopic exploration of the small bowel revealed a large, calcified 3.5 cm × 3 cm gallstone with evidence of pressure necrosis; segmental bowel resection with stapled anastomosis was performed and patient recovered appropriately after surgery. Cholecystectomy was not performed due to multiple co-morbidities and absence of gallbladder stones. However, she presented two months later with signs and symptoms of SBO. A repeat abdominal CT showed dilated bowel with no clear transition point. This was suspected to be due to adhesions. After an initial conservative treatment which produced mild improvement, laparotomy was performed which revealed a second large non-calcified gallstone and necrotic small bowel with a pocket of abscess. *Conclusion.* The most sensitive diagnostic tool for GSI is enhanced abdominal CT but dilemma arises when GSI is not detected on CT. A high index of suspicion and further exploration are required in order not to miss other vital findings.

1. Introduction

Gallstone ileus (GSI) is a rare form of bowel obstruction that occurs in 0.4–1.5% of patients with cholelithiasis [1]. Gallstones (>2 cm) are thought to enter the duodenum through a cholecystoduodenal fistula which forms as a rare complication of gallstone disease. GSI is an important complication of gallstone disease since it is often underreported and poorly managed.

Gallstones which enter the GI tract through a cholecystoduodenal fistula often become mechanically obstructed at the ileum due to its reduced diameter and the ileocecal valve. Patients present with small bowel obstruction symptoms including severe abdominal pain, nausea, vomiting, and abdominal distention. Differential diagnosis is completed by CT scans that reveal the presence of calcified gallstones in the lumen of the bowel at the transition point. Treatment includes minimally invasive surgery if possible or laparotomy to remove the stones and resect bowel if indicated. We report an interesting case of recurrent GSI that was not detected by CT scan but diagnosed intraoperatively. The clinical presentation, investigative findings, and management are discussed along with relevant literatures.

2. Case Report

A forty nine-year-old female presented to the emergency department due to episodes of sudden cramping, epigastric pain and nausea 2 months following endoscopic retrograde

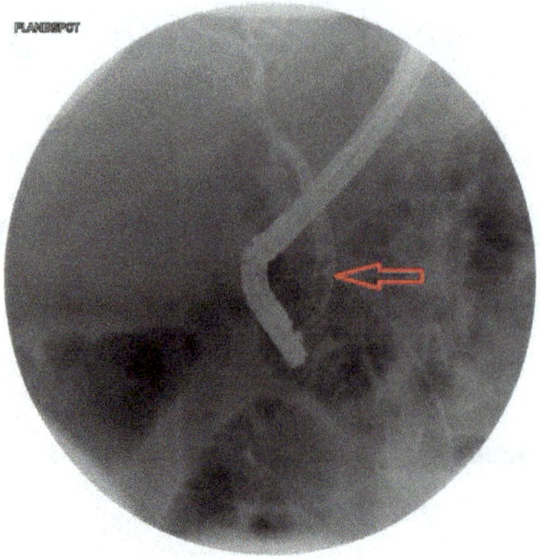

Figure 1: ERCP shows multiple stones in the common bile duct (red arrow).

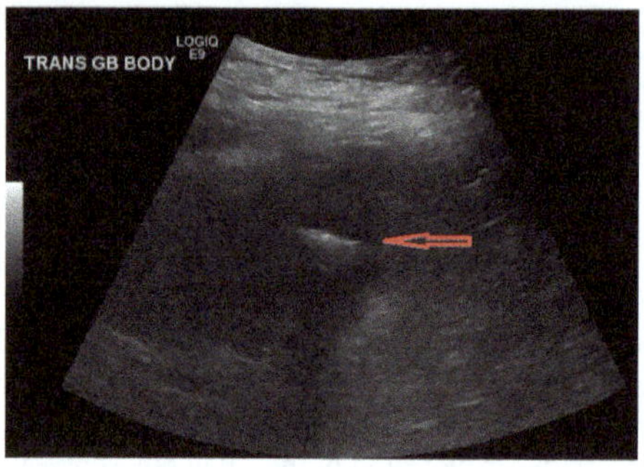

Figure 2: Abdominal ultrasound depicting a large stone in the gallbladder (red arrow).

cholangiopancreatography (ERCP) where three gallstones were removed from the common bile ducts (Figure 1). Before she underwent ERCP and endoscopic sphincterotomy, right upper quadrant abdominal ultrasound done on account of obstructive jaundice showed a noninflammed gallbladder with a large stone and a dilated common bile duct (Figure 2). Her past medical history was also notable for severe aortic stenosis, pulmonary hypertension, diabetes, unstable angina, and morbid obesity with BMI of 60 kg/m^2. Given her comorbidities, the plan during her ERCP visit was to perform her cholecystectomy at the same time she will undergo her gastric bypass, after optimizing her cardiopulmonary disease. At presentation, her abdominal computed tomography (CT) revealed evidence of small bowel obstruction with clear evidence of gallstone ileus (Figure 3). A cholecystoduodenal fistula was also present (Figure 4). Evidence of a decompressed gallbladder (Figure 5) and a clear transition point were noted. She was taken to the OR for laparoscopic exploration and small bowel examination. The segment that had the stone was identified and exteriorized through a small midline incision; the bowel was necrotic due to pressure ischemia; thus segmental bowel resection was performed with stapled anastomosis (Figure 6). A large, calcified 3.5 cm × 3 cm gallstone was found in the small bowel impacted at 60 cm proximal to the ileocecal valve (Figure 3) with evidence of pressure necrosis to the bowel. The bowel was examined via laparoscopy from the Ligament of Treitz to the ileocecal valve with no evidence of additional stones. Patient recovered appropriately after surgery and was discharged home.

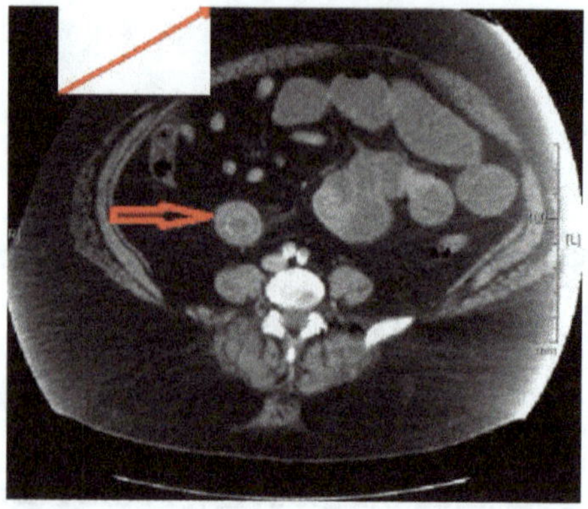

Figure 3: Contrast CT scan depicting gallstone in bowel (short red arrow).

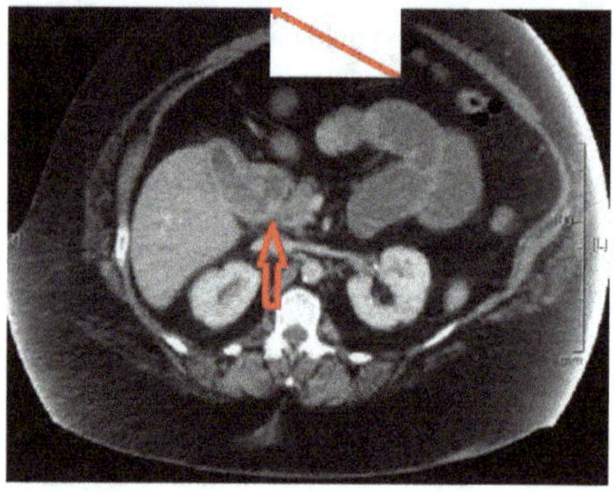

Figure 4: Contrast CT scan depicting cholecystoduodenal fistula (short red arrow).

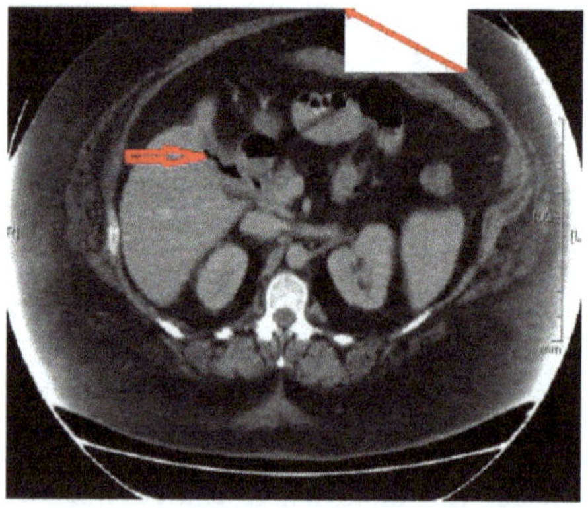

Figure 5: CT contrast scan depicting decompressed GB and air in GB, verifying that a stone was released (short red arrow).

A month later, she presented with signs and symptoms of small bowel obstruction. On physical exam, her abdomen was distended but with no tenderness. Patient was also noted to be in septic shock requiring vasopressors and unable to tolerate surgery; she was treated conservatively with Gastrografin challenge test (50 ml of water mixed with 100 ml of Gastrografin

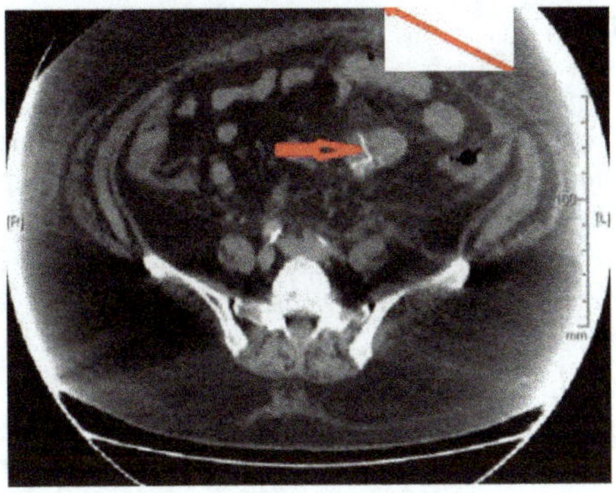

FIGURE 6: CT contrast scan depicting bowel anastomosis after 1st surgery (short red arrow).

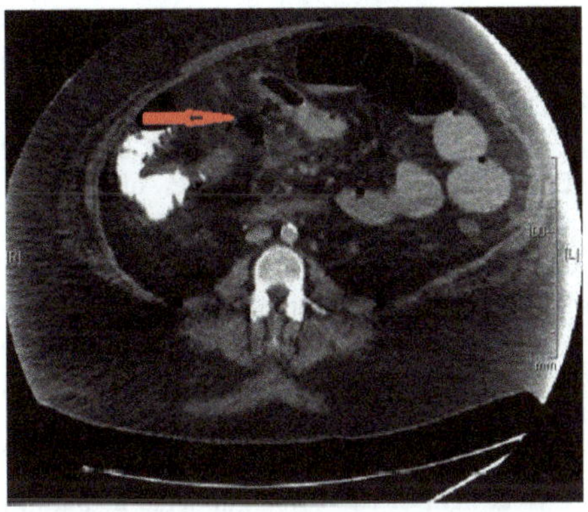

FIGURE 7: CT contrast scan depicting free air in pocket of abscess where bowel was perforated (short red arrow).

and given through the nasogastric tube, followed by abdominal X-ray in eight hours), which revealed contrast in the colon. Her symptoms completely resolved; she tolerated oral intake and was discharged from the hospital.

Patient presented again one month later with similar symptoms. At this presentation, she had an abdominal CT scan, which showed dilated bowel with no clear transition point. She was treated conservatively for five days with mild improvement where she tolerated liquids but not solid food. During the same hospital stay, she developed sudden severe abdominal pain, shortness of breath, tachycardia, and hypoxia. Another CT scan was performed with pulmonary embolism (PE) protocol which was negative for PE, but positive for free air (Figure 7). Patient was taken back to the OR for laparotomy, which revealed a second large non-calcified gallstone in the ileum impacted at the ileocecal valve distal to the previous anastomosis and perforated necrotic small bowel with a pocket of abscess. An intraoperative diagnosis of recurrent GSI was made. The abdomen was washed out; bowel resected; but anastomosis could not be performed given the severe inflammation. Patient was brought back to the OR for washout and closure; again, bowel anastomosis could not be performed, nor could the bowel be brought out as an end ileostomy due to severe obesity and shortened thickened mesentery. The bowel was placed in the upper part of the midline incision and the wound closed around it. Patient recovered appropriately and was discharged home. Subsequently, patient underwent elective surgery for cholecystectomy, takedown and primary repair of cholecystoduodenal fistula, bile duct exploration, suture repair of extra hepatic bile duct, and takedown of ileostomy with primary anastomosis.

3. Discussion

Gallstone ileus (GSI) is defined as bowel obstruction resulting from the impaction of one or more gallstones due to a cholecystoduodenal fistula. It is an uncommon complication of cholecystolithiasis; a rare cause of obstruction; and accounts for 1% to 4% of cases of mechanical obstruction of the bowel [2]. There are six factors known to cause a fistula: foreign body, radiation, inflammation, epithelialization, neoplasia, and distal obstruction. Risk factors for cholecystolithiasis include obesity and middle age, and it is also noted that females carry a greater risk.

Enhanced abdominal CT with contrast is considered the most helpful tool for diagnosis of gallstone ileus, as it is highly sensitive, specific, and accurate [3]. The findings of CT include obstruction of the small intestine, ectopic gallstones, pneumobilia, and gallbladder abnormalities. The information obtained with CT such as the site of obstruction, the size of the impacted gallstone, and the migration of the gallstone are important for determining whether conservative treatment is appropriate. The goals of treating GSI should be to relieve the intestinal obstruction quickly and to minimize morbidity and mortality. Once a gallstone has impacted within the small bowel and caused ileus, it rarely passes out spontaneously through the intestine [4, 5], though reports indicate that gallstones smaller than 25 mm usually pass through spontaneously [6].

The surgical dilemma in this case lies in the fact that despite the occurrence of a second bowel obstruction, GSI was not clearly noted in the CT scan. In addition, a decompressed gallbladder was not noted as well. It is accepted that the second stone was not calcified which is why it was not detected on the CT scan. It is recommended that these be checked upon initial surgery to prevent recurrent gallstones. Although the bowel was examined in the initial surgery for presence of additional stones in this case, it is probable that the second stone was in the gallbladder or duodenum. While the limitations of bowel examination by laparoscopy cannot be discounted, laparotomy was avoided in the initial surgery due to her significant cardiopulmonary disease and BMI. Recurrence of GSI can happen if the cholecystoduodenal fistula has not been closed, and this is more likely if a second stone is present in the gallbladder. It is fairly controversial in the literature whether to proceed with cholecystectomy or not in the presence of a cholecystoduodenal fistula, but there are substantial data to avoid cholecystectomy due to the high morbidity, though it is not considered a contraindication [7, 8]. Recurrence of GSI has been reported in 5–8% of patients [9], and 50% of all recurrences have been reported to occur within one month of the initial operation, while the remainder do so within 2 years [1, 10]. Methods to prevent recurrence involve cholecystectomy to prevent further bowel impaction, and closure of cholecystoduodenal fistula. In this case, the presence of gallstones after initial endoscopic management of CBD stones should have prompted laparoscopic cholecystectomy before considering a bariatric operation, but this could not be done at the time due to the patient's severe comorbidities. Additionally, the symptoms of small bowel obstruction that occurred one month after GSI laparoscopic management should have led to consideration of a priority treatment of the cholecystoduodenal fistula, but the cholecystoduodenal fistula was not addressed during that presentation because the patient was in septic shock on vasopressors and unable to tolerate surgery. In three cases previously described in the literature, the cholecystoduodenal fistula was completely mobilized with a combination of blunt and sharp dissection and divided using the endoscopic linear stapling device [11]. In two other cases, after division of the cystic duct and cystic artery, the gallbladder was dissected from the liver bed, leaving just the fistulous connection to the duodenum [11]. Then division of the fistula was completed using the same stapling device. All five patients had uneventful postoperative course. The hospital stay of the five patients ranged from 5 to 10 days [11].

4. Conclusion

Enhanced abdominal CT remains the most helpful diagnostic tool for GSI. Disproportionate symptoms and signs of a small bowel obstruction, in a patient with a history of gallstone disease or previous GSI, should alert the surgeon to suspect GSI as a possible cause despite the absence of radiologic findings. Further exploration is indicated to detect the presence of other vital findings such as noncalcified gallstones in the small bowel, pressure necrosis, bowel perforation, and abscess formation. Surgery is often indicated to relieve intestinal obstruction quickly and to minimize morbidity and mortality.

Abbreviations

GSI: Gallstone ileus
SBO: Small bowel obstruction
CT: Computed tomography
ERCP: Endoscopic retrograde cholangiopancreatography
BMI: Body mass index
PE: Pulmonary embolism.

Authors' Contributions

Osagiede O, Colibaseanu D and Jrebi N designed the report, analyzed the data and wrote the manuscript; Jrebi N performed the surgical procedure; Jrebi N and Pacurari P collected the clinical data and imaging information. All authors read and approved the final manuscript.

References

[1] J. R. Apollos and R. V. Guest, "Recurrent gallstone ileus due to a residual gallstone. A case report and literature review," *International Journal of Surgery Case Reports*, vol. 13, pp. 12–14, 2015.

[2] A. A. Ayantunde and A. Agrawal, "Gallstone ileus: diagnosis and management," *World Journal of Surgery*, vol. 31, no. 6, pp. 1294–1299, 2007.

[3] C. Y. Yu, C. C. Lin, R. Y. Shyu et al., "Value of CT in the diagnosis and management of gallstone ileus," *World Journal of Gastroenterology*, vol. 11, no. 14, pp. 2142–2147, 2005.

[4] A. Farooq, B. Memon, and M. A. Memon, "Resolution of gallstone ileus with spontaneous evacuation of gallstone," *Emergency Radiology*, vol. 14, no. 6, pp. 421–423, 2007.

[5] T. Miyasaka, H. Yoshida, H. Makino, M. Watanabe, E. Uchida, and E. Uchida, "Response of gallstone ileus to conservative therapy," *Journal of Nippon Medical School*, vol. 81, no. 6, pp. 388–391, 2014.

[6] Y. Kasahara, H. Umemura, S. Shiraha, T. Kuyama, K. Sakata, and H. Kubota, "Gallstone ileus. Review of 112 patients in the Japanese literature," *The American Journal of Surgery*, vol. 140, no. 3, pp. 437–440, 1980.

[7] F. Carlei, E. Lezoche, D. Lomanto et al., "Cholecystoenteric fistula is not a contraindication for laparoscopic cholecystectomy: report of five cases treated by laparoscopic approach," *Surgical Laparoscopy Endoscopy*, vol. 7, no. 5, pp. 403–406, 1997.

[8] F. J. Moreno Ruiz, A. del Rey Moreno, R. M. Suescun Garcia et al., "Treatment of cholecystoduodenal fistula in the era of laparoscopy," *Revista Española de Enfermedades Digestivas*, vol. 93, no. 11, pp. 715–720, 2001.

[9] N. Hayes and S. Saha, "Recurrent gallstone ileus," *Clinical Medicine & Research*, vol. 10, no. 4, pp. 236–239, 2012.

[10] M. P. Doogue, C. K. Choong, and F. A. Frizelle, "Recurrent gallstone ileus: underestimated," *Australian and New Zealand Journal of Surgery*, vol. 68, no. 11, pp. 755–756, 1998.

[11] A. Latic, F. Latic, M. Delibegovic, J. Samardzic, D. Kraljik, and S. Delibegovic, "Succcessful laparoscopic treatment of cholecystoduodenal fistula," *Medicinski Arhiv*, vol. 64, no. 6, pp. 379–380, 2010.

43

Denture Impaction Causing an Upper Esophageal Diverticulum

Shireen Samargandy, Hani Marzouki, Talal Al-Khatib, and Mazin Merdad

Department of Otolaryngology-Head and Neck Surgery, King Abdulaziz University, Jeddah, Saudi Arabia

Correspondence should be addressed to Shireen Samargandy; shireensamargandy@gmail.com

Academic Editor: Yoshihiro Moriwaki

Background. Dentures are a common cause of inadvertent foreign body ingestion particularly in the elderly. Due to their radiolucent nature, they often present a diagnostic challenge to care providing physicians. *Case Presentation.* A 66-year-old female presented to our otolaryngology clinic with a 2-year history of dysphagia. Her physical examination was unremarkable. Computed tomography scan of the neck and barium swallow suggested Zenker diverticulum. She was planned for endoscopic diverticulotomy; however, during surgery, a foreign body was incidentally found and retrieved, which was a partial lower denture. The diverticulum resolved thereafter, and the patient's symptoms abated. *Conclusion.* The authors recommend evaluating the esophagus endoscopically first in cases of upper esophageal diverticular formation, even when planning an open repair approach, to rule out any concealed foreign bodies.

1. Introduction

Accidental foreign body (FB) ingestion is a common problem in children and certain elderly populations. Among edentulous populations with compromised mental status or neurological disabilities, dentures are a frequent cause of FB impaction in the esophagus. Dentures are notoriously challenging to diagnose due to their radiolucent nature. Although the use of radiopaque substances in denture manufacturing has been recommended, such materials have yet to be successfully used without compromising denture quality. Hence, there is often a delay in the diagnosis and management of patients with impacted dentures, predisposing them to higher risks of complications such as esophageal perforation, diverticulum or fistula formation, or obstruction of the bowel. A rise in the rate of complications from 3.2% to 23.5% was reported when comparing patients managed after 24 hours with ones managed after 48 hours [1]. There are several described cases of denture impaction in the aerodigestive tracts in literature; however, only a small number of cases presented with diverticular formation. Here we present a special case of prolonged esophageal denture impaction that was diagnosed as Zenker diverticulum and later discovered to be a denture embedded in the patient's upper esophagus.

2. Case Presentation

A 66-year-old female presented to the otolaryngology clinic at our institution with a 2-year history of dysphagia to solids and liquids that was unprogressive in course. Her complaint was associated with mild odynophagia and unmeasured weight loss, as well as occasional coughing, aspirations, and regurgitation. Her past medical and surgical history was unremarkable.

On examination, the patient looked well but slightly underweight. She had no issues in phonation or respiration. There was no neck tenderness or swelling. Her oral exam was unremarkable except for being partially edentulous and having a missing single lower incisor tooth. Flexible laryngoscopy was performed in clinic and was normal.

Prior to her presentation at our institution, the patient had a computed tomography (CT) scan of the neck done in another hospital which showed a well-defined air-filled space at the level of the cricopharyngeus (CP) muscle measuring 13x19x37 millimeters. The report suggested Zenker diverticulum. She was referred to our tertiary care center for surgical management.

On admission, the patient's vital signs and basic laboratory blood investigations were within normal limits. Her

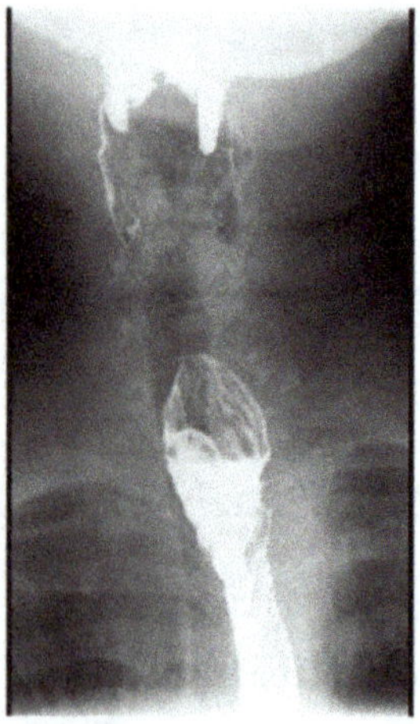

FIGURE 1: Barium swallow showing a left paramedian diverticulum with mild indentation on the trachea.

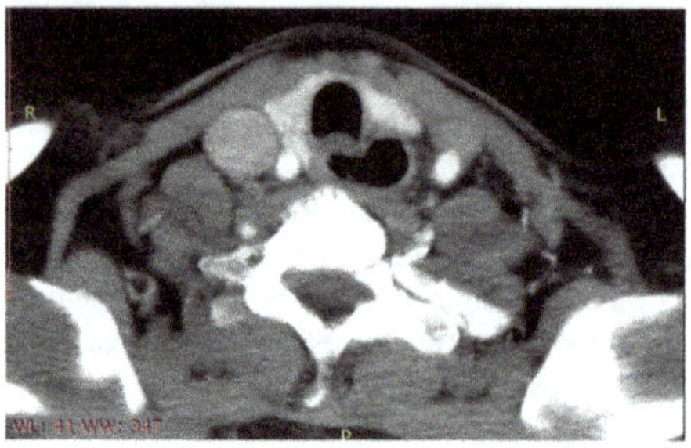

FIGURE 2: Axial CT scan image of the neck with contrast confirming the diverticulum arising from the midline that is directed towards the left side.

chest X-ray was unremarkable. A barium swallow revealed a left paramedian diverticulum located at the thoracic inlet (Figure 1). The previous CT was reviewed, and the radiologist confirmed the presence of a cricopharyngeal diverticulum arising from the midline and directed towards the left side consistent with Zenker diverticulum (Figure 2).

Considering the patient's clinical scenario and imaging studies, the patient was offered definitive surgery in the form of endoscopic diverticulotomy, with the possibility of converting to an open approach if endoscopic exposure was inadequate.

In the operating room, a Weerda scope was advanced orally to the level of the CP muscle. We were not able to visualize a clear CP bridge; however, a large cavity was seen at the level of the muscle with a free edge of a FB seen within. A zero-degree telescope was used to enhance visualization. The distal part of the FB was embedded in the esophageal wall. After gentle blunt dissection, it was successfully removed using long forceps (Figure 3) and was a removable partial lower incisor denture (Figure 4). Inspection of the esophagus after retrieval revealed minimal injury to the esophageal wall and complete resolution of the pouch.

Postoperatively, the patient was well, and her symptoms abated. She was kept under observation for the first 24 hours where her vital signs remained stable. Her diet progressed

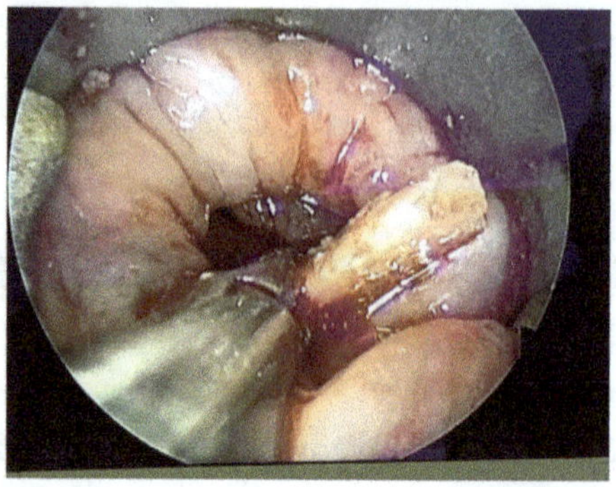

FIGURE 3: Endoscopic image of the foreign body retrieval.

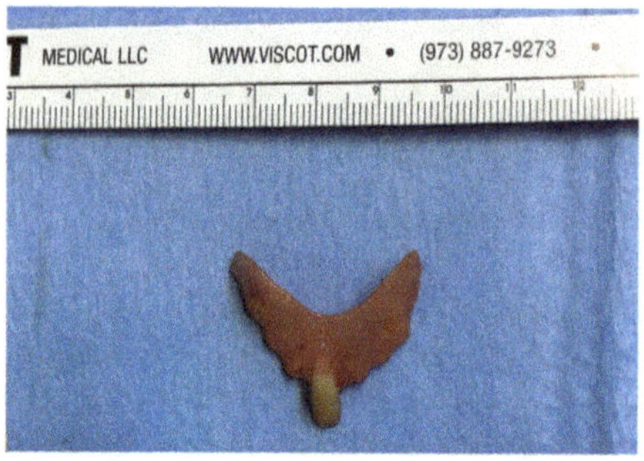

FIGURE 4: Removable partial lower incisor denture measuring 3 centimeters.

from soft to regular on the second day, after which she was discharged.

3. Discussion

Accidental ingestion of foreign bodies is a problem often faced in the emergency department with acute symptoms or, less frequently, in clinics with insidious presentations. Accidental ingestion and impaction of dental prostheses have been previously reported in literature. The incidence of esophageal denture impaction among FB ingestions ranged between 0.4% and up to 17.6%, and the most common site of impaction was the esophagus [2]. Certain high-risk groups have been mentioned in the literature including patients with confused mental status, alcohol inebriation, general anesthesia, medication overdoses, and neurological diseases such as seizure disorder [3, 4]. However, a systematic review by Kent et al. evaluated published reports of denture swallowing or aspiration over 15 years and concluded that 56% of patients did not have any predisposing factors. They also noted that most retrieved dentures were damaged or loose [5].

Patients with inadvertent denture swallowing may present with a clear history of the ingestion incident with or without additional complaints. They may also have no recollection of the accident and present instead with other vague symptoms that can resemble Zenker diverticulum. The most common symptoms upon presentation are throat discomfort, dysphagia, odynophagia, and persistent FB sensation [1, 6, 7]. The most reliable clinical signs indicative of FB entrapment in the cervical esophagus were neck tenderness and pooling of saliva in the pyriform sinuses [3, 5, 7, 8]. Our patient had no positive signs on clinical examination or flexible fiberoptic laryngoscopy.

The majority of case reports and retrospective studies documenting unintentional denture swallowing reported acute ingestions with patients often presenting within the span of 48 hours [6–8]. However, there were case reports with prolonged denture impactions varying in duration from days to years [3, 4]. Longer durations of denture entrapment have been linked with increased frequency of various complications stressing the importance of early intervention [1, 3]. Some late complications are life threatening such as fistula formation with major vessel erosion, major bronchus fistulas, abscess formation, or bowel perforation. Other possible complications include acute laryngeal edema and stricture or diverticular development [4, 7]. Fortunately, our patient only had a relatively minor complication of pulsion diverticulum formation after a lengthy 2-year course of impaction that resolved immediately after FB extraction.

There are several classifications for pharyngeal/esophageal diverticula.

One of the commonly encountered types of diverticula is Zenker diverticulum, which is an acquired false pulsion diverticulum located just adjacent to the CP muscle that forms because of increased pressure in the pharynx during deglutition leading to herniated mucosa and submucosa through a muscular wall defect. In contrast, our patient had a true pulsion type diverticulum just below the CP muscle bearing a higher resemblance to a Killian Jamieson diverticulum.

The majority of dentures are created from a synthetic resin acrylic termed polymethyl methacrylate. This material is radiolucent, making the diagnosis of impacted dentures more problematic [9]. They may or may not possess a metal attachment/clasp, and delays in discovery occur more often with unclasped dentures. Despite numerous reports of this problem, a radio-opaque denture material alternative has yet to be commercially available possibly due to their increased vulnerability to crack or break [9]. With that in mind, we can logically deduce that lateral neck radiographs would be rarely helpful. If they are performed, however, there are possible signs reported which include air in the esophagus, FB shadow, and salivary pooling with fluid level, in addition to losing the cervical lordosis [10]. Water-soluble contrast studies of the upper gastrointestinal tract would be ideal to detect the location of impaction and presence of a diverticulum and to diagnose other possible causes of dysphagia such as strictures. The utilization of barium studies in cases of suspected FB ingestion has been less favored in the literature as they can make the following endoscopy more challenging by coating the FB. CT imaging offers some advantages over other radiological techniques by its superiority in detecting acrylic based dentures and potential complications [8].

Initially, our patient's management plan included endoscopic diverticulotomy for a Zenker diverticulum; however, it was aborted upon discovery and removal of the culprit FB. There are several approaches for the removal of impacted dental prostheses: observation, endoscopic or open surgical retrieval. Although there had been reports of cases where dentures passed spontaneously, there is limited value for a watchful waiting approach in cases of denture impaction due to their high complication rates [7]. Our present case was managed successfully with endoscopic extraction of the ingested dental prosthesis. Ultimately, the method of removing the FB largely depends on clinical judgment.

4. Conclusion

When managing certain patients with dysphagia and odynophagia, a high index of suspicion for FB ingestion is needed even with prolonged symptoms. Emphasis on enquiring about dentures is particularly of value in the elderly, and thorough examination of the oral cavity and dentition is essential. Even though most dentures are radiolucent, imaging studies could still aid in the diagnosis, particularly studies of the upper gastrointestinal tract and CT radiography. Lateral neck radiographs might be useful in detecting radiopaque clasps on dental prostheses. When managing a suspected CP level diverticulum, including Zenker diverticulum, the authors recommend first evaluating the upper esophagus endoscopically, even when planning an open approach, to rule out any concealed FBs.

Abbreviations

FB: Foreign body
CT: Computed tomography
CP: Cricopharyngeus.

Disclosure

The study was conducted at King Abdulaziz University Hospital, Jeddah, Saudi Arabia.

Authors' Contributions

Shireen Samargandy contributed to data collection and manuscript preparation. Mazin Merdad, Hani Marzouki, and Talal Al-Khatib contributed to manuscript reviewing.

References

[1] P. Singh, A. Singh, P. Kant, B. Zonunsanga, and A. S. Kuka, "An impacted denture in the oesophagus—an endoscopic or a surgical emergency—a case report," *Journal of Clinical and Diagnostic Research*, vol. 7, no. 5, pp. 919-920, 2013.

[2] P. Nandi and G. B. Ong, "Foreign body in the esophagus: review of 2394 cases," *British Journal of Surgery*, vol. 65, no. 1, pp. 5–9, 1978.

[3] G. A. Dar, F. A. Ganie, M. Ishaq et al., "Prolonged impacted denture in the esophagus: a case report and review of the literature," *The Journal of the American Dental Association*, vol. 3, no. 1, pp. 32–35, 2015.

[4] S. Hashmi, J. Walter, W. Smith, and S. Latis, "Swallowed partial dentures," *Journal of the Royal Society of Medicine*, vol. 97, no. 2, pp. 72–75, 2004.

[5] S. J. Kent, J. Mackie, and T. V. Macfarlane, "Designing for safety: implications of a fifteen year review of swallowed and aspirated dentures," *Journal of Oral & Maxillofacial Research*, vol. 7, no. 2, p. e3, 2016.

[6] O. G. Nwaorgu, P. A. Onakoya, O. A. Sogebi, D. D. Kokong, and O. O. Dosumu, "Esophageal impacted dentures," *Journal of the National Medical Association*, vol. 96, no. 10, pp. 1350–1353, 2004.

[7] T. O. Adedeji, A. O. Olaosun, O. A. Sogebi, and J. E. Tobih, "Denture impaction in the oesophagus experience of a young ENT practice in Nigeria," *Pan African Medical Journal*, vol. 18, p. 330, 2014.

[8] S. N. Bandyopadhyay, S. Das, S. K. Das, and A. Mandal, "Impacted dentures in the oesophagus," *The Journal of Laryngology & Otology*, vol. 128, no. 5, pp. 468–474, 2014.

[9] G. M. Brauer, "The desirability of using radio-opaque plastics in dentistry—a status report," *The Journal of the American Dental Association*, vol. 102, pp. 347–349, 1981.

[10] J. Marais, R. Mitchell, and A. J. A. Wightman, "The value of radiographic assessment for oropharyngeal foreign bodies," *The Journal of Laryngology & Otology*, vol. 109, no. 5, pp. 452–454, 1995.

44

Esophageal Dieulafoy Lesion: A Rare and Potentially Fatal Entity

Eoghan P Burke

Royal College of Surgeons Ireland, Dublin, Ireland

Correspondence should be addressed to Eoghan P Burke; eoghanburke@rcsi.ie

Academic Editor: Yoshifumi Nakayama

A 35-year-old gentleman presented acutely to the emergency department with large volume haematemesis and melena. Following adequate initial resuscitation, the patient underwent emergency upper gastrointestinal endoscopy which revealed a dilated tortuous submucosal vessel which was actively bleeding at the midpoint of the esophagus. This was consistent with a Dieulafoy lesion. However, its position in the midpoint of the esophagus is rare. Our patient recovered well following intervention.

1. Introduction

Dieulafoy lesions are a rare but important cause of massive gastrointestinal (GI) bleeding. They account for less than 2% of gastrointestinal bleeds but have a significant risk of morbidity and mortality secondary to delayed diagnosis and treatment [1]. The underlying pathophysiology of these lesions is poorly understood. They are classified as dilated tortuous histologically normal submucosal arteries [2]. They classically occur in the stomach on the lesser curvature but have been reported in the colon, duodenum, and rarely in the esophagus as in our report [3]. Patients typically present with acute onset large volume haematemesis and/or melena. Unlike bleeding from a Mallory-Weiss tear, bleeding from a Dieulafoy lesion is not typically associated with preceding retching or vomiting [4]. Diagnosis usually involves endoscopy although there is a growing role for angiography particularly if suspicion remains following a normal endoscopic evaluation. Endoscopy has the added advantage of being therapeutic as well as diagnostic [5].

2. Case Presentation

A 35-year-old gentleman presented acutely to the emergency department with haematemesis and melena. He had no past medical or surgical history and was not taking any regular medications. He worked as a secondary school teacher. Of note, he had no risk factors or diagnosis of liver disease, cirrhosis, or portal hypertension. The haematemesis and melena occurred acutely with no preceding vomiting. He had been attending a choir rehearsal with his class of students when the bleeding occurred. On clinical examination, he was noted to be of normal BMI. He was hypotensive and tachycardic in the emergency department, and laboratory investigations were significant for a haemoglobin of 8 g/dl. The massive transfusion protocol was activated, and he was prepared for emergency endoscopy. At esophagogastroduodenoscopy, he was found to be actively bleeding from a visible dilated tortuous vessel at the midpoint of the esophagus. The bleeding was pulsatile in nature. The findings were consistent with a Dieulafoy lesion (Figure 1).

He remained stable with no further bleeds. The patient was counselled on the need for further evaluation to determine whether a definitive procedure was required to excise this vessel completely given its high risk of rebleeding. However, he refused further investigations/interventions. He was discharged home well.

3. Discussion

Dieulafoy's lesion was initially described by Gallard in 1884 as "military aneurysms of the stomach." However, it became synonymous with the French surgeon Dr Georges Dieulafoy in 1898 when he more accurately characterised them during his investigation of fatal upper gastrointestinal haemorrhage in three young asymptomatic men [6].

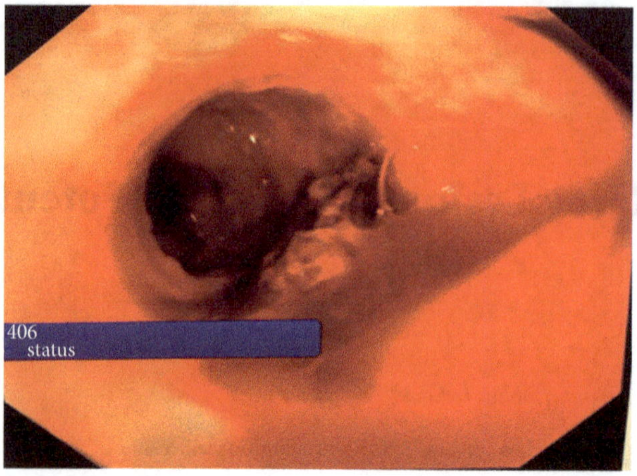

Figure 1: EGD image of active bleeding from a visible dilated tortuous vessel at the midpoint of the esophagus. His bleeding was controlled using endoclips and haemostatic powder (Figure 2).

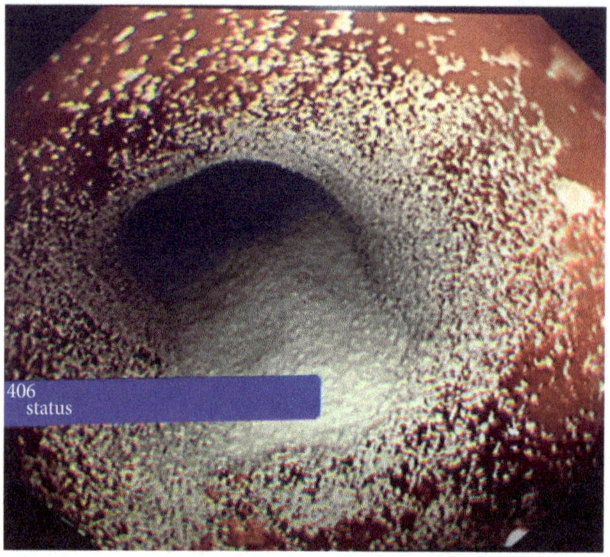

Figure 2: EGD image postsuccessful haemostasis using dual therapy of endoclips and haemostatic powder.

These lesions are classically found in the stomach predominantly on the lesser curvature. The precise reason for this remains controversial. Some have attributed it to the fact that the submucosal blood supply in this region of the stomach arises directly from the right and left gastric arteries which run adjacent to the lesser curvature suspended in the hepatogastric ligament and so do not have to transit a significant distance prior to reaching their end-organ [7]. However up to 1/3 of Dieulafoy lesions may occur outside the stomach, predominantly in the duodenum and colon. The aetiology for these lesions, at sites other than the lesser curvature of the stomach, remains unclear [8].

The underlying pathophysiology for the development of these lesions is poorly understood. These lesions are histologically normal, when analysed in resected specimens, but maintain a larger calibre in comparison with adjacent blood vessels. It is well documented that a normal artery of the gastrointestinal tract will narrow as it traverses the wall of the organ it is supplying [9]. This, however, is not the case in Dieulafoys lesions as these vessels maintain the same patency throughout their course. As these vessels remain larger in diameter within the submucosa, they may cause damage to the overlying mucosa secondary to forceful pulsation. Should the overlying mucosa breakdown these vessels are then exposed and subject to trauma and thus haemorrhage, often without any proceeding symptoms [10].

These lesions are reported as being rare in the esophagus [11]. A literature review performed on PubMed using the following search string: ((Dieulafoy Lesion) AND (Dieulafoy's Lesion)) AND (Oesophagus OR esophagus) yielded 32 results. On review of the abstracts of these reports, 10 were found to pertained to Dieulafoy's lesions in the oesophagus presenting with upper GI bleeding and were published in the English language with abstracts available. Table 1 reviews these previous reports. It remains unclear, however, whether this is due to under diagnosis. These vascular abnormalities can present with massive upper gastrointestinal haemorrhage and can be fatal if haemostasis

TABLE 1: Summary of previously published case reports and case series pertaining to Dieulafoy lesions in the oesophagus.

Publication	Demographics	Presentation	Site of lesion	Treatment and outcome
Inayat, F., Ullah, W., Hussain, Q. and Hurairah, A., 2017. Dieulafoy's lesion of the oesophagus: a case series and literature review. Case Reports, 2017, p. bcr2016218100.			3 patients	
	53 years old caucasian male.	1 week history of melena	Distal oesophagus	Adrenaline injection and haemoclips
	68 years old Caucasian male	Admitted following RTA, on day 2 of admission developed fresh rectal bleeding	Distal oesophagus	Haemoclips
	80 years old Caucasian male	2-day history of haematemesis	Distal oesophagus	All three patients recovered well and were discharged home with no further intervention
Nemakayala, D.R., rai, M.P., Yam, J.L. and Laird-Fick, H., 2018. Dieulafoy's lesion in the oesophagus: A rare cause of upper gastrointestinal Bleeding. Case Reports, 2018, pp. bcr-2017.	55 years old Caucasian male.	3-day history of melena and a presyncopal episode	Distal oesophagus	Adrenaline injection and gold probe cautery Discharged home with no further intervention
Ertekin, C., Barbaros, U., Taviloglu, K., Guloglu, R. and Kasoglu, A., 2002. Dieulafoy's lesion of esophagus. Surgical Endoscopy And Other Interventional Techniques, 16 [1], pp. 219–219.	25-year-old female	Haematemesis and melena	Distal oesophagus	Band ligation Discharged home with no further intervention
El Hajj, I.I., Malik, S. and McGrath, K.M., 2010. Endoscopic clipping of Dieulafoy's lesion in the upper esophagus. Digestive and Liver Disease, 42 [2], pp. 155–156.	61-year-old male	Haematemesis.	Upper oesophagus	Haemoclip Discharged home with no further intervention
Benatta, M.A. and Grimaud, J.C., 2017. Band ligation for a gastroesophageal junction Dieulafoy's lesion. The Pan African medical journal, 26.	24-year-old male	Haematemesis	OGJ	Band ligation Discharged home with no further intervention
Yoshida, T., Adachi, K., Tanioka, Y., Sasaki, T., Ono, S., Hanada, H., Esaki, T., Yagawa, T., Takeo, S., Saiki, Y. and Harada, T., 2004. Dieulafoy's lesion of the esophagus correctly diagnosed and successfully treated by the endoscopic injection of N-butyl-2-cyanoacrylate. Endoscopy, 36(02), pp. 183–185.	74-year-old male	Haematemesis and melena	Distal oesophagus	Injected with N-butyl-2-cyanoacrylate Discharged home with no further intervention
Ho, K.M., 2004. Use of Sengstaken-Blakemore tube to stop massive upper gastrointestinal bleeding from Dieulafoy's lesion in the lower oesophagus. Anaesthesia and intensive care, 32 [5], pp. 711–714.	71-year-old male	Haematemesis	Distal oesophagus	Adrenaline injection and bipolar diathermy Further bleed controlled with Sengstaken–Blakemore tube Repeat OGD did not identify a bleeding point Discharged home with no further intervention
Malliaras, G.P., carollo, A. and Bogen, G., 2016. Esophageal Dieulafoy's lesion: An exceedingly rare cause of massive upper GI bleeding. Journal of surgical case reports, 2016 [6], p.rjw074.	55-year-old male	Haematemesis	Distal oesophagus	Adrenaline and haemoclip placement Discharged home with no further intervention
Thimmapuram, J., Shah, M. and Srour, J., 2011. Esophageal Dieulafoy lesion: An unusual cause of GI bleeding. Gastrointestinal endoscopy (Print), 73 [5], pp. 1055–1056.	55-year-old male	Haematemesis	Mid oesophagus	Adrenaline injection and haemoclip application Discharged home with no further intervention

Table 1: Continued.

Publication	Demographics	Presentation	Site of lesion	Treatment and outcome
Abraham, P., Mukerji, S.S., Desai, D.C. And Joshi, A.G., 2004. Dieulafoy lesion in mid-esophagus with esophageal varices. Indian journal of gastroenterology: official journal of the Indian Society of Gastroenterology, 23 [6], pp. 220–221.	54-year-old male	Haematemesis	Distal oesophagus	Band ligation

cannot be obtained. If identified they can often be managed effectively with standard endoscopic techniques.

These lesions are under recognized and should be considered in all cases of acute GI bleeding.

References

[1] M. Baxter and E. Aly, "Dieulafoy's lesion: current trends in diagnosis and management," *The Annals of The Royal College of Surgeons of England*, vol. 92, no. 7, pp. 548–554, 2010.

[2] R. A. Chaer and W. S. Helton, "Dieulafoy's disease," *Journal of the American College of Surgeons*, vol. 196, no. 2, pp. 290–296, 2003.

[3] G. Marangoni, A. B. Cresswell, W. Faraj, H. Shaikh, and M. J. Bowles, "An uncommon cause of life-threatening gastrointestinal bleeding: 2 synchronous Dieulafoy lesions," *Journal of Pediatric Surgery*, vol. 44, no. 2, pp. 441–443, 2009.

[4] Y. T. Lee, R. S. Walmsley, R. W. L. Leong, and J. J. Y. Sung, "Dieulafoy's lesion," *Gastrointestinal Endoscopy*, vol. 58, no. 2, pp. 236–243, 2003.

[5] K. Suresh, D. Ortolano, A. Ashiq, and S. Patel, "An interesting case of gastrointestinal bleeding resulting from Dieulafoy's lesion," *American Journal of Medical Case Reports*, vol. 8, no. 4, pp. 110-111, 2020.

[6] G. L. Juler, H. G. Labitzke, R. Lamb, and R. Allen, "The pathogenesis of Dieulafoy's gastric erosion," *American Journal of Gastroenterology*, vol. 79, no. 3, 1984.

[7] G. Anagnostopoulos, S. Foley, and K. Ragunath, "Dieulafoy lesion in the duodenum," *The New Zealand Medical Journal (Online)*, vol. 118, no. 1225, 2005.

[8] P. Katsinelos, I. Pilpilidis, G. Paroutoglou et al., "Dieulafoy-like lesion of the colon presenting with massive lower gastrointestinal bleeding," *Surgical Endoscopy And Other Interventional Techniques*, vol. 18, no. 2, p. 346, 2004.

[9] M. J. Morowitz, R. Markowitz, B. M. Kamath, and D. von Allmen, "Dieulafoy's lesion and segmental dilatation of the small bowel: an uncommon cause of gastrointestinal bleeding," *Journal of Pediatric Surgery*, vol. 39, no. 11, pp. 1726–1728, 2004.

[10] C. Contardo, "Upper gastrointestinal bleeding related to dieulafoy lesion," *Revista de gastroenterologia del Peru: organo oficial de la Sociedad de Gastroenterologia del Peru*, vol. 20, no. 4, pp. 422–429, 2000.

[11] F. Inayat, W. Ullah, Q. Hussain, and A. Hurairah, "Dieulafoy's lesion of the oesophagus: a case series and literature review," *BMJ Case Reports*, vol. 2017, Article ID bcr2016218100, 2017.

45

Colorectal Cancer Related to Chronic *Strongyloides stercoralis* Infection

M. Sava,[1,2] T. Huynh,[3] A. Frugoli,[3] L. Kong,[4] M. Salehpour,[5] and B. Barrows[6]

[1]*Western University of Health Sciences, Ventura, CA, USA*
[2]*Community Memorial Health Systems, Graduate Medical Education, Ventura, CA, USA*
[3]*Community Memorial Health Systems, Graduate Medical Education, Department of Internal Medicine, Ventura, CA, USA*
[4]*Community Memorial Health Systems, Graduate Medical Educations, Department of Hematology Oncology, Ventura, CA, USA*
[5]*Community Memorial Hospital, Department of General Surgery, Ventura, CA, USA*
[6]*Community Memorial Hospital, Department of Pathology, Ventura, CA, USA*

Correspondence should be addressed to T. Huynh; thuynh3@cmhshealth.org

Academic Editor: Haruhiko Sugimura

The majority of individuals with *Strongyloides stercoralis* (*S. stercoralis*) colitis are clinically asymptomatic. Symptomatic individuals may complain of nonspecific gastrointestinal symptoms, such as abdominal pain, intermittent or persistent diarrhea, nausea, or loss of appetite. In addition, skin manifestations such as recurrent urticaria can occur. If infection is not diagnosed and left untreated, it can lead to chronic inflammation of the gastrointestinal tract. It is well documented that chronic colitis such as inflammatory bowel disease can predispose individuals to colorectal cancer. Additionally, there is evidence of chronic parasitic infections inducing the development of cancers in other organs within the gastrointestinal tract. In this case vignette, we describe a case of chronic *Strongyloides stercoralis* infection in a Peruvian woman presenting with colorectal cancer.

1. Introduction

Strongyloidiasis is caused by *S. stercoralis*, a soil-transmitted helminth, endemic in tropical and subtropical regions including Latin America, sub-Saharan Africa, and Southeast Asia [1–3]. Worldwide, between 30 and 100 million people are infected. However, in the United States, a series of small studies in select populations have shown that between 0% and 6.1% of persons sampled were infected by *S. stercoralis* [4]. The presence of infection is greater for immigrants to the United States. The total prevalence of *S. stercoralis* is likely underestimated because of the low sensitivity of testing, nonspecific symptoms, and no clear guidelines for testing in nonendemic areas. *S. stercoralis* infection can persist for decades in a single patient due to its autoinfection life cycle. Infectious agents, including parasites, often have oncogenic potential. According to Parkin et al., the global health burden of infection associated with cancer in 2002 included 17.8% of the malignancy burden. The infections associated with malignancy range from chronic bacterial infections, such as *Helicobacter pylori*, viral etiologies including viral hepatitis, and, in rare cases, flukes or parasites can also contribute to cancer development [5]. Multiple studies have reported that *S. stercoralis* may be a cofactor in HTLV-1-related T-cell lymphoma in endemic areas [6, 7]. In addition, a number of case reports have described the occurrence of gastrointestinal cancer with *S. stercoralis* infection, suggesting that the parasite may be a risk factor for gastrointestinal malignancy [3, 5, 8, 9]. Contrary to this, some hypothesize that gastrointestinal malignancy is a risk for infection.

This case vignette describes a rare parasitic infection with review of microbe-associated malignancy literature and suggests possible hypotheses for an association between chronic *S. stercoralis* infection and colorectal cancer.

2. Case Report

A 70-year-old Peruvian female with a history of gastroesophageal reflux disease, osteoporosis, and hyperlipidemia was admitted for worsening abdominal pain and nonbloody diarrhea with associated weight loss and early satiety. The patient first noticed an increase in her vague abdominal pain with diarrhea after she returned from a trip to Peru about six weeks prior. She frequently travels to Peru to visit family at least biannually. She reported chronic intermittent non-specific symptoms of abdominal pain and bloating for years. Upon return from her recent trip, she was prescribed sulfamethoxazole and trimethoprim for a total of three days for possible traveler's diarrhea and her symptoms subsided. The following week, she developed upper abdominal pain that gradually became more severe. It was worse with direct pressure and relieved with rest. She also had unintentional weight loss of five pounds in the last month. Her last colonoscopy was done in 2012 (nearly 7 years prior, in Peru), which was unremarkable except for diverticulosis without polyps. She has no family history of colon polyps, colorectal cancer, celiac disease, or inflammatory bowel disease (IBD).

Physical exam was notable for subumbilical and right lower quadrant tenderness. A complete blood count with differential revealed normocytic anemia (hemoglobin 10.9 g/dL) and peripheral eosinophilia (13.1%). Laboratory studies revealed iron deficiency, albumin 3.4 g/dL, and CEA 2.1. A stool PCR panel was positive for enteroaggregative *Escherichia coli* (EAEC) and enteropathogenic *Escherichia coli* (EPEC). Stool ova and parasite (O&P) examination was positive for *S. stercoralis*, and a fecal occult blood test was also positive. Review of medical records revealed new-onset anemia for the last year and intermittent eosinophilia (19%) for the last 3 years, with multiple health care visits for gastrointestinal complaints.

The patient underwent computed tomography (CT) of the abdomen and pelvis with intravenous contrast, which demonstrated marked irregularity of the right ascending colon and sigmoid with heterogeneous enhancing right colonic mass (~7 cm) with a few small adjacent lymph nodes (Figure 1). There was colo-colonic intussusception with associated submucosal edema. She underwent follow-up colonoscopy that demonstrated a nearly obstructing pedunculated mass with malignant appearance in the right ascending colon near the cecum (Figure 2), a 10 mm sessile polyp in the descending colon, and moderate diverticulosis of the left colon. The colonic mass was biopsied in multiple areas, and the polyp excised. Biopsy of the mass revealed invasive adenocarcinoma, and the descending colon polyp was found to be a tubulovillous adenoma.

Given the patient's stool exam was positive for *S. stercoralis* with gastrointestinal symptoms, the patient was treated with ivermectin 200 μg/kg on day one and repeated 24 hours later, with an additional dose at two weeks. Due to the size of the obstructing mass with risk of colon perforation, the patient underwent exploratory laparotomy with right hemicolectomy and reanastomosis (Figure 3). Pathologic evaluation of the specimen revealed stage IIIB with poorly differentiated adenocarcinoma with lymphovascular invasion, perineural invasion, and 3 of 38 lymph nodes involved. Sections of the uninvolved colon were unremarkable and showed no inflammation or other features suggestive of *S. stercoralis* infection (Figure 4(a)). Histologic examination of the mass showed sheet-like architecture of the malignant cells with scattered foci of gland formation, consistent with poorly differentiated adenocarcinoma (Figure 4(b)). Sections of the carcinoma also demonstrated numerous tumor infiltrating lymphocytes and scattered lymphocyte aggregates at the periphery of the tumor consistent with a Crohn's-like inflammatory response. Mismatch repair protein immunohistochemistry for possible hereditary nonpolyposis colon cancer (HNPCC) showed absent nuclear expression of MLH1 and PMS2. However, the MLH1 methylation study was positive for hypermethylation (59.4%; ref <20%), and a BRAF V600E mutation was identified by molecular studies, consistent with sporadic adenocarcinoma (not associated with HNPCC). Up to 15% of colon cancers show altered expression of mismatch repair proteins correlating with microsatellite instability in tumor cells. However, the majority of these cases are due to sporadic loss of MLH1 expression as a result of somatic/epigenetic inactivation of MLH1 (promoter hypermethylation). The presence of BRAF V600E mutation is helpful since this mutation has been found in sporadic microsatellite unstable tumors, but not in HNPCC-associated cancers [10]. Risks and benefits of oral chemotherapy with capecitabine and oxaliplatin and IV chemotherapy with oxaliplatin were discussed, including adjuvant therapy.

3. Discussion

S. stercoralis infection in humans starts with infectious filariform larvae penetrating the skin, entering venous circulation, and migrating to the lungs [4]. The organisms are then carried to the pharynx and swallowed [4]. This cycle can be accelerated by ingestion of contaminated water containing filariform larvae. In the small intestine, the larvae develop into adult females, which reproduce asexually and release eggs into the gastrointestinal tract [4, 11]. The persistence of *S. stercoralis* infection is due to the parasite's unusual capability to undergo an autoinfective cycle in absence of reinfection [12]. Autoinfection is characterized by the ability of rhabditiform larvae in the large intestine to transform into infectious filariform larvae, then penetrate the intestinal mucosa, and migrate to other organs including the lungs, restarting the cycle [4]. Another peculiarity of *S. stercoralis* is its capacity to cause hyperinfection syndrome, as a result of uncontrolled overproliferation of filariform larvae in stool and sputum, leading to the clinical manifestation of larval migration with development or exacerbation of gastrointestinal and pulmonary symptoms [3]. Hyperinfection syndrome primarily occurs in immunocompromised individuals and can have a high mortality rate (approaching 100%) if not diagnosed and treated [13]. Patients with *S. stercoralis* infection may have a variety of symptoms involving the gastrointestinal tract (abdominal pain and diarrhea), skin (itching and urticaria), and respiratory tract (asthma-like symptoms and dyspnea) [4]. In a meta-analysis, urticaria showed a strong association with *S. stercoralis* infection, while diarrhea and abdominal pain had a weaker association [12].

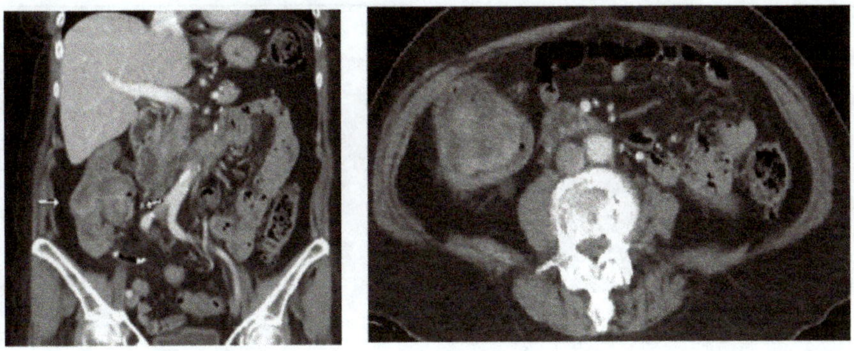

(a) (b)

FIGURE 1: Right ascending mass in ascending colon CT. (a) (Arrows) colo-colonic intussusception with associated submucosal edema. (b) Right colonic mass measuring approximately 7 cm.

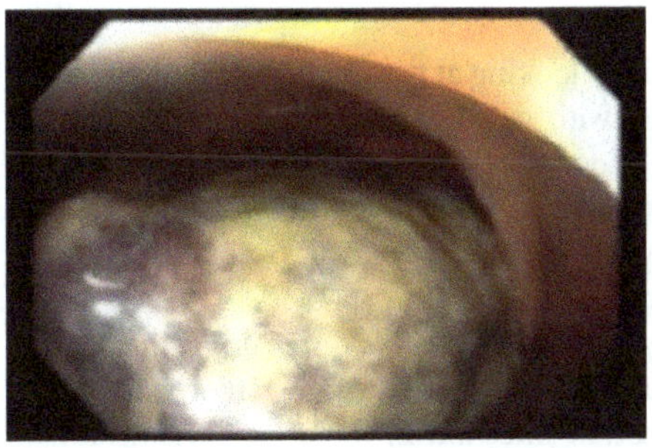

FIGURE 2: Images from colonoscopy demonstrating pedunculated large mass in the cecum.

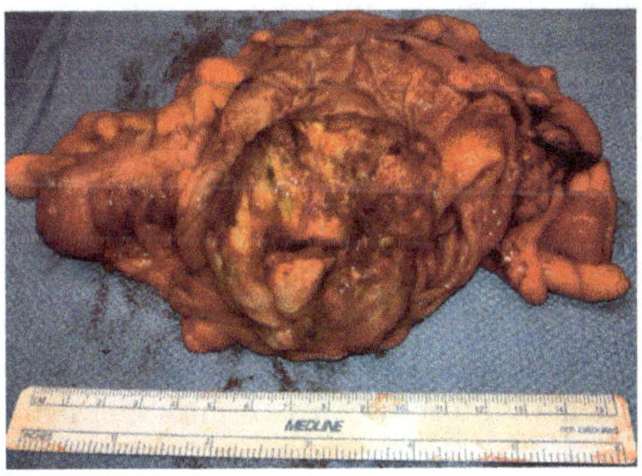

FIGURE 3: Gross pathologic specimen demonstrating a large tumor.

The gold standard for the diagnosis of strongyloidiasis is serial stool examination. Routine stool examination identifies up to 30% of cases because of low infectious burden and intermittent larval excretion. Thus, repeat stool collection of multiple samples can increase the sensitivity of the test to 80–90%. Eosinophilia is an important marker in nematode parasite infections and is common with strongyloidiasis. The eosinophil count may be normal in patients with severe strongyloidiasis or immunosuppression [11]. The patient in our case report demonstrated absolute eosinophilia (up to 1000/μL; ref 0–500/μL) and a positive stool O&P examination, which aided in making the diagnosis, so appropriate treatment could be started. We suggest that the parasitic load was high enough to stimulate the immune system to increase production of eosinophils in this patient.

The connection between infection and malignancy is well studied. Knoll et al. in their expert review reported that "infections are estimated to be responsible for up to 25% to 50% of all cancers that occur in humans." In their 18 Pearl review, they provide examples of infections caused by viruses, bacteria, parasites, and fungi with their contribution to the development of malignancy. A summary of the prior research investigating infection-associated malignancy risk states infections can promote carcinogenesis by three main mechanisms: chronic inflammation due to the persistence of an infectious agent in the host; insertion of oncogenes into the host genome; and reduced immune surveillance as a result of immunosuppression [14]. Two of the most well-known flukes or parasites associated with carcinogenesis include *Schistosoma haematobium* infection and its association with cancer of the urinary bladder; and the liver flukes, *Clonorchis sinensis* and *Opisthorchis viverrini*, which are associated with cholangiocarcinoma of the liver [15]. Despite the classification of these specific parasites as carcinogens, no correlation has been proposed for *S. stercoralis* in colorectal cancer. *S. stercoralis* colitis often remains asymptomatic for decades, predisposing individuals to chronic inflammation of the gut and colon. Mucosal damage caused by parasites, their eggs, or secreted products can lead to restorative hyperplasia of damaged tissue. Additionally, *S. stercoralis*, like other parasites, could have immunomodulating capabilities that alter the immune response between Th1 and Th2 signaling, which would provide a microenvironment that hinders immune surveillance [16]. This immune modulation has been well documented with other parasites including protozoa such as *Toxoplasma gondii* and *Trypanosoma cruzi* as outlined by Callejas et al. [15]. Physical damage and/or immunomodulation may create a microenvironment conducive to the development of neoplasia [5]. A large cohort study of 5209 cancer patients investigated the association of coinfection with *S. stercoralis* and HTLV-1 with cancer and showed that *S. stercoralis* infection was associated with an increased occurrence of liver cancer and lymphoma [7]. A proposed mechanism for this interaction suggests the *S. stercoralis* antigen may stimulate HTLV-1-

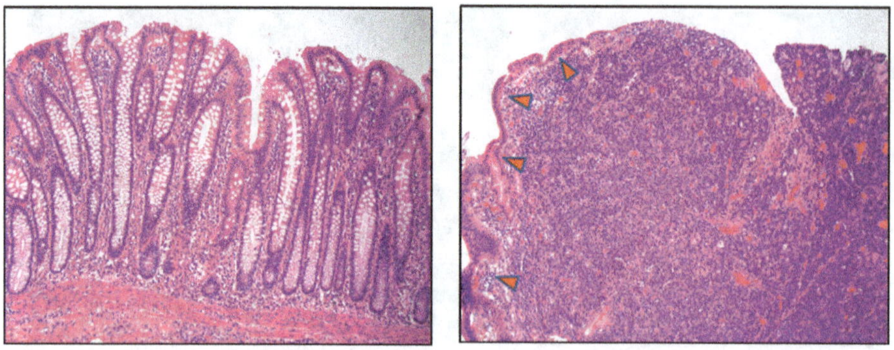

(a) (b)

Figure 4: (a) Uninvolved colon from the colectomy specimen with minimal reactive changes and no significant acute or chronic inflammation (100× magnification). (b) Colon mass from the colectomy specimen showing poorly differentiated invasive adenocarcinoma with superficial ulceration, sheet-like architecture, and minimal gland formation undermining adjacent reactive colonic epithelium (arrowheads).

infected cell replication by activating the IL-2/IL-2R system in dually infected patients, potentially fostering the development of adult T-cell leukemia in this population [17]. A case report describing a Korean patient presenting with both *S. stercoralis* infection and early gastric adenocarcinoma showed *S. stercoralis* adults and eggs associated with gastric adenocarcinoma and adenoma tissues suggesting a possible causative role of *S. stercoralis* infection [8]. Another case report identified *S. stercoralis* in a duodenal biopsy from a patient found to have colorectal cancer, which also suggests a potential correlation between *S. stercoralis* and cancer development [3]. An association between colorectal cancer with chronic *S. stercoralis* has also been reported in a Columbian patient case report [18]. Hirata et al. demonstrated an increased prevalence of *S. stercoralis* infection in patients with biliary tract cancer compared to control patients, suggesting *S. stercoralis* infection as a risk factor for malignancies in the hepato-pancreato-biliary system [9]. The associations between parasitic infections and human cancers are well documented. Two parasites, *S. haematobium and O. viverrini*, are definitive causes of cancer while *S. mansoni, S. japonicum,* and *Clonorchis sinensis* are well known to be associated with cancer. However, studies demonstrating the correlation between *S. stercoralis* infection and cancer are rare in the literature.

In our case, we were able to detect *S. stercoralis* larvae in the patient's stool samples; however, we were unable to detect eggs or worms in the patient's surgical biopsy or colorectal adenocarcinoma (after the first dose of ivermectin was administered). Review of outpatient records did demonstrate chronic GI complaints. Our observations and the aforementioned studies suggest that *S. stercoralis* infection, leading to chronic inflammation, may not only serve as a cofactor for induction of HTLV-1 lymphoma but may also stimulate induction of colon carcinogenesis by direct epithelial injury and/or activation of the host immune response. However, additional research is needed to identify specific mechanisms concerning the role of *S. stercoralis* infection in colon carcinogenesis [15]. An alternative argument includes that patients with immunosuppression are at higher risk of developing parasitic infection. The study conducted by Machado et al. addresses the alternative hypothesis by looking at the frequency of *S. stercoralis* infection in patients with gastrointestinal cancer versus other types of cancer (bladder, breast, melanoma, lung, and uterus). The study shows that the diagnosis of *S. stercoralis* infection was significantly higher in patients with gastrointestinal cancer than in non-gastrointestinal cancer patients [19]. In another study evaluating the prevalence of *S. stercoralis* infection in patients being treated for cancer, it was shown that the overall prevalence of *S. stercoralis* infection in these patients was low [6].

4. Conclusion

Strongyloides stercoralis infection is among the most neglected and elusive parasitic conditions worldwide. Our case report is among the few cases that support an association between gastrointestinal cancer and chronic *S. stercoralis* infection. We propose that chronic *S. stercoralis* infection may be a risk factor for gastrointestinal cancer. Further research to clarify the mechanism of increased cancer risk is needed to emphasize the importance of ruling out *S. stercoralis* infection in cancer patients of endemic areas, particularly those with gastrointestinal malignancy.

References

[1] R. M. Genta, "Global prevalence of strongyloidiasis: critical review with epidemiologic insights into the prevention of disseminated disease," *Clinical Infectious Diseases*, vol. 11, no. 5, pp. 755–767, 1989.

[2] D. M. Parkin, "The global health burden of infection-associated cancers in the year 2002," *International Journal of Cancer*, vol. 118, no. 12, pp. 3030–3044, 2006.

[3] C. Catalano, J. Aron, R. Bansal, and A. Leytin, "Colorectal cancer associated with *Strongyloides stercoralis* colitis," *ACG Case Reports Journal*, vol. 4, no. 1, p. e104, 2017.

[4] Centers for Disease Control and Prevention, *Strongyloides Epidemiology and Risk Factors*, Centers for Disease Control and Prevention, Atlanta, GA, USA, 2018.

[5] B. J. Vennervald and K. Polman, "Helminths and malignancy," *Parasite Immunology*, vol. 31, no. 11, pp. 686–696, 2009.

[6] A. Safdar, K. Malathum, S. J. Rodriguez, R. Husni, and K. V. Rolston, "Strongyloidiasis in patients at a comprehensive cancer centre in the United States," *Cancer*, vol. 100, no. 7, pp. 1531–1536, 2004.

[7] T. Tanaka, T. Hirata, G. Parrott et al., "Relationship among *Strongyloides stercoralis* infection, human T-cell lymphotropic virus type 1 infection, and cancer: a 24-year cohort inpatient study in Okinawa, Japan," *The American Journal of Tropical Medicine and Hygiene*, vol. 94, no. 2, pp. 365–370, 2016.

[8] A. N. Seo, Y.-K. Goo, D.-I. Chung, Y. Hong, O. Kwon, and H.-I. Bae, "Comorbid gastric adenocarcinoma and gastric and duodenal *Strongyloides stercoralis* infection: a case report," *The Korean Journal of Parasitology*, vol. 53, no. 1, pp. 95–99, 2015.

[9] T. Hirata, K. Kishimoto, N. Kinjo, A. Hokama, F. Kinjo, and J. Fujita, "Association between *Strongyloides stercoralis* infection and biliary tract cancer," *Parasitology Research*, vol. 101, no. 5, pp. 1345–1348, 2007.

[10] E. Domingo, R. C. Niessen, C. Oliveira et al., "BRAF-V600E is not involved in the colorectal tumorigenesis of HNPCC in patients with functional MLH1 and MSH2 genes," *Oncogene*, vol. 24, no. 24, pp. 3995–3998, 2005.

[11] D. Greaves, S. Coggle, C. Pollard, S. H. Aliyu, and E. M. Moore, "Strongyloides stercoralis infection," *BMJ*, vol. 347, no. jul30 3, p. F4610, 2013.

[12] F. Tamarozzi, E. Martello, G. Giorli et al., "Morbidity associated with chronic *Strongyloides stercoralis* infection: a systematic review and meta-analysis," *The American Journal of Tropical Medicine and Hygiene*, vol. 100, no. 6, pp. 1305–1311, 2019.

[13] C. S. Lam, M. K. H. Tong, K. M. Chan, and Y. P. Siu, "Disseminated strongyloidiasis: a retrospective study of clinical course and outcome," *European Journal of Clinical Microbiology & Infectious Diseases*, vol. 25, no. 1, pp. 14–18, 2006.

[14] S. Khurana, M. L. Dubey, and N. Malla, "Association of parasitic infections and cancers," *Indian Journal of Medical Microbiology*, vol. 23, no. 2, p. 74, 2005.

[15] B. E. Callejas, D. Martínez-Saucedo, and L. I. Terrazas, "Parasites as negative regulators of cancer," *Bioscience Reports*, vol. 38, no. 5, 2018.

[16] L. J. Knoll, D. A. Hogan, J. M. Leong, J. Heitman, and R. C. Condit, "Pearls collections: what we can learn about infectious disease and cancer," *PLoS Pathogens*, vol. 14, no. 3, Article ID e1006915, 2018.

[17] M. Satoh, H. Toma, K. Sugahara et al., "Involvement of IL-2/IL-2R system activation by parasite antigen in polyclonal expansion of CD4+25+ HTLV-1-infected T-cells in human carriers of both HTLV-1 and *S. stercoralis*," *Oncogene*, vol. 21, no. 16, pp. 2466–2475, 2002.

[18] C. Tomaino, C. Catalano, M. Tiba, and J. Aron, "Su2012: a first case report of colorectal cancer associated with chronic *Strongyloides stercoralis* colitis and the complex management decisions that follow," *Gastroenterology*, vol. 148, no. 4, pp. 1–S575, 2015.

[19] E. R. Machado, E. M. Teixeira, M. d. r. F. Gonçalves-pires, Z. M. Loureiro, R. A. Araújo, and J. M. Costa-Cruz, "Parasitological and immunological diagnosis of *Strongyloides stercoralis* in patients with gastrointestinal cancer," *Scandinavian Journal of Infectious Diseases*, vol. 40, no. 2, pp. 154–158, 2008.

46

Esophageal Gastrointestinal Stromal Tumor with Rare Intracranial Metastasis

José Carvalho ,[1] Margarida Teixeira,[2] Francisco Teixeira Silva,[1] Alexandra Esteves,[1] Carlos Ribeiro,[1] and Diana Guerra[1]

[1]*Serviço de Medicina Interna, ULSAM—Hospital de Santa Luzia, Viana Do Castelo, Portugal*
[2]*Serviço de Anatomia Patológica, Hospital de Braga, Braga, Portugal*

Correspondence should be addressed to José Carvalho; med06053@hotmail.com

Academic Editor: Hirotada Akiho

Introduction. Gastrointestinal stromal tumors (GISTs) are mesenchymal tumors and constitute the largest group of nonepithelial digestive neoplasms. However, they do not represent more than 1% of primary digestive tumors. They commonly metastasize to the liver and peritoneum, but brain metastases are extremely rare. *Clinical Case.* A 76-year-old woman with a diagnosis of esophageal GIST with liver and lung metastases for 13 years, medicated with imatinib, is presented. She was brought to the emergency department after falling and due to changes in behavior and vertigo with 24 hours of evolution. On physical examination, she presented changes in behavior, dysarthria, dysmetria on the right, gait imbalance, and no motor or sensory deficits. On brain computed tomography and posteriorly on magnetic resonance, 2 lesions were observed, left frontal and right cerebellar, compatible with metastatic lesions. After contribution of neurosurgery, histology was obtained that confirmed the lesions were GIST metastases. Imatinib was maintained, and whole brain radiotherapy was performed. After 6 months, she died. *Discussion.* The rarity of GIST brain metastases is noteworthy, and because of that, there is not enough experience to be certain of the best treatment. Our patient lived for 13 years with excellent disease control with imatinib, but the fact that it does not cross the blood-brain barrier makes it not useful in preventing or treating brain lesions. New tyrosine kinase inhibitors that may cross the blood-brain barrier could be the answer to these cases.

1. Introduction

Gastrointestinal stromal tumors (GISTs) are mesenchymal tumors and constitute the largest group of nonepithelial digestive neoplasms; however, they do not represent more than 1% of primary digestive tumors [1]. They are more commonly found in the stomach, jejunum, and ileum and rarely arise from the esophagus [2].

GISTs may present with malignant behavior, depending on the mitotic rate, primary site, size, and metastases, in up to 30%. When there are metastases, they commonly are found in the liver and peritoneum. Brain metastases are extremely rare [2].

Imatinib, a tyrosine kinase inhibitor (TKI), used to treat GISTs with outstanding success, does not cross the blood-brain barrier and seems to have a limited role in treating patients with intracranial metastases [3, 4].

We present a case of an esophageal GIST treated with imatinib with success, but that presented later with rare intracranial metastasis.

2. Clinical Case

A 76-year-old woman with a diagnosis of esophageal GIST with liver and lung metastases for 13 years, medicated with imatinib 400 mg per day, was brought to the emergency department after falling. She presented changes in behavior, dysarthria, dysmetria of the right limbs, and gait imbalance with 24 hours of evolution. She had no sensory or motor deficits.

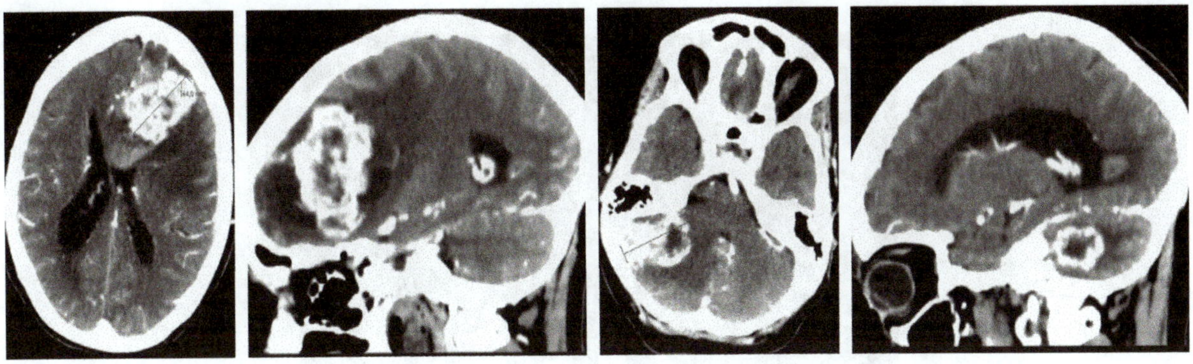

Figure 1: Enhanced CT scan showing 2 lesions with halo of edema, left frontal and right cerebellar. The frontal lesion had an associated bleeding area of 3 cm in diameter.

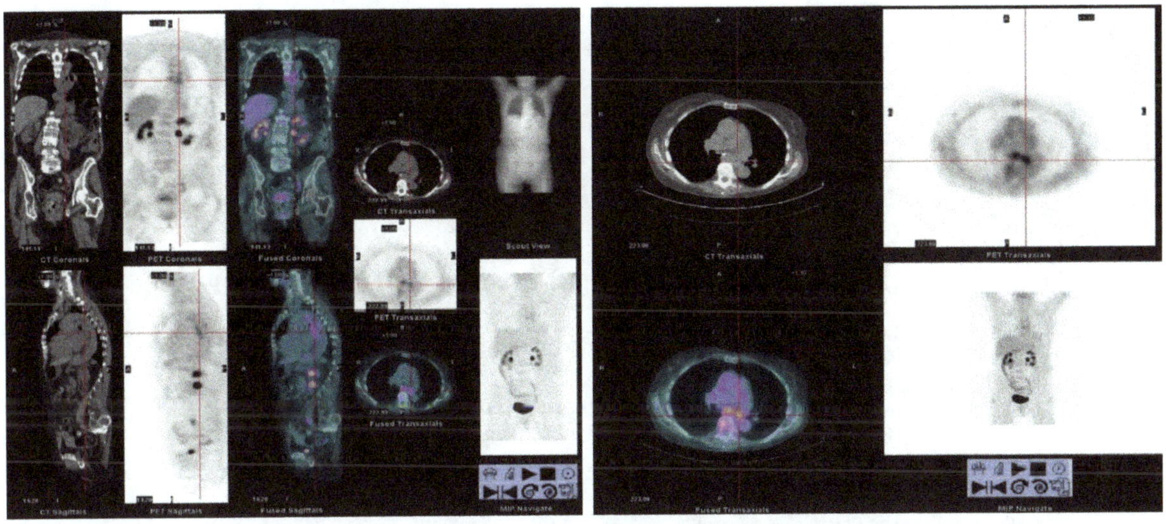

Figure 2: PET-CT showing an already-known metabolically active esophageal lesion, with possible adjacent ganglion metastasis.

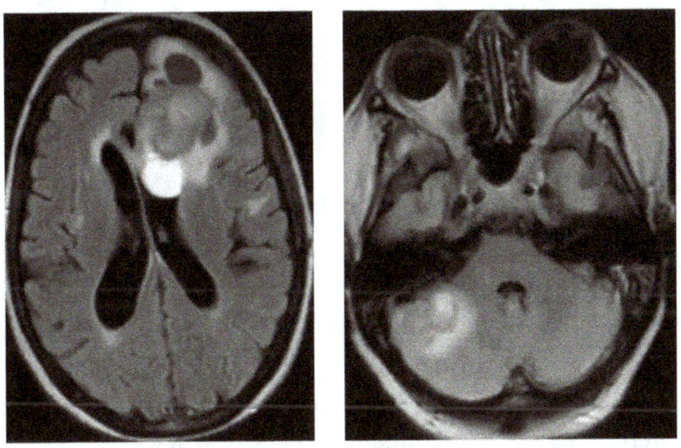

(a) (b)

Figure 3: Continued.

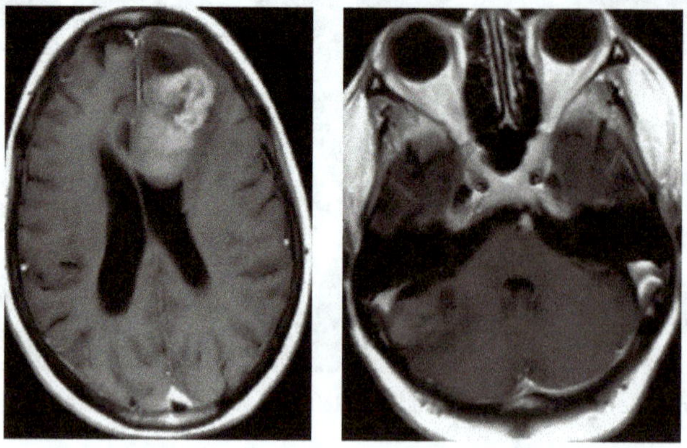

(c) (d)

Figure 3: MRI showing the same lesions seen in the CT scan, suggestive of metastases. (a), (b) T2-FLAIR; (c), (d) contrast-enhanced T1-weighted.

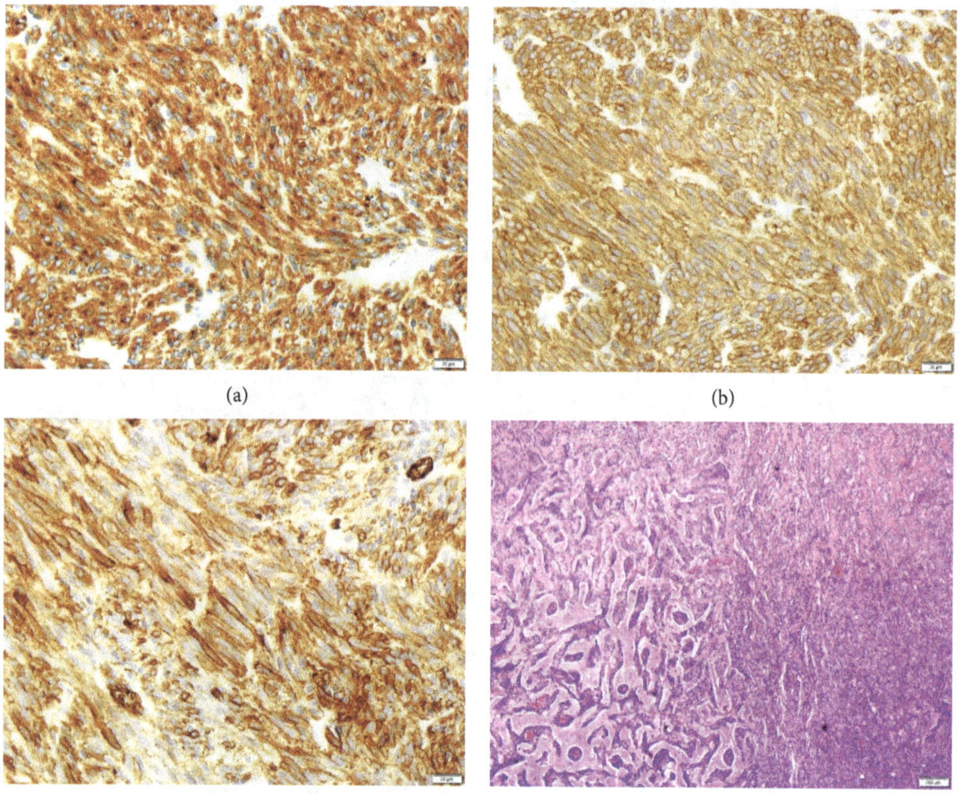

(a) (b) (c) (d)

Figure 4: Spindle cell neoplasm with an immunohistochemical study showing positivity for CD117 (a), DOG1 (b), and CD34 (c).

On brain computed tomography (CT), 2 contrast capturing lesions with halo of edema were observed, left frontal and right cerebellar. The frontal lesion had an associated bleeding area of 3 cm in diameter. The findings were suggestive of metastatic lesions (Figure 1).

Thirteen years earlier, she was started on imatinib with an excellent result, with resolution of lung and liver metastases, maintaining only a stable esophageal thickening over the years.

As GIST brain metastases are rare and to better characterize the lesions, a positron emission tomography computed tomography (PET-CT) and a magnetic resonance imaging (MRI) of the brain were obtained. PET-CT described an already known metabolically active esophageal lesion, with possible adjacent ganglion metastasis (Figure 2). MRI confirmed the 2 lesions as being compatible with brain metastases (Figure 3).

After contribution of neurosurgery, an excisional biopsy of the frontal lesion was performed and histology was obtained, showing a spindle cell neoplasm whose immunohistochemical study showed positivity for CD117, DOG1, and CD34, being compatible with GIST metastasis (Figure 4).

The treatment option was to maintain imatinib and perform whole brain radiotherapy, but without improvement. Her clinical state progressively deteriorated until she died approximately 6 months after the first admission.

3. Discussion

The rarity of GIST brain metastases is noteworthy [2, 5, 6]. Only few cases are described in the literature, and because of that, there is lack of experience and evidence to be certain of the best treatment [2]. Our patient lived for 13 years with excellent disease control with imatinib, but the fact that it does not cross the blood-brain barrier makes it not useful in preventing or treating brain lesions.

There is one case [3] that describes reduction of brain lesions with the use of sunitinib, another TKI, that penetrates the blood-brain barrier, but with such few cases, it is difficult to prove its advantage in relation to resection or radiotherapy. Nevertheless, TKI that may cross the blood-brain barrier could deserve research in the future.

References

[1] I. Judson and G. Demetri, "Advances in the treatment of gastrointestinal stromal tumours," *Annals of Oncology*, vol. 18, no. 10, pp. 20–24, 2007.

[2] M. Prabhek, V. M. Srinivasan, A. Srivatsan et al., "Gastrointestinal stromal tumor with intracranial metastasis: case presentation and systematic review of literature," *BMC Cancer*, vol. 19, no. 1, p. 1119, 2019.

[3] H. Takeuchi, H. Koike, T. Fujita, H. Tsujino, and Y. Iwamoto, "Sunitinib treatment for multiple brain metastases from jejunal gastrointestinal stromal tumor: case report," *Neurologia Medico-Chirurgica*, vol. 54, no. 8, pp. 664–669, 2014.

[4] T. Tanaka, "Gastrointestinal stromal tumors with intracranial metastasis: treatment strategy and review of the literature," *Brain Metastases from Primary Tumors*, Academic Press, Cambridge, MA, USA, pp. 213–224, 2016.

[5] H. Naoe, E. Kaku, Y. Ido et al., "Brain metastasis from gastrointestinal stromal tumor: a case report and review of the literature," *Case Reports in Gastroenterology*, vol. 5, no. 3, pp. 583–589, 2011.

[6] K. Sato, T. Tanaka, N. Kato, T. Ishii, T. Terao, and Y. Murayama, "Metastatic cerebellar gastrointestinal stromal tumor with obstructive hydrocephalus arising from the small intestine: a case report and review of the literature," *Case Reports in Oncological Medicine*, vol. 2014, Article ID 343178, 6 pages, 2014.

47

Intestinal Pseudo-Obstruction as the Initial Clinical Presentation in Systemic Lupus Erythematosus: A Rare and Severe Disorder

Akwe Nyabera, Mohanad Elfishawi, Francisco Cuevas, Fahad Riaz, and Adriana Abrudescu

NYC Health + Hospitals/ Queens, Jamaica, NY, USA

Correspondence should be addressed to Akwe Nyabera; nyaberaa@nychhc.org

Academic Editor: Shiro Kikuchi

Intestinal pseudo-obstruction (IPO) is a rarely recognized complication of systemic lupus erythematosus (SLE). We present a 36-year-old African American female, with only known past medical history of anemia, admitted for frequent vomiting, abdominal distension, abdominal pain, diarrhea, and fever that had been ongoing for 5 days. Laboratory results revealed leukopenia and thrombocytopenia. Imaging revealed dilated small bowel loops, abdominal ascites, as well as mild bilateral hydroureteronephrosis without obstructing calculus. Serologic testing confirmed a diagnosis of SLE. The patient was placed on immunosuppressive therapy and responded well. IPO has previously been described as a rare finding in patients with SLE, with bilateral hydroureteronephrosis and lupus interstitial cystitis having been noted as common concomitant factors. One must have a high level of suspicion to recognize it as being one of the initial clinical presentations. Early recognition and appropriate management preclude unnecessary invasive procedures that do not take into account the pathophysiology of the condition and allow for appropriate management and return of peristaltic function.

1. Introduction

Systemic lupus erythematosus-related intestinal pseudo-obstruction was initially reported in the 1970s [1]. It is more common in Asian populations and usually presents with signs and symptoms of large or small bowel obstruction in the absence of mechanical obstruction. This results in decreased flow of abdominal contents and may be complicated by perforation, ischemia, and infarction [1, 2]. IPO is only seen in 1.96% of patients with SLE. Of these 1.96% patients, only approximately 57.6% present with it as the initial manifestation [2]. The pathophysiology of IPO in SLE remains unclear; however, one possible mechanism includes systemic autoimmune processes targeting smooth muscle cells, supported by the high concomitant lupus cystitis and hydroureteronephrosis, with the latter witnessed in up to 63.6% of cases [3, 4]. Other theories that have been postulated include vasculitis leading to chronic bowel ischemia as well as intrinsic muscle dysmotility affecting the muscularis propria [4, 5]. An understanding of the pathophysiology and appropriate treatment is vital for favorable outcomes.

2. Case Report

A 36-year-old African American female presented with abdominal distension, diarrhea, nausea, and vomiting that had been ongoing for a week. Her past medical history was only significant for anemia. However, when questioned further, she also described a history of ankle pain and a dark rash behind her ears that had been present for 3 weeks. She had initially presented to the ED with similar complaints two days prior to admission and was discharged home with metronidazole and ciprofloxacin under the impression of bacterial gastroenteritis. However, she returned when her symptoms progressively worsened.

Physical examination revealed a distended abdomen with normoactive bowel sounds that was nontender to palpation. Laboratory results revealed elevated acute phase reactants, anemia, and acute renal insufficiency. A 2-view abdominal X-ray showed dilated loops of small bowel suggestive of small bowel obstruction (Figure 1); however, there was no obvious transition point or visible obstruction. Computed tomography (CT) scan findings showed small bowel thickening and were also notable for bilateral hydroureteronephrosis and moderate intra-abdominal ascites (Figures 2(a), 2(b)). Initial treatment was targeted at IPO in the setting of enteritis, and she was treated conservatively via nasogastric tube insertion, administration of antibiotics: vancomycin, meropenem, and doxycycline, as well as nil per os (NPO) status.

Her kidney function continued to worsen with an increase in her creatinine level from a baseline of 0.75 mg/dL to 4.55 mg/dL. Urinalysis was negative for blood and protein. CT scans showed persistent bilateral ureter hydronephrosis, and renal Lasix scan revealed decreased renal flow and function bilaterally, with no obstruction in either kidney. Given the fact that the urinalysis was negative for blood and protein, the observed acute renal failure was determined to be less likely due to lupus nephritis and more likely to be secondary to the bilateral hydroureteronephrosis, frequently associated with lupus interstitial cystitis. Another factor taken into consideration was her reduced oral intake and frequent vomiting which may have contributed to the acute kidney injury. Insertion of bilateral ureteral stents for the hydroureteronephrosis was discussed; however, due to the lack of visible obstruction, the procedure was foregone.

Further rheumatologic workup showed elevated antinuclear antibody (1 : 1280), double-stranded DNA antibody (>1000 IU/mL), anti-Smith antibody (>8 AI), erythrocyte sedimentation rate (ESR) (106 mm/hr) and C-reactive protein (CRP) (51.4 mg/L), low C3 complement (27 mg/dL) and low C4 complement (4 mg/dL), as well as positive direct antiglobulin test IGG, positive anti-cardiolipin antibody, negative anti-beta-2-glycoprotein I antibody, negative lupus anticoagulant, negative rheumatoid factor, and negative SSA and SSB. Total WBC count was (3.67 K/μL) with decreased absolute lymphocyte count of (0.72 K/μL). Additionally, persistent thrombocytopenia was also observed, with a platelet cell count drop to (44 K/μL), indicating lupus thrombocytopenia and involvement of multiple systems.

The patient was treated with intravenous methylprednisolone 1 gm daily for 5 days and continued on maintenance steroid therapy which was slowly tapered and switched to oral methylprednisolone. She also received 5 days of intravenous immunoglobulin therapy (IVIG) at 400 mg/kg/day for persistent thrombocytopenia, with an improvement in her platelet count. This, in addition to aggressive electrolyte repletion, enteral nutrition, and antibiotics, showed a notable improvement in her IPO, renal failure, and ascites, with marked changes noted on repeat CT scan performed prior to discharge (Figure 3).

The patient was then discharged on oral methylprednisolone with follow-up in the rheumatology clinic and later started on hydroxychloroquine 200 mg daily twice daily and mycophenolate mofetil (CellCept) 1 gm twice daily as steroid-sparing agent. SLE workup at the six-month clinic visit revealed normal levels of Smith antibody (0.5 AI), C3 complement (111 mg/dL), and C4 complement (33 mg/dL) and negative dsDNA antibody. All her bowel symptoms fully resolved and did not recur.

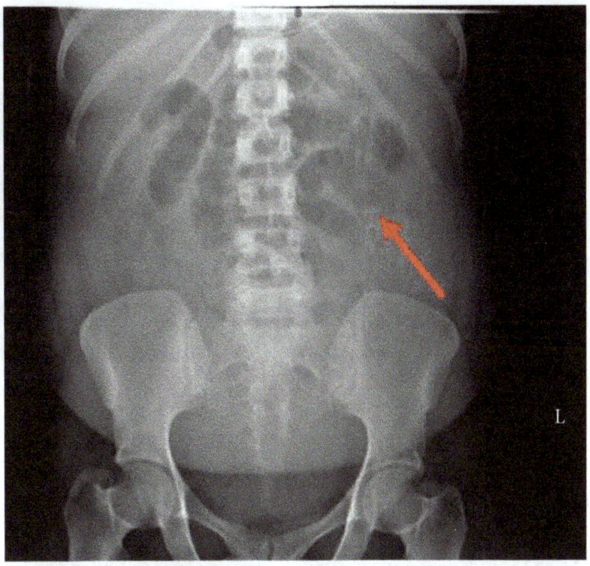

FIGURE 1: 2-view abdominal X-ray showing dilated loops of small bowel.

3. Discussion

Gastrointestinal manifestations such as esophageal hypomotility, malabsorption, mesenteric vasculitis, and pancreatitis are common in patients with SLE [6]. We present a rare case of IPO as one of the initial symptoms of active SLE. In an 11-year longitudinal study conducted by Zhang et al, they found that, amongst 4331 patients with SLE, IPO was present in 1.96%, with an in-hospital fatality rate of 7.1%. IPO was the initial presenting factor in approximately 57.6% of these patients with a rate of misdiagnosis of 78%. Another two studies that took into account both newly diagnosed SLE and previously known cases indicated that IPO was the initial presenting symptom 50% and 41% of the time [2, 5].

Signs and symptoms include abdominal distension, diarrhea, nausea, vomiting, weight loss, or constipation. From a review of the literature, diagnosis of lupus after manifestation of symptoms can range from anywhere between 2 and 25 days in active SLE and up to 3 years in inactive SLE [7]. Laboratory tests are often helpful in the diagnosis of SLE. In the study by Zhang et al. they found that, when compared, laboratory findings revealed that positive ANA, elevated CRP, hypoalbuminemia, hypocomplementemia, positive anti-SSA antibodies, and positive anti-SSB antibodies were more common in patients with IPO-related SLE [2]. Our patient's laboratory results were significant for a high titer antinuclear antibody (1 : 1280), double-stranded DNA antibody (>1000 IU/mL), and anti-Smith antibody (>8 AI).

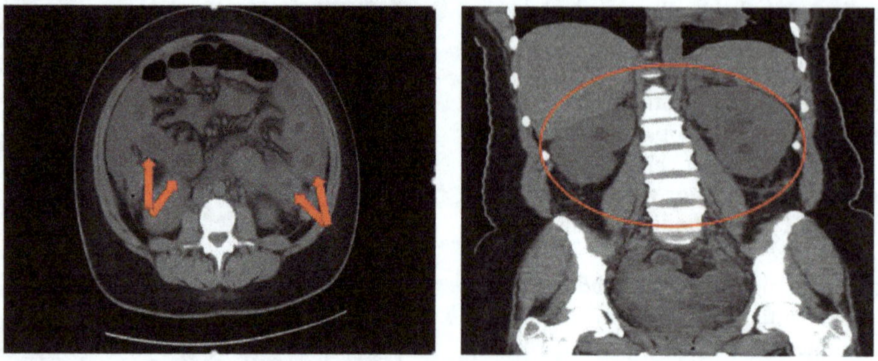

(a) (b)

Figure 2: Abdominal CT scan showing small bowel thickening (a), bilateral hydroureteronephrosis (b), and moderate intra-abdominal ascites.

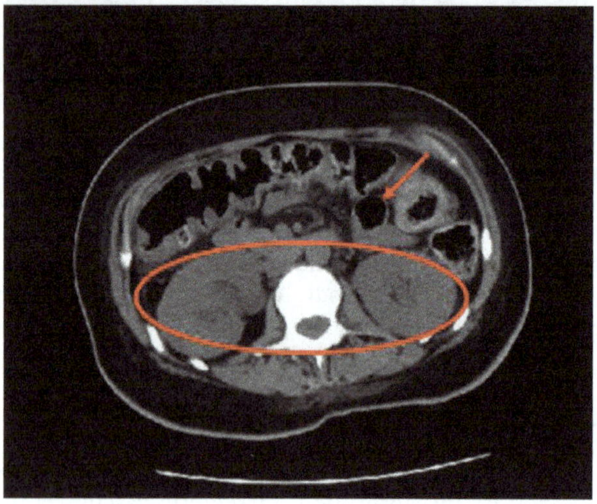

Figure 3: Resolution of previously seen hydronephrosis (red circle), dilated loops of bowel (red arrow), and ascites.

Several imaging modalities such as abdominal X-ray, CT scan, voiding cystourethrogram, and renal Lasix scan may be used to provide further insight into the condition. On imaging, our patient was noted to have diffusely dilated viscera, small bowel thickening, abdominal ascites, and concomitant bilateral hydroureteronephrosis in the absence of any identifiable structural obstruction. Hydroureteronephrosis is a finding that has been noted in up to two-thirds of patients with IPO-related SLE, and more rarely, in some cases, hepatobiliary involvement in the form of megacholedochus has also been observed [2, 4, 7].

The pathogenic mechanism remains unclear; however, several theories have been put forth in the literature. The involvement of the gastrointestinal, hepatobiliary, and genitourinary systems suggests possible associated smooth muscle dysmotility secondary to vasculitis and immune complex deposition in the intestinal tract and bladder vessels [3, 8, 9]. Common autoantigens in the gastrointestinal wall and bladder may be responsible. A strong link between hydroureteronephrosis, interstitial cystitis, and intestinal pseudo-obstruction has previously been observed [3, 9]. Indeed lupus interstitial cystitis is associated with hydroureteronephrosis in up to 92% of cases [10]. This is because of distal ureteral obstruction at the ureterovesical junction secondary to bladder inflammation and edema, as well as detrusor muscle spasm in the setting of inflammation [11]. Histological examination reveals edema and inflammation of the submucosa associated with a high amount of eosinophilic infiltration. Necrosis and loss of myocytes in the muscularis propria and atrophy of the mucosa is also observed. A few studies have found abnormalities of innervation and occasional vasculitis in the absence of thrombosis [4, 7, 8, 12].

As with our patient, medical management of IPO-related SLE is attained with immunosuppressive therapy combined with corticosteroids. Prognosis of the disease often depends on the presence of vital organ involvement [2, 13]. Depending on the severity of the symptoms, high-dose IV pulse corticosteroids can be used initially, switched to oral therapy, and then tapered off gradually. These measures in combination with adequate supportive care (oral antibiotics, parenteral nutrition, and adequate hydration) often result in a favorable prognosis, with the resolution of the IPO and urinary symptoms [4, 5]. It is important to note that, on review of the literature, several studies describe patients undergoing surgical intervention, such as exploratory laparotomy and insertion of ureteral stents; however, these procedures provide no additional benefits, are unnecessary, and put the patient at an increased risk for complications [2, 4, 7, 13].

In conclusion, IPO has been recognized as a rare complication of SLE. It commonly occurs with associated urinary tract involvement, and a high clinical suspicion is required to diagnose it. Early diagnosis confers a more favorable prognosis, allowing for appropriate medical management and avoidance of unnecessary surgical intervention.

Authors' Contributions

Dr. Akwe Nyabera wrote the first draft of the manuscript. Study concept and design were agreed upon by Dr. Akwe Nyabera and Dr. Francisco Cuevas. Critical revision of the manuscript was done by Dr. Adriana Abrudescu, Dr. Mohanad Elfishawi, Dr. Fahad Riaz, Dr. Francisco Cuevas, and Dr. Akwe Nyabera.

References

[1] Q. Huang, W. Lai, C. Yuan et al., "Predictors of intestinal pseudo-obstruction in systemic lupus erythematosus complicated by digestive manifestations: data from a Southern China lupus cohort," *Lupus*, vol. 25, no. 3, pp. 248–254, 2016.

[2] L. Zhang, D. Xu, H. Yang et al., "Clinical features, morbidity, and risk factors of intestinal pseudo-obstruction in systemic lupus erythematosus: a retrospective case-control study," *The Journal of Rheumatology*, vol. 43, no. 3, pp. 559–564, 2016.

[3] S. Mukhopadhyay, S. Jana, M. Roy et al., "Lupus cystitis: an unusual presentation of systemic lupus erythematosus," *Indian Journal of Nephrology*, vol. 24, no. 5, pp. 308–311, 2014.

[4] F. D. Park, J. K. Lee, G. D. Madduri, and P. Ghosh, "Generalized megaviscera of lupus: refractory intestinal pseudo-obstruction, ureterohydronephrosis and megacholedochus," *World Journal of Gastroenterology*, vol. 15, no. 28, pp. 3555–3559, 2009.

[5] A. Alexopoulou, A. Andrianakos, and S. P. Dourakis, "Intestinal pseudo-obstruction and ureterohydronephrosis as the presenting manifestations of relapse in a lupus patient," *Lupus*, vol. 13, no. 12, pp. 954–956, 2004.

[6] P. A. Hill, K. M. Dwyer, and D. A. Power, "Chronic intestinal pseudo-obstruction in systemic lupus erythematosus due to intestinal smooth muscle myopathy," *Lupus*, vol. 9, no. 6, pp. 458–463, 2000.

[7] P. Jin, X. Ji, H. Zhi et al., "A review of 42 cases of intestinal pseudo-obstruction in patients with systemic lupus erythematosus based on case reports," *Human Immunology*, vol. 76, no. 9, pp. 695–700, 2015.

[8] S. Lee and R. Thundyil, "A frequently missed entity in systemic lupus erythematosus (SLE): intestinal pseudo-obstruction (IpsO)," *Medical Journal of Malaysia*, vol. 72, no. 6, pp. 374-375, 2017.

[9] J. Moriuchi, Y. Ichikawa, M. Takaya et al., "Lupus cystitis and performation of the small bowel in a patient with systemic lupus erythematosus and overlapping syndrome," *Clinical and Experimental Rheumatology*, vol. 7, pp. 533–536, 1989.

[10] A. Shimizu, A. Tamura, O. Tago, M. Abe, Y. Nagai, and O. Ishikawa, "Lupus cystitis: a case report and review of the literature," *Lupus*, vol. 18, no. 7, pp. 655–658, 2009.

[11] R. W. Orth, M. H. Weisman, A. H. Cohen, L. B. Talner, D. Nachtsheim, and N. J. Zvaifler, "Lupus cystitis: primary bladder manifestations of systemic lupus erythematosus," *Annals of Internal Medicine*, vol. 98, no. 3, pp. 323–326, 1983.

[12] A. Maruyama, T. Nagashima, M. Iwamoto, and S. Minota, "Clinical characteristics of lupus enteritis in Japanese patients: the large intestine-dominant type has features of intestinal pseudo-obstruction," *Lupus*, vol. 27, no. 10, pp. 1661–1669, 2018.

[13] F.-J. Zhang, J. Zhang, L. Zhou, A. Wang, and X. Li, "Intestinal pseudo-obstruction as the initial manifestation of systemic lupus erythematosus," *American Journal of Emergency Medicine*, vol. 37, pp. 176.e1–176.e2, 2019.

48

Burkitt Lymphoma of the Duodenum: An Uncommon Phenomenon

Fahad Malik, Manuel Gonzalez, and Wahib Zafar

Internal Medicine, Richmond University Medical Center, Staten Island, NY 10310, USA

Correspondence should be addressed to Fahad Malik; fahadimalik@live.com

Academic Editor: Hirotada Akiho

Burkitt lymphoma is an aggressively growing tumor commonly found in African children, involving the jaw and facial bones. Most non-Hodgkin lymphoma tumors involve extra nodal sites like the nervous system and gastrointestinal tract. A rare variant of this type of lymphoma is found in immunocompromised patients specifically in the gastrointestinal tract with accompanying gastrointestinal symptoms. Burkitt lymphoma is a malignancy that has commonly presented in GI tract but rarely in the duodenum. This clinical variant can commonly involve stomach, ileum, and cecum. However, there is very limited data available regarding the duodenal growth of this tumor. Duodenal involvement of Burkitt lymphoma is extremely rare and accounts for < 1% of all lymphomas. We present a case report of an older patient with a duodenal Burkitt lymphoma diagnosed by biopsy. A high suspicion should be present while treating immunocompromised patients with chronic abdominal symptoms especially with complications such as bleeding or occult positive testing. Early endoscopy intervention with biopsy can help identity and treat these conditions with improved outcomes for the patients.

1. Introduction

Burkitt lymphoma is an aggressively growing tumor commonly found in African children, involving the jaw and facial bones. A rare variant of this type of lymphoma is found in HIV positive or immunocompromised patients specifically in the gastrointestinal tract with accompanying gastrointestinal symptoms. This clinical variant can commonly involve stomach, ileum, and cecum. However, there is limited data available regarding the duodenal growth of this tumor. Duodenal involvement of Burkitt lymphomas is extremely rare and accounts for < 1% of all lymphomas. We present a case of an older adult with duodenal Burkitt lymphoma diagnosed by biopsy due to the chronic abdominal pain.

2. Case History

A 39-year-old male, with no significant previous medical history, presented to the emergency department for evaluation of severe diarrhea. He complained of continued lightheadedness, severe abdominal tenderness, watery diarrhea with semi-formed dark stools five to seven times daily, and unintentional weight loss of about twenty pounds in the past three months due to loss of appetite. The patient described the severity of the abdominal pain as 10/10, intermittent, burning, and located in the right lower quadrant and having no correlation with food intake. He was a nonsmoker and nonalcoholic but admitted to binge drinking at times on the weekends. He also admitted to having unprotected sex occasionally with multiple female partners in the past few years. He worked as a full time employee in a restaurant. The family history revealed carcinoma in the grandmother which was not worked up.

Physical examination revealed a young looking male of average build resting comfortably in bed. Lung examination revealed no abnormalities and cardiac examination was normal. Skin examination was unremarkable. The patient had no palpable lymph nodes. Abdominal examination revealed mild epigastric tenderness on deep palpation but no hepatosplenomegaly or rebound tenderness. Rectal examination revealed normal sphincter tone with heme occult positive stool.

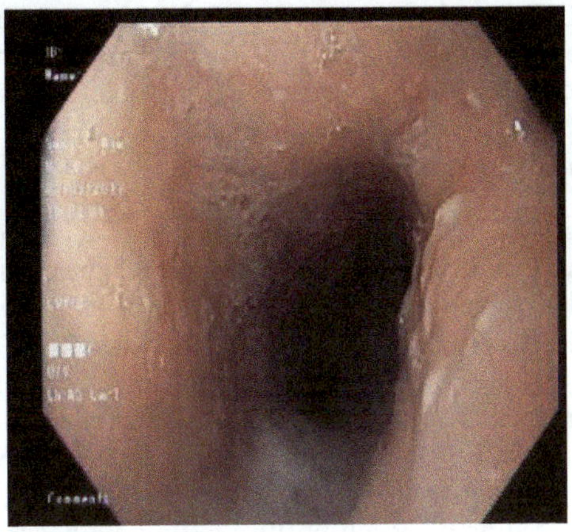

FIGURE 1: Candidiasis.

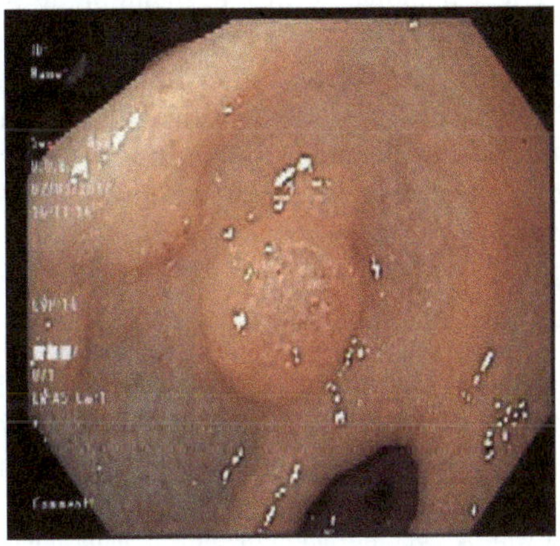

FIGURE 2: Ulcerated nodule in antrum.

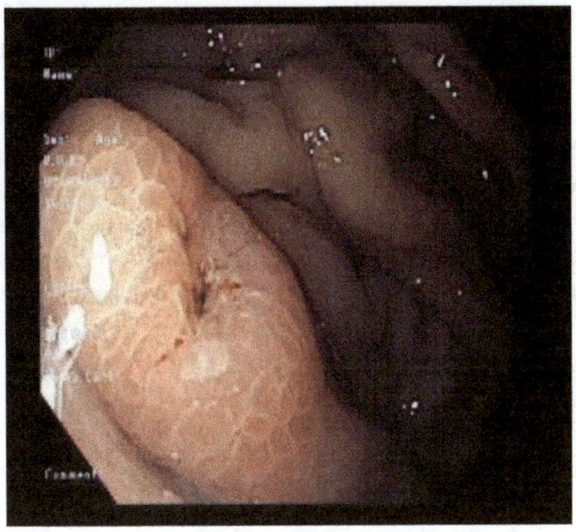

FIGURE 3: Ulcerated nodule in the gastric body.

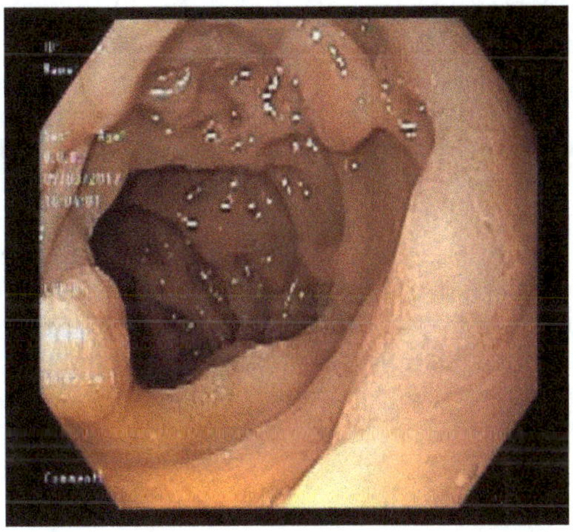

FIGURE 4: Nodules in the 2nd part of duodenum.

Abnormal laboratory findings included the following: complete blood count, hemoglobin 6.6g/dl; hct 20.7%; MCV 89.1 fl; on chemistry, Na 134 mmol/L; chloride 107 mmol/L; lactate dehydrogenase 1060 U/L; bicarbonate 25 mmol/L; anion gap 13.2;AST 59 u/l, ALT 30 u/l, uric acid 10.5 mg/dl, total protein 7.3 g/dl; albumin 1.9g/dl; vitamin B12 >2000 pg/mL; iron studies revealed microcytic anemia with iron 16mcg/dl; TIBC 213mcg/L; % saturation 7.5%; transferrin 163 mg/dL; ferritin 26 ng/mL; white blood count, platelets, potassium, magnesium, phosphorus, renal function, lactic acid, alkaline phosphatase, total bilirubin, direct bilirubin, and lipase were normal; urinalysis, urine cultures, and blood cultures x2 were negative. HIV-1 antibody was positive. This was a new diagnosis for the patient. CD4 count was 126 cells/mcl.

Chest X-ray and ultrasound of the abdomen were essentially normal. Esophagogastroduodenoscopy showed esophageal candidiasis (Figure 1) and multiple nodules in the antrum (Figure 2), along with nodules in the body of the stomach with central erosions and nonbleeding ulcerations. One large nodule found to be in the body of the stomach with central ulceration which was healing and nonbleeding at the time. This was assumed to be the culprit of iron deficiency microcytic anemia (Figure 3). The second part of duodenum was filled with multiple nodules without erosions or active bleeding (Figure 4). Pathology of the gastric mucosa showed atypical lymphoid proliferation which is typical for reactive gastropathy. The biopsy of the duodenum was consistent with Burkitt lymphoma.

The pathology report revealed that the small intestinal mucosal region was infiltrated by multiple clusters of atypical B-lymphocytes. These atypical lymphocytes cells were positive for CD20, CD79a, PAX5, CD10 weakly, BCL6, and cMYC and negative for MUM1, BCL2, CD5, CD23, CD30, cyclin D1, CD138, kappa, and lambda. CD20, PAX5, and CD79 positivity indicated a B-cell lineage origin. MYC and BCL6 positivity along with negative BCL2 markers indicated oncologic cell proliferation unlikely from benign hyperplasia. The proliferation index was calculated to be 90-100% for ki67/mib1 indicating a very high proliferation rate. This report also included mitotic figures and multiple focal macrophages. Fluorescence in situ hybridization results interpretation was also consistent with 68% of the cells having a positive signal pattern with MYC-IGH [t (8; 14)] fusion.

The hallmark of Burkitt lymphoma is the presence of MYC-IGH rearrangement. This report was strongly consistent with Burkitt lymphoma.

The patient was initially treated with Fluconazole for candidiasis and pantoprazole for ulcerations. The patient underwent a complete work-up including a bone marrow biopsy, lumbar puncture, and complete body imaging for staging purposes along with further work-up for acquired immune deficiency syndrome. The patient was diagnosed with Burkitt lymphoma of stage IV-B as per Ann Arbor staging system for lymphoma grading due to lymphocytic infiltration to bone marrow. The HAART regimen (Truvada/Raltegravir) and prophylactic treatment for opportunistic organisms began once the CD4 count of 126 resulted. An Ommaya reservoir shunt and port was placed for the patient to begin chemotherapy. He was treated rophylactically with allopurinol to prevent tumor lysis syndrome. He was started on an anthracycline based chemotherapy regimen. Intrathecal methotrexate was started as part of R-hyper-CVAD (Rituximab, Cyclophosphamide with Mesna, Dexamethasone, Doxorubicin, and Vincristine) and Neupogen was given as required. The patient continued having multiple episodes of diarrhea while undergoing inpatient chemotherapy treatment which began resolving within 3 days of chemotherapy and the patient finally began to have an improved quality of life. The patient was discharged after a total of 12 days from the hospital and currently continues to follow up for outpatient chemotherapy. He was scheduled for a colonoscopy to complete gastrointestinal work-up on multiple occasions but due to neutropenia from chemotherapy it had to be postponed.

3. Discussion

Lymphomas are commonly grouped as Hodgkin's lymphomas or non-Hodgkin's lymphomas. Of all the adult non-Hodgkin's lymphomas, only 1-2% are Burkitt lymphoma [1, 2]. Burkitt lymphomas are further classified into endemic, sporadic, or immunocompromised related Burkitt lymphoma. Sporadic Burkitt lymphoma accounts for 1-2% of all adult lymphomas [3, 4]. The immunodeficiency related Burkitt lymphoma usually is held accountable for over 30% of lymphomas in immunocompromised patients but very few cases have ever been reported specifically in the duodenal region of the gastrointestinal tract. Burkitt lymphoma is known to be an aggressive B-cell lymphocytic malignant tumor that has commonly presented in the gastrointestinal tract mainly in stomach but rarely in the duodenum [5–7].

The hallmark of Burkitt lymphoma is the presence of MYC-IGH 8:14 rearrangements. Our patient demonstrated negative kappa and lambda chains but flow cytometry immunophenotyping can have multiple variations in Burkitt lymphoma. Therefore, the MYC-IGH 8:14 rearrangements are diagnostic even in the event of having lack of light chain expressions [8–10]. Burkitt lymphoma is well known to be an aggressively growing tumor; nonetheless, if appropriately treated with HAART and chemotherapy, it has shown to quickly respond to treatment. HAART and chemotherapy (hyper-CVAD and Methotrexate) combined can significantly improve outcomes in patients like in our patient. It is still uncertain whether this regimen would improve the overall prognosis for immunocompromised related Burkitt lymphoma [11, 12].

Across all variants, Burkitt lymphoma of the duodenum the immunocompromised subtype is extremely rare and very limited literature is currently present. Duodenal involvement of Burkitt lymphomas likely accounts for less than 1% of all cases as there are only a few cases to be studied for reference [1–3]. In conclusion, a high suspicion of lymphomas should be present while treating immunocompromised patients with chronic abdominal symptoms especially with complications such as bleeding or occult positive testing. Early endoscopy intervention with biopsy can help identify these conditions and improve outcomes for the patients [2, 5, 7]. Burkitt lymphoma is a malignancy that has commonly presented in gastrointestinal tract but rarely in the duodenum. As survival rates of AIDs patients improve due to more effective antiviral treatments, more cases of duodenum lymphomas will be described in literature, and we can better assess the implications of lymphomas according to anatomical location.

References

[1] K. A. Blum, G. Lozanski, and J. C. Byrd, "Adult Burkitt leukemia and lymphoma," *Blood*, vol. 104, no. 10, pp. 3009–3020, 2004.

[2] M. Corti, M. F. Villafañe, L. Souto, R. Schtirbu, M. Narbaitz, and M. D. D. Soler, "Burkitt's lymphoma of the duodenum in a patient with AIDS," *Journal of the Brazilian Society of Tropical Medicine*, vol. 40, no. 3, pp. 338–340, 2007.

[3] G. Erkan, M. Çoban, A. Çalıskan et al., "A burkitt's lymphoma case mimicking crohn's disease: A case report," *Case Reports in Medicine*, vol. 2011, Article ID 685273, 4 pages, 2011.

[4] C. Hu, C. Lin, H. Chien, K. Yeh, and R. Chien, "Primary duodenal Burkitt lymphoma presenting as sessile, button-like bleeding polyps," *Advances in Digestive Medicine*, vol. 2, no. 1, pp. 33–36, 2015.

[5] J. R. Carvalho, L. Carrilho-Ribeiro, A. Zagalo, F. C. Medeiros, C. Ferreira, and J. Velosa, "A rare case of burkitt's lymphoma of the duodenal bulb," *Annals of Gastroenterology*, vol. 29, no. 2, pp. 230–232, 2016.

[6] K. Matsueda, I. Fujita, J. Horii, and T. Toyokawa, "Burkitt lymphoma of the duodenum," *Internal Medicine*, vol. 57, no. 10, pp. 1493-1494, 2018.

[7] A. M. Onder and J. Reeves-Garica, "The endoscopic and computed tomographic appearance of Burkitt's lymphoma of the stomach with follow-up studies," *International Pediatrics*, vol. 18, no. 1, pp. 55–57, 2003.

[8] K. Kelemen, R. M. Braziel, K. Gatter, T. C. Bakke, S. Olson, and G. Fan, "Immunophenotypic variations of Burkitt lymphoma," *American Journal of Clinical Pathology*, vol. 134, no. 1, pp. 127–138, 2010.

[9] J. A. Ferry, "Burkitt's lymphoma: clinicopathologic features and differential diagnosis," *The Oncologist*, vol. 11, no. 4, pp. 375–383, 2006.

[10] Z. Kaleem, B. A. Zehnbauer, G. White, and M. M. Zutter, "Lack of expression of surface immunoglobulin light chains in B-Cell non-hodgkin lymphomas," *American Journal of Clinical Pathology*, vol. 113, no. 3, pp. 399–405, 2000.

[11] J. Cortes, D. Thomas, A. Rios et al., "Hyperfractionated cyclophosphamide, vincristine, doxorubicin, and dexamethasone and highly active antiretroviral therapy for patients with acquired immunodeficiency syndrome-related burkitt lymphoma/leukemia," *Cancer*, vol. 94, no. 5, pp. 1492–1499, 2002.

[12] D. A. Thomas, S. Faderl, S. O'Brien et al., "Chemoimmunotherapy with hyper-CVAD plus rituximab for the treatment of adult Burkitt and Burkitt-type lymphoma or acute lymphoblastic leukemia," *Cancer*, vol. 106, no. 7, pp. 1569–1580, 2006.

Ciliated Hepatic Foregut Cyst: A Report of a Case Incidentally Discovered during Transplant Evaluation

Thomas Enke,[1] **Wuttiporn Manatsathit**,[2] **Shaheed Merani**,[3] **and Kurt Fisher**[4]

[1]*The University of Nebraska Medical Center, NE, USA*
[2]*Division of Gastroenterology and Hepatology, University of Nebraska Medical Center, Omaha, NE, USA*
[3]*Department of Transplant Surgery, University of Nebraska Medical Center, Omaha, NE, USA*
[4]*Department of Pathology, University of Nebraska Medical Center, Omaha, NE, USA*

Correspondence should be addressed to Thomas Enke; thomas.enke@unmc.edu

Academic Editor: Hideto Kawaratani

Ciliated hepatic foregut cyst (CHFC) is a rare benign cyst of the liver derived from an embryonic remnant of foregut epithelium. CHFC is typically asymptomatic and is found incidentally. Recent reports of malignant transformation may warrant surgical removal of CHFC. We present the case of a 54-year-old male who was discovered to have a CHFC while undergoing kidney transplant evaluation.

1. Introduction

Ciliated hepatic foregut cyst (CHFC) is a rare benign cyst of the liver derived from an embryonic remnant of foregut epithelium [1]. Patients with CHFC are almost always asymptomatic and mostly incidentally found on abdominal imaging. Although CHFC is benign and generally appears as a simple cyst on imaging, it has been reported to mimic appearance of hepatic cystic neoplasm on cross sectional imaging and rarely reported to be associated with malignancy [2]. With increasing utilization of abdominal cross images, and advancement in computerized tomography (CT) and magnetic resonance imaging (MRI), incidental hepatic cysts are increasingly detected, yet CHFC remains extremely uncommon [3]. Herein, we present a case of CHFC resembling a hepatic cystic neoplasm detected during kidney transplant evaluation.

2. Case Report

A 54-year-old male with end stage renal disease undergoing kidney transplant evaluation presented to hepatology clinic for further evaluation of a hepatic cyst. The cyst was incidentally found on abdominal CT, and the patient was completely asymptomatic. A noncontrast abdominal CT scan revealed a 2.3 cm lesion of low attenuation in segment IVa of the liver. Additional workup including, bilirubin, ALT, AST, GGT, hepatitis B, C, and HIV screening were unremarkable. A subsequent contrast enhanced abdominal magnetic resonance imaging (MRI) scan confirmed a 2.8 cm hypodense cyst with a 1.7 cm solid component in the posterior aspect of the cyst with enhancement. A follow-up contrast enhanced MRI was performed, which demonstrated persistent of solid component (Figure 1).

Considering the persistent 1.7 cm solid component in the cyst, concern of hepatic cystic neoplasm was entertained. Additionally, immunosuppression after kidney transplant may facilitate progression of a neoplastic process if left untreated. Therefore, the decision was made to proceed with surgical resection. A laparoscopic approach was initially performed, which revealed a superficial hepatic cyst within segment IV of the liver, consistent with prior imaging. Given the location of the cyst, it was decided to convert to an open surgical approach. A tan, thin-walled, mucin-filled cyst (2.7 x 2.0 x 1.1 cm) was removed via cyst enucleation without complication (Figure 2). The patient received hemodialysis post-operative day (POD) 1, was advanced to a general diet POD 2, and was discharged home on POD 3. Histology revealed a ciliated pseudostratified epithelium consistent with a CHFC (Figure 3).

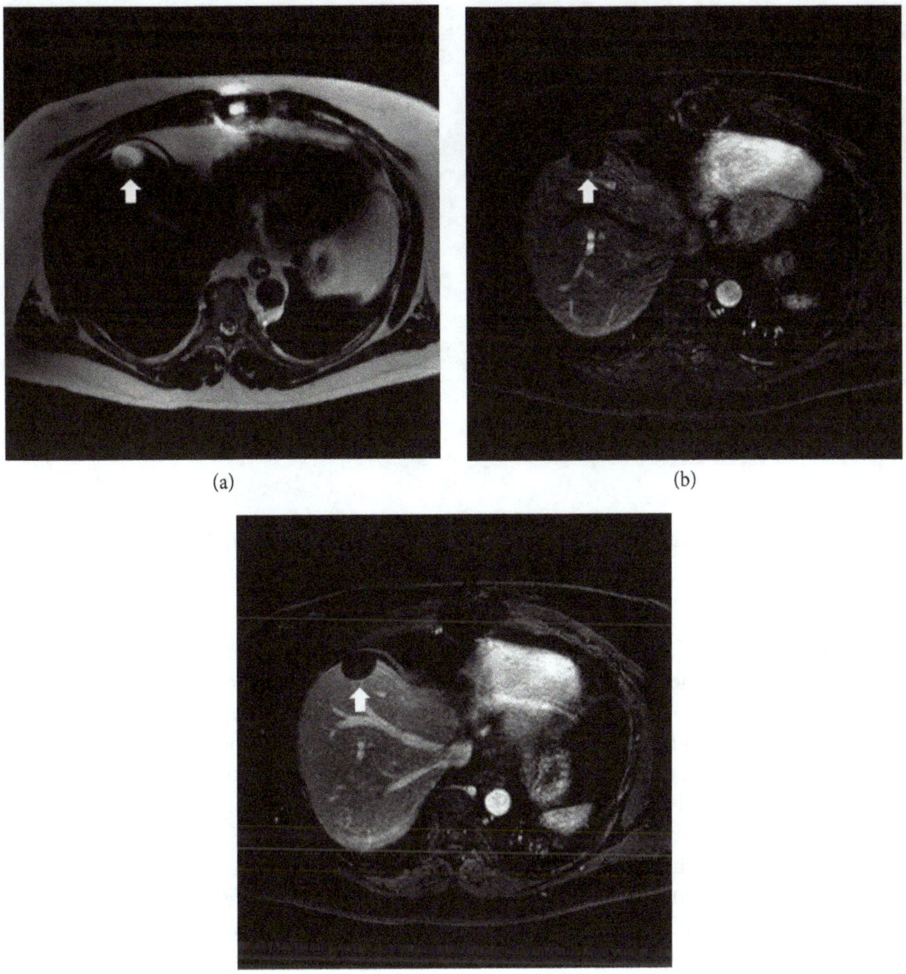

(a) (b) (c)

FIGURE 1: Transverse abdominal MRI of hepatic cyst. (a) T2-weighted image. (b) Arterial phase following intravenous contrast. (c) Venous phase following intravenous contrast.

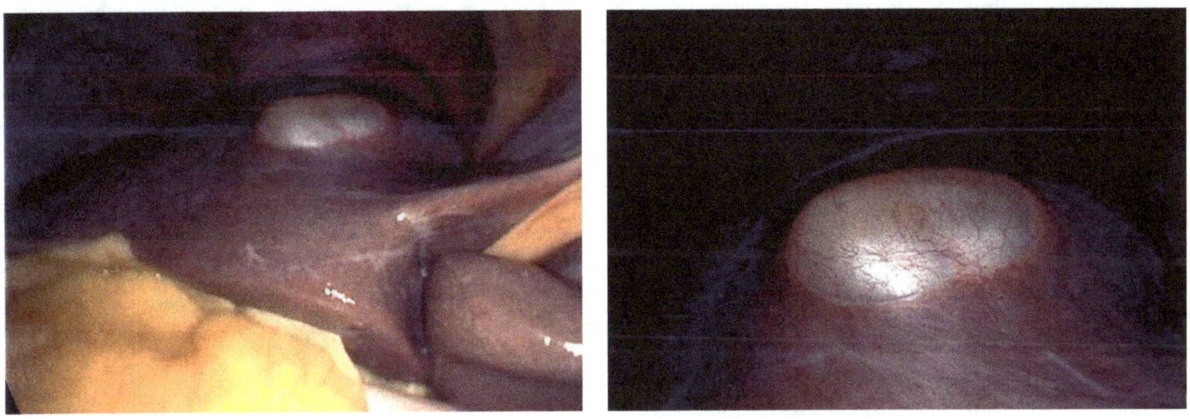

FIGURE 2: Intra-operative view of ciliated hepatic foregut cyst.

3. Discussion

CHFC is a rare benign hepatic cyst originally described by Wheeler and Edmonson as a cystic remnant of foregut epithelium similar to bronchogenic and esophageal cysts [1]. A literature review discovered 109 reported cases since 1964. Histologically, CHFCs classically consist of 4 layers, including a ciliated pseudostratified columnar epithelium, subepithelial connective tissue, a smooth muscle layer, and an outer fibrous capsule [1]. CHFCs are typically discovered during the fifth

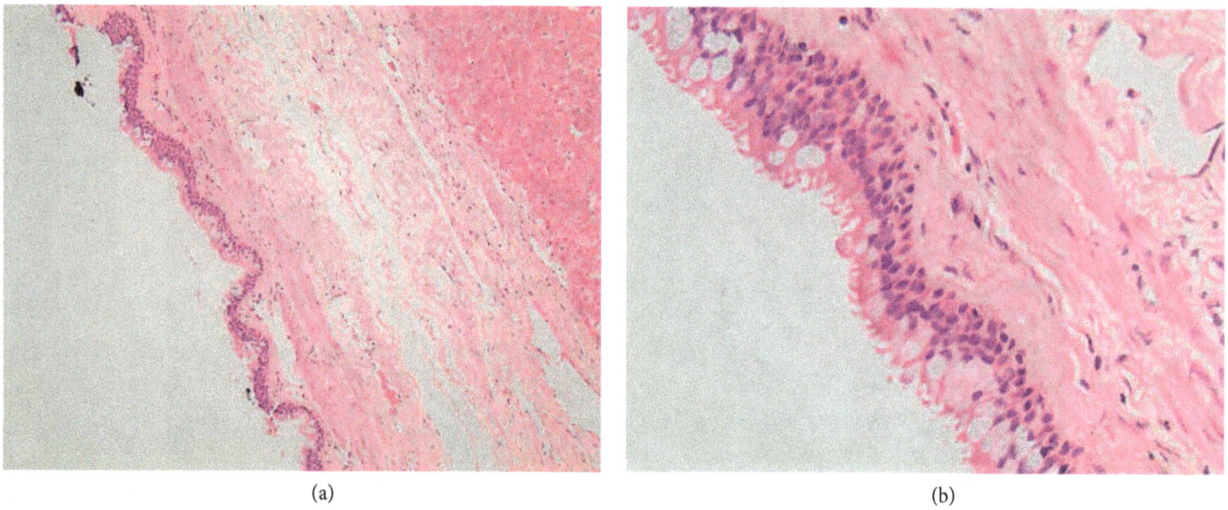

FIGURE 3: Histological sample of ciliated hepatic foregut cyst with hematoxylin and eosin staining. (a) Low power magnification. (b) High-power magnification.

decade of life, but may present at any age [2–4]. Most patients are asymptomatic at time of diagnosis. When symptomatic, the majority present with right upper quadrant abdominal pain [2, 3]. However, a few cases of CHFCs causing jaundice from biliary obstruction have been reported [5, 6]. Classically, CHFCs are located in the left lobe of the liver, specifically segment IV, but can present within the right lobe as well [2, 3]. Additionally, extrahepatic locations, such as the gallbladder and extrahepatic biliary system, have been reported [2, 6–8].

Radiographic imaging is usually insufficient for diagnosis given the variability in appearance. Typically, CHFCs are small (<4 cm), subcapsular, unilocular, and fluid-filled, but may present with findings suggestive of solid debris as seen in the above patient [2, 3, 10, 11]. Ultrasound evaluation usually reveals a hypoechoic cyst and hyperdense without contrast enhancement on CT imaging [10]. Large variability is seen on MRI T1-weighted imaging, but CHFCs are nearly exclusively hyperintense on T2-weighted imaging [3, 10, 11]. The variety of imaging findings provide for a large differential which includes, simple cysts, mucinous cystic neoplasm (MCN), pyogenic abscess, amebic abscess, hydatid cyst, intrahepatic pseudocyst, biliary cystadenoma, and cystadenocarcinoma [12].

Definitive diagnosis is made through histology which reveals a pseudostratified columnar epithelium, subepithelial connective tissue layer, smooth muscle layer, and outer fibrous capsule [1]. Presence of cartilage and respiratory glands would be suggestive of a bronchogenic cyst and are absent in CHFCs. Fine needle aspiration (FNA) cytology may provide for a non-surgical diagnosis with reports of a positive predictive value of 76% [3, 13]. The finding of pseudostratified squamous epithelium in a mucoid background is nearly diagnostic, given the absence of other liver pathology with similar cytology [13].

Although CHFCs were originally believed to be benign, more recent reports of CHFCs undergoing malignant transformation have challenged that dogma [14, 16]. Rates of malignant transformation were reported to range from 3% to 5% with squamous cell carcinoma being the most common malignancy [2, 3]. Size appears to be the largest risk factor for malignant transformation in CHFCs [2, 3]. Rates of malignant transformation are lower than those seen in MCN, which may be as high as 10% [17]. The role of carbohydrate antigen (CA) 19-9, and/or carcinoembryonic antigen (CEA) as a marker of malignant progression in CHFC does not appear helpful. There have been reports of patients with CHFC discovered to have elevated serum CEA, and elevated intra-cystic CEA and CA19-19 in the absence of malignancy [6, 16]. The current management of CHFC remains controversial. Given the potential risk of malignant transformation, most agree that surgical excision, increasingly performed through a laparoscopic approach, should be performed if the cyst is greater than 4–5 cm, symptomatic, growing, or possesses wall abnormalities on imaging [18, 19]. In the absence of radiographic features concerning for malignancy, a more conservative approach with serial imaging could be considered given the overall low risk of malignant transformation, particularly when lacking the above features.

CHFC is a rare cyst, but has been more frequently diagnosed in recent years. Given the potential for malignant transformation, it is an important diagnosis to consider in the setting of a hepatic cyst. Due to the limited number of cases, further characterization and understanding of the disease is important.

References

[1] C. Ambe, L. Gonzalez-Cuyar, S. Farooqui, N. Hanna, and S. C. Cunningham, "Ciliated hepatic foregut cyst: 103 cases in the world literature," *Open Journal of Pathology*, vol. 2, no. 3, pp. 45–49, 2012.

[2] S. Sharma, A. Corn, V. Kohli, H. I. Wright, A. Sebastian, and N. Jabbour, "Ciliated hepatic foregut cyst: an increasingly diagnosed condition," *Digestive Diseases and Sciences*, vol. 7, no. 6, pp. 581–589, 2008.

[3] D. A. Wheeler and H. A. Edmondson, "Ciliated hepatic foregut cyst," *The American Journal of Surgical Pathology*, vol. 8, no. 6, pp. 467–470, 1984.

[4] P. Betalli, D. Gobbi, E. Talenti, R. Alaggio, P. Gamba, and G. F. Zanon, "Ciliated hepatic foregut cyst: from antenatal diagnosis to surgery," *Pediatrc Radiology*, vol. 38, no. 2, pp. 230–232, 2008.

[5] H. Kiyochi, K. Okada, K. Iwakawa et al., "Ciliated hepatic foregut cyst with obstructive jaundice," *Case Reports in Gastroenterology*, vol. 2, no. 3, pp. 479–485, 2008.

[6] K. C. Bishop, C. M. Perrino, M. B. Ruzinova, and E. M. Brunt, "Ciliated hepatic foregut cyst: a report of 6 cases and a review of the English literature," *Diagnostic Pathology*, vol. 10, no. 1, Article ID 81, 2015.

[7] O. S. Al Beteddini, N. K. Amra, and E. Sherkawi, "Ciliated foregut cyst in the triangle of calot: the first report," *Surgical Case Reports*, vol. 2, no. 1, Article ID 20, 2016.

[8] J. Cottreau, A. Costa, M. Walsh, and T. Arnason, "Ciliated foregut cyst of the common hepatic duct: an unusual mimic of a type II choledochal cyst," *International Journal of Surgical Pathology*, vol. 24, no. 7, pp. 644–647, 2016.

[9] T. Koletsa, V. Tzioufa, A. Michalopoulos, S. Apostolidis, B. Papadopoulos, and P. Hytiroglou, "Ciliated hepatic foregut cyst communicating with the gallbladder," *Virchows Archiv*, vol. 446, no. 2, pp. 200–201, 2005.

[10] M. Boumoud, A. Daghfous, H. Maghrebi et al., "Imaging features of ciliated hepatic foregut cyst," *Diagnostic and Interventional Imaging*, vol. 96, no. 3, pp. 301–303, 2015.

[11] K. Ansari-Gilani and J. Modaresi Esfeh, "Ciliated hepatic foregut cyst: report of three cases and review of imaging features," *Gastroenterology Report*, vol. 5, no. 1, pp. 75–78, 2017.

[12] A. A. Borhani, A. Wiant, and M. T. Heller, "Cystic hepatic lesions: a review and an algorithmic approach," *American Journal of Roentgenology*, vol. 203, no. 6, pp. 1192–1204, 2014.

[13] K. J. Kaplan, M. Escobar, M. Alonzo, and J. W. Berlin, "Ciliated hepatic foregut cyst: report of a case on fine-needle aspiration," *Diagnostic Cytopathology Banner*, vol. 35, no. 4, pp. 245–249, 2007.

[14] J. M. Wilson, R. Groeschl, B. George et al., "Ciliated hepatic cyst leading to squamous cell carcinoma of the liver–a case report and review of the literature," *International Journal of Surgery Case Reports*, vol. 4, no. 11, pp. 972–975, 2013.

[15] X. Zhang, Z. Wang, and Y. Dong, "Squamous cell carcinoma arising in a ciliated hepatic foregut cyst: case report and literature review," *Pathology–Research and Practice*, vol. 205, no. 7, pp. 498–501, 2009.

[16] Z. Ben Ari, O. Cohen-Ezra, J. Weidenfeld et al., "Ciliated hepatic foregut cyst with high intra-cystic carbohydrate antigen 19–9 level," *World Journal of Gastroenterology*, vol. 20, no. 43, pp. 16355–16358, 2014.

[17] Y. Nakayama, Y. Kato, S. Okubo et al., "A case of mucinous cystic neoplasm of the liver: a case report," *Surgical Case Reports*, vol. 1, no. 1, p. 9, 2015.

[18] M. D. Goodman, G. Z. Mak, J. P. Reynolds, A. D. Tevar, and T. A. Pritts, "Laparoscopic excision of a ciliated hepatic foregut cyst," *Journal of the Society of Laparoendoscopic Surgeons*, vol. 13, no. 1, pp. 96–100, 2009.

[19] J. Saravanan, G. Manoharan, S. Jeswanth, and P. Ravichandran, "Laparoscopic excision of large ciliated hepatic foregut cyst," *Journal of Minimal Access Surgery*, vol. 10, no. 3, pp. 151–153, 2014.

Synchronous Gastric Adenocarcinoma and Diffuse Large B-Cell Lymphoma in the Pelvis: A Rare Case Presentation

Evangelia Pliakou, Dimitra-Ioanna Lampropoulou, Nikolaos Soupos, and Gerasimos Aravantinos

Second Department of Medical Oncology, General Oncology Hospital of Kifissia "Agioi Anargiroi", Athens, Nea Kifissia 14564, Greece

Correspondence should be addressed to Evangelia Pliakou; evangeliaplk@hotmail.com

Academic Editor: Tetsuo Hirata

Multiple primary cancer (MPC) is defined as more than one primary tumour diagnosed at the same patient, either simultaneously or sequentially. Its incidence is low and varies in reporting among medical centers. Diffuse large B-cell lymphoma (DLBCL) is the most common subtype of non-Hodgkin lymphoma (NHL) while gastric cancer (GC) is the fifth most frequently diagnosed malignancy. The aim of this article is to present a rare case of a female patient who was diagnosed with two synchronous malignancies, an adenocarcinoma of the stomach (SRCC) and an aggressive extranodal NH lymphoma (DLBCL) within 2 months. Given the fact that there is an expanding availability of more sensitive diagnostic and screening methods, we aim to increase surveillance amongst medical doctors and provide valuable information for further systematic analysis and identification of such rare cases of concurrent malignancies.

1. Introduction

Multiple primary cancer (MPC) is a distinct clinical entity that refers to cases in which more than one primary tumours are diagnosed at the same patient, either simultaneously or sequentially. Synchronous multiple primary cancer (SMPC) is characterised by two or more primary tumours diagnosed within six months [1]. Its incidence is low, and it has been connected with a substantial variation among medical centers; the synchronous presentation of a solid tumour with a hematological malignancy is even less common. Currently, the expanding availability of more sensitive screening methods has contributed to increasing diagnosis of multiple primaries.

Diffuse large B-cell lymphoma (DLBCL), an aggressive type of lymphoma, is the most common subtype of non-Hodgkin lymphoma (NHL), accounting for approximately 30% of all NHL cases [2, 3]. Immunotherapy and chemotherapy remain the most widely used and effective treatment options. Gastric cancer (GC) is the fifth most frequently diagnosed type of malignancy and the fourth cause of cancer death worldwide. In 2020, it newly occurred in 1.09 million people and caused about 769 000 deaths worldwide [4]. The incidence of signet ring cell carcinoma (SRCC) subtype has been constantly increasing, displaying less sensitivity to chemotherapy and a very low 5-year survival rate. Surgical resection and lymphadenectomy remain the gold standard in GC treatment [5]. In this article, we describe a rare case of DLBCL and gastric adenocarcinoma coexisting in an immunocompetent patient; our aim is to increase surveillance amongst medical doctors and provide further information for the diagnosis of SMPC.

2. Case Presentation

A 68-year-old female patient presented to a community hospital with a history of epigastralgia, abdominal fullness, and gastroesophageal reflux over the past months. Her medical history was significant for hypothyroidism (under thyroid hormone replacement therapy) and dyslipidemia.

The patient was a 45 pack-year smoker (approximately one and a half pack per day). When asked about her family history, she reported that her father was diagnosed with bone cancer while her brother was diagnosed with laryngeal cancer (no further information available). The patient had also suffered from intermittent epigastric discomfort for several years without seeking any medical attention. Fever, night sweats, and weight loss were absent. Upon admission for further medical examination and lab tests, the patient was diagnosed with grade 1 anaemia; none other was significant from the routine hematology and biochemistry tests apart from hepatitis B virus (HBV) surface antigen which resulted positive. Subsequently, the patient was referred for endoscopy: the initial esophagogastroduodenoscopy revealed mucosal edema in the pyloric antrum with the presence of erosion. Furthermore, an irregularly elevated area with edema and redness was noted in the lesser curvature; the *Campylobacter*-like organism test (CLO test) was negative. A second endoscopy, performed about a week later, showed deterioration with some extraphytic ulcerous lesions and greater edema in the lesser curvature. The biopsies revealed a poorly differentiated signet ring cell carcinoma (adenocarcinoma of diffuse type), and the patient was referred to our medical oncology department, for cancer staging and initiation of neoadjuvant therapy. In the meanwhile, the patient suffered from lower back, pelvis, and right hip pain, which was continuously deteriorating to the point that she was unable to walk or stand still (ECOG performance status 3). Magnetic resonance imaging (MRI) and computed tomography (CT) scans were performed, revealing gastric wall thickening in the propyloric area as well as small lymph nodes <10 mm nearby. Furthermore, we found a large, soft-tissue osteolytic mass (97 mm × 76 mm × 97 mm) in the right sacroiliac joint which invaded into the sacrum, the ilium, and the cervical spine at the S1–S4 level. There was no evidence of ascites, peritoneal or liver metastasis. Since adenocarcinoma is not common to metastasize in these areas as an osteolytic lesion, we speculated that the origin of the mass required further investigation. Interestingly, the biopsy from the mass revealed the presence of a lymphoproliferative disease, compatible with DLBCL (CK7–, CD20+, CD-3–, CD138–, CD5–, TDT–, CD10–, bcl6+, MUM1+, bcl2+, c-myk+, ki67: 100%). Thus, the diagnosis of DLBCL with a concurrent gastric adenocarcinoma was confirmed. However, a few days later, while being hospitalized, the patient underwent emergency surgery twice due to gastrointestinal perforation; no treatment was administered due to poor performance status. She was also admitted twice in the intensive care unit (ICU) and eventually died as a result of complications, about three months after the diagnosis of the synchronous malignancies.

3. Discussion

According to Fukuda et al., only 16 cases of synchronous gastric cancer and extranodal DLBCL were previously reported; interestingly, only two of them were diagnosed in female patients, like in our case [6]. The underlying mechanisms for developing lymphoma, especially DLBCL, and a concurrent nonhematological malignancy remain unknown. There is, however, evidence supporting a correlation between the development of both tumours; these include immune function alterations, the presence of pathogens, molecular/biological abnormalities, genetic predisposition, or an underlying immunodeficiency. Inaba et al. linked the treatment of primary gastric lymphoma, especially DLBCL, with an increased risk for developing gastric adenocarcinomas [7]. Moreover, an Argentine study concluded that 32% of MPC patients had a family history of cancer [8]. Indeed, our patient had also a significant family history of cancer (both father and brother died of malignancies). Furthermore, other risk factors have been associated with MPCs such as tobacco, alcohol intake, infections (e.g., EBV), and immunosuppression as well as toxic effects related to treatment. The prognosis of MPC patients can be evaluated independently and depends on the stage of each cancer.

Currently, no consensus regarding the management of synchronous gastric adenocarcinoma and lymphoma exists. Thus, decision-making regarding the optimal treatment strategy can be quite challenging. Prioritizing treatment in such patients is crucial, and certain factors must be taken into consideration, such as the stage of each tumour, response to therapy, and performance status. These difficulties in therapy are discussed in detail in a prospective descriptive study conducted by Babu et al., in which lung carcinoma and gastrointestinal malignancies were the most common MPCs [9]. DLBCL typically presents as a rapidly progressing lymphoma, resulting in symptomatic disease that could be fatal without treatment. Thus, DLBCL treatment should be administered immediately upon diagnosis not only due to the aggressive behavior of this malignancy but also because of the high remission rate. Once lymphoma is controlled, treatment for the gastric carcinoma should be initiated based on the patient's condition.

Another topic for consideration is the cumulative toxicities that may develop during MPC treatments; thus, a multidisciplinary approach is crucial for ensuring the optimal effect.

The accurate diagnosis and management of synchronous malignancies can be challenging due to their rare occurrence. Given that it is impractical and not always feasible to obtain a biopsy from every suspicious lesion, the awareness of the different biological behaviors between a gastrointestinal tumour and a lymphoma is critical towards the diagnosis and treatment. After all, the accuracy of the diagnosis is based on the biopsy of the lesion under suspicion. Therefore, if the appearance of new lesions challenges the routine metastatic rule, as happened in our case, the possibility of synchronous multiple primary cancer should be further investigated.

The patient gave fully informed written consent to the publication of this report.

References

[1] C. S. Warren and O. Gates, "Multiple primary malignant tumors: a survey of the literature and a statistical study," *American Journal of Cancer*, vol. 16, pp. 1358–1414, 1932.

[2] National Cancer Institute, "Surveillance, epidemiology, and end results: cancer stat facts: NHL—diffuse large B-cell lymphoma (DLBCL)," 2022, https://seer.cancer.gov/statfacts/html/dlbcl.html/.

[3] L. H. Sehn and G. Salles, "Diffuse large B-cell lymphoma," *New England Journal of Medicine*, vol. 384, no. 9, pp. 842–858, 2021.

[4] H. Sung, J. Ferlay, R. L. Siegel et al., "Global cancer statistics 2020: GLOBOCAN estimates of incidence and mortality worldwide for 36 cancers in 185 countries," *CA: A Cancer Journal for Clinicians*, vol. 71, no. 3, pp. 209–249, 2021.

[5] R. Sitarz, M. Skierucha, J. Mielko, J. Offerhaus, R. Maciejewski, and W. P. Polkowski, "Gastric cancer: epidemiology, prevention, classification, and treatment," *Cancer Management and Research*, vol. 10, pp. 239–248, 2018.

[6] S. Fukuda, T. Wakasa, H. Hanamoto et al., "Synchronous gastric cancer and primary lymphoma of right adrenal gland: a case report," *Clinical Journal of Gastroenterology*, vol. 14, no. 5, pp. 1350–1357, 2021.

[7] K. Inaba, R. Kushima, N. Murakami et al., "Increased risk of gastric adenocarcinoma after treatment of primary gastric diffuse large B-cell lymphoma," *BMC Cancer*, vol. 13, no. 1, p. 499, 2013.

[8] S. L. Ares, S. Polo, L. Ezcurdia et al., "Multiple primary cancer in adults," *Journal of Clinical Oncology*, vol. 24, Article ID 16027, 2006.

[9] G. Babu, V. Asati, K. C. Lakshmaiah et al., "Every distant deposit is not a metastasis: synchronous primaries do exist," *Indian Journal of Cancer*, vol. 56, no. 1, pp. 70–73, 2019.

51

Squamous Cell Papilloma of the Esophagus: A Case Series Highlighting Endoscopic and Histologic Features

Dustin J. Uhlenhopp,[1] Kristin M. Olson,[2] and Tagore Sunkara[3]

[1]*Department of Internal Medicine, MercyOne Des Moines Medical Center, Des Moines, IA, USA*
[2]*Division of Gastroenterology and Hepatology, University of Nebraska Medical Center, Omaha, NE, USA*
[3]*Department of Gastroenterology and Hepatology, MercyOne Des Moines Medical Center, Des Moines, IA, USA*

Correspondence should be addressed to Dustin J. Uhlenhopp; dustin.j.uhlenhopp@gmail.com

Academic Editor: Hideto Kawaratani

Esophageal squamous papillomas are rare epithelial lesions typically discovered incidentally during EGD. Their prevalence is estimated to be less than 0.01% in the general population. We present three cases of esophageal squamous papillomas identified histologically. It may be possible to identify these lesions macroscopically. One study provided a positive predictive value of 88% for squamous papilloma utilizing the triad of exophytic growth, wart-like projections, and surface vessel crossing seen on narrow band imaging during endoscopy. The etiology is unclear. Chronic mucosal irritation from GERD or esophagitis is the prevailing theory of pathogenesis, but HPV has been detected in some lesions. The malignant potential of these lesions is considered controversial. There are documented cases demonstrating complications with squamous cell carcinoma, so we recommend removal of all esophageal squamous papillomas; however, the small absolute number of cases documented in the literature makes drawing any associations or conclusions between esophageal squamous papillomas and squamous cell carcinoma difficult. Further research is needed regarding treatment and surveillance. This case series helps contribute to the small but growing literature of this rare finding.

1. Introduction

Esophageal squamous papillomas (ESPs) are rare epithelial lesions typically discovered incidentally during esophagogastroduodenoscopy (EGD). The occurrence in patients undergoing EGD is less than 0.45% [1] but was noted to make up 4.5% of all esophageal lesion biopsies at one medical center during a 15-year period [2], and the prevalence in the general population, inferred from autopsy, is less than 0.01% [3]. We present a case series of 3 patients found to have ESPs discovered over a one year period of approximately 600 EGDs, which is consistent with the incidence reported in the literature. Most patients are asymptomatic unless the lesion is large. The most common symptom from a squamous papilloma is dysphagia. A majority of these lesions are found in the distal one-third of the esophagus. Though rare, there are case reports demonstrating ESP complications with squamous cell carcinoma [3–6].

2. Cases

2.1. Case 1. A 53-year-old male with history of alcohol abuse presented with new-onset seizure/syncope, six painless maroon stools, and coffee-ground emesis. The patient admitted to frequent diclofenac use and ketorolac injections. He did not have a history of varices. Vital signs demonstrated tachycardia (heart rate 111 beats/min) and hypotension (79/59 mmHg). Physical exam revealed pale conjunctiva, dry mucous membranes, and maroon colored stool. He was found to be anemic with a hemoglobin of 7.9 G/dL and had an elevated INR of 1.2. He was transfused two units of packed red blood cells and was started on a pantoprazole drip.

Once stabilized, initial EGD revealed an island of tissue growth in the mid-esophagus and a bleeding duodenal ulcer that was injected with epinephrine, cauterized with gold probe and clipped. Biopsy of the esophageal lesion was deferred to outpatient follow-up given the severity of the patient's presenting condition. He had no further signs of gastrointestinal bleeding. Two weeks later, a repeat EGD was performed. Biopsies were taken of the stomach mucosa and mid-esophageal mass (see Figure 1). Gastric biopsy demonstrated mild chronic gastritis without dysplastic changes or *Helicobacter pylori*. Esophageal biopsy demonstrated findings consistent with squamous papilloma (see Figures 2 and 3).

2.2. Case 2. A 61-year-old female with history of uncontrolled diabetes mellitus type 2 complicated by gastroparesis, prior esophageal dilation, and ileostomy was being evaluated with endoscopy as outpatient for worsening dysphagia. EGD was significant for a small nodule in the proximal esophagus (see Figure 4), normal GEJ (gastroesophageal junction), mild gastritis, and normal duodenum. Gastric biopsy demonstrated mild chronic gastritis without dysplastic changes or *Helicobacter pylori*. Esophageal biopsy demonstrated findings consistent with squamous papilloma.

2.3. Case 3. A 54-year-old female with history of fibromyalgia, chronic opioid dependency, cyanocobalamin deficiency, vitamin D deficiency, and GERD with previously noted Los Angeles class C esophagitis was being evaluated with endoscopy as outpatient for dysphagia and abdominal pain. EGD was significant for an exophytic wart-like growth in the distal esophagus, minimally irregular *Z*-line noted at GEJ, mild gastritis without ulcers, and normal duodenum. GEJ biopsy demonstrated focal intestinal metaplasia suggestive of Barrett's esophagus without dysplastic changes. Esophageal biopsy demonstrated findings consistent with squamous papilloma (see Figures 5 and 6).

3. Discussion

Squamous papilloma of the esophagus is a rare lesion. Its macroscopic appearance is similar to other, less benign growths (verrucous squamous cell carcinoma, granulation tissue, or papillary leukoplakia). Other differential considerations should include fibrovascular polyp, inflammatory fibroid polyp, leiomyoma, and malignant melanoma [10]. Narrow band imaging (NBI) can further evaluate a squamous papilloma during endoscopy as microvessels within the lesion will not be dilated [11]. Based on a study of 41 esophageal polypoid lesions, the triad of exophytic growth, wart-like projections, and surface vessel crossing seen on NBI during endoscopy can provide a positive predictive value of 88.2% for squamous papilloma [7]. The study noted the whitish color of squamous papillomas does not help differentiate from other lesions.

Squamous papilloma cases usually consist of a small (<5 mm) solitary lesion that is found incidentally while evaluating a patient for abdominal pain or reflux [8, 9, 11]. Histological evaluation classically demonstrates a fibrovascular core branching out from the lamina propria forming finger-like projections without invasion into the submucosa completely surrounded by marked neutrophil infiltration and covered by acanthotic squamous epithelium [1, 7–9].

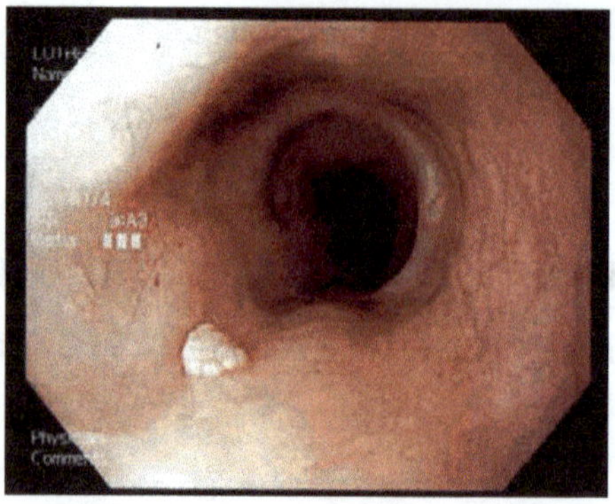

Figure 1: Esophageal squamous papilloma in Case 1. Esophageal squamous cell papilloma is an exophytic growth with wart-like projections on conventional endoscopy. Its whitish color is a poor differentiator from other lesions [7].

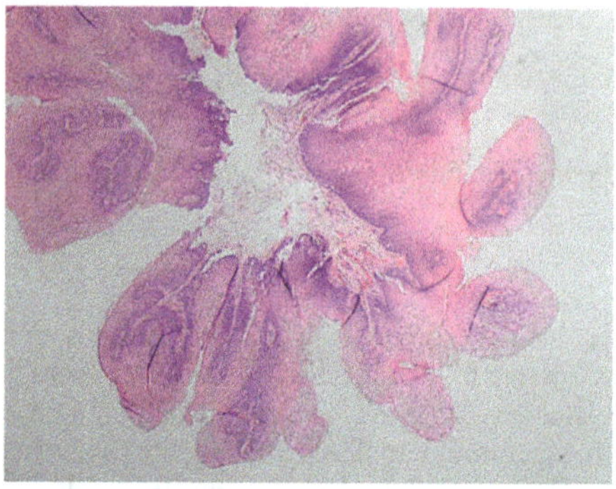

Figure 2: Esophageal squamous papilloma in Case 1. Lesion is diagnosed pathologically with hematoxylin and eosin stain demonstrating a fibrovascular core branching out from the lamina propria forming finger-like projections without invasion into the submucosa surrounded by marked neutrophil infiltration and covered by acanthotic squamous epithelium (H&E, *x*20) [1, 7–9].

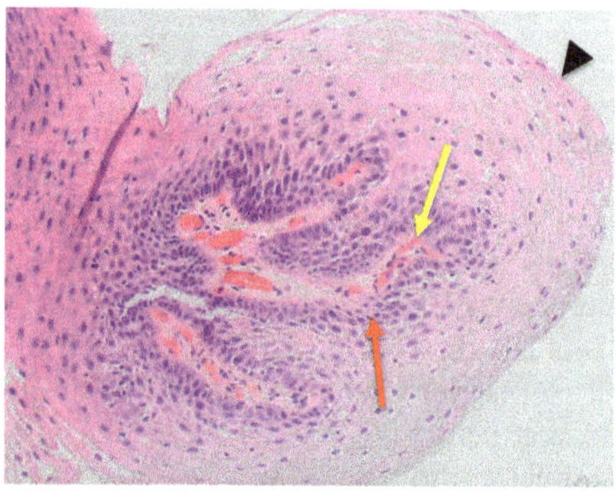

Figure 3: Esophageal squamous papilloma in Case 1. A fibrovascular core branching out from the lamina propria forming finger-like projections (yellow arrow) without invasion into the submucosa surrounded by marked neutrophil infiltration (red arrow) and covered by acanthotic squamous epithelium (black arrowhead) can be seen (H&E, *x*100).

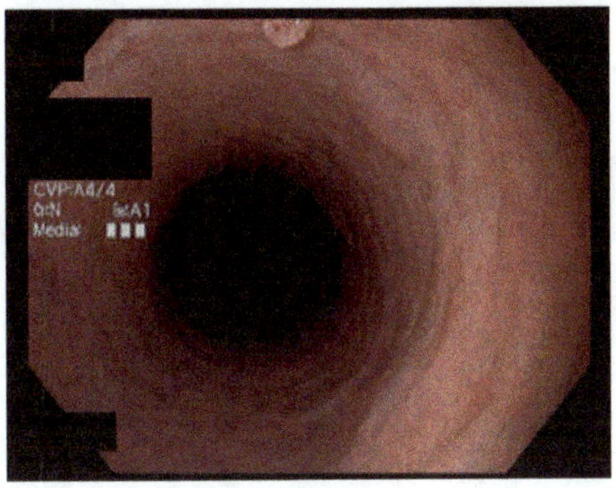

FIGURE 4: Partially visible esophageal squamous papilloma in Case 2 demonstrating exophytic growth with wart-like projections.

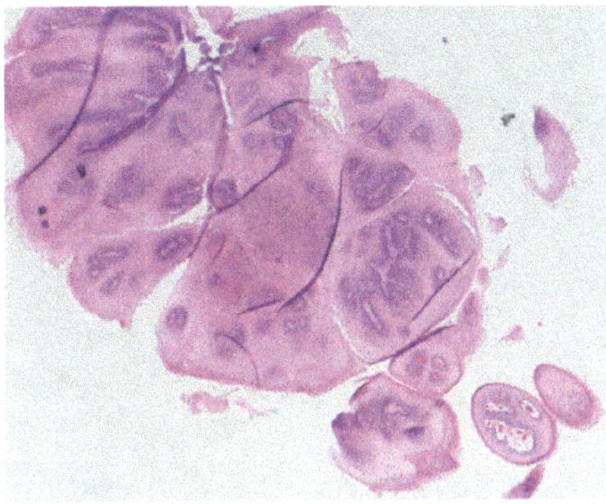

FIGURE 5: Esophageal squamous papilloma in Case 3. Note is made of fibrovascular cores branching out from the lamina propria forming finger-like projections surrounded by marked neutrophil infiltration and covered by acanthotic squamous epithelium (H&E, x20).

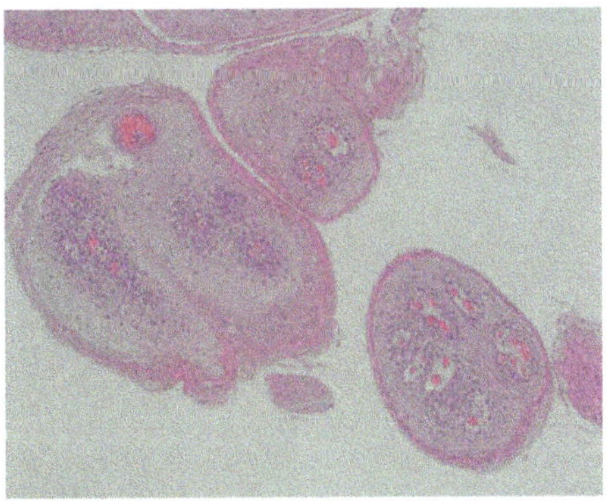

FIGURE 6: Esophageal squamous papilloma in Case 3. Several fibrovascular cores branching out from the lamina propria with finger-like projections can be seen without invasion into the submucosa. These are surrounded by marked neutrophil infiltration and covered by acanthotic squamous epithelium (H&E, x100).

The etiology is unclear. Chronic mucosal irritation from GERD or esophagitis is the prevailing theory of pathogenesis, but HPV (human papillomavirus)—strongly associated with cervical, anal, and oropharyngeal cancers (depending on viral serotype)—has been detected in some lesions [1, 4]. A study comparing clinicopathological characteristics of Japanese patients to western countries identified 38 esophageal squamous papillomas (ESPs) in 35 patients over a period of 13 years and noted four tumors in four female patients (10.5%) tested positive for HPV subtype 6 [1]. A study evaluating HPV in 18 patients with 19 cases of ESPs in a Mexican cohort identified HPV in almost 80% of ESPs utilizing amplified chromogenic in situ hybridization or PCR though all cases exhibited low expression of cell-cycle markers [9].

There have been several other studies with HPV-positive ESP results ranging from 0 to 64% and with different esophageal lesion location distribution curves indicating that differences in detection methods or possibly geographical/environmental exposure factors may play a role in prevalence [1]. Our three cases did not test positive for HPV.

Complications with squamous cell carcinoma (SCC) have been reported [3–6]; however, the small absolute number of cases makes drawing any associations or conclusions between ESP and SCC difficult [12]. Review of the literature seems to suggest malignant potential appears highest in cases where the patient is symptomatic and has multiple lesions (papillomatosis), or a particularly large lesion [5, 6].

The gold standard for evaluation is biopsy. There are various proposed therapies for squamous papillomas including forceps biopsy resection, cautery, radiofrequency ablation, mucosectomy for larger lesions, and potentially esophagectomy if presentation is extreme and does not respond to more conservative therapy [4, 5, 11, 13, 14]. Future research is needed regarding treatment and surveillance for these lesions. Though rare, there are documented cases demonstrating malignant potential, so we recommend removal of esophageal squamous papillomas.

Disclosure

A portion of this work has been published previously as an abstract at the American College of Gastroenterology Annual Scientific Meeting on October 25, 2019, in San Antonio, TX.

References

[1] K. Takeshita, S.-I. Murata, S. Mitsufuji et al., "Clinicopathological characteristics of esophageal squamous papillomas in Japanese patients-with comparison of findings from western countries," *Acta Histochemica Et Cytochemica*, vol. 39, no. 1, pp. 23–30, 2006.

[2] T. Terada, "A clinicopathologic study of esophageal 860 benign and malignant lesions in 910 cases of consecutive esophageal biopsies," *International Journal of Clinical and Experimental Pathology*, vol. 6, no. 6, pp. 191–198, 2013.

[3] T. Attila, A. Fu, N. Gopinath, C. J. Streutker, and N. E. Marcon, "Esophageal papillomatosis complicated by squamous cell carcinoma," *Canadian Journal of Gastroenterology*, vol. 23, no. 6, pp. 415–419, 2009.

[4] J. Y. Cho, D. Y. Cheung, T. J. Kim, and J. K. Kim, "A case of esophageal squamous cell carcinoma in situ arising from esophageal squamous papilloma," *Clinical Endoscopy*, vol. 52, no. 1, pp. 72–75, 2019.

[5] M. C. D'Huart, J. B. Chevaux, A. M Bressenot et al., "Prevalence of esophageal squamous papilloma (ESP) and associated cancer in northeastern France," *Endoscopy International Open*, vol. 3, no. 3, pp. E101–E106, 2015.

[6] J. Reynoso, R. E. Davis, W. W. Daniels, Z. T. Awad, Z. Gatalica, and C. J. Filipi, "Esophageal papillomatosis complicated by squamous cell carcinoma in situ," *Diseases of the Esophagus*, vol. 17, no. 4, pp. 345–347, 2004.

[7] M.-W. Wong, M.-J. Bair, S.-C. Shih et al., "Using typical endoscopic features to diagnose esophageal squamous papilloma," *World Journal of Gastroenterology*, vol. 22, no. 7, pp. 2349–2356, 2016.

[8] E. Kim, M. F. Byrne, and F. Donnellan, "Endoscopic mucosal resection of esophageal squamous papillomatosis," *Canadian Journal of Gastroenterology*, vol. 26, no. 11, pp. 780–782, 2012.

[9] O. L. Bohn, L. Navarro, J. Saldivar, and S. Sanchez-Sosa, "Identification of human papillomavirus in esophageal squamous papillomas," *World Journal of Gastroenterology*, vol. 14, no. 46, pp. 7107–7111, 2008.

[10] S. A. Tabatabaei, N. A. Moghadam, M. Ahmadinejad, A. Mirmohammadsadeghi, H. Masoudpour, and P. Adibi, "Giant esophageal squamous papilloma: a case report," *Journal of Digestive Diseases*, vol. 10, no. 3, pp. 228–230, 2009.

[11] S.-J. Tsai, C. C. Lin, and C. W. Chang, "Benign esophageal lesions: endoscopic and pathologic features," *World Journal of Gastroenterology*, vol. 21, no. 4, pp. 1091–1098, 2015.

[12] B. Jideh, M. Weltman, Y. Wu, and C. H. Chan, "Esophageal squamous papilloma lacks clear clinicopathological associations," *World Journal of Clinical Cases*, vol. 5, no. 4, pp. 134–139, 2017.

[13] G. d. Genio, F. Del Genio, and P. Schettino, "Esophageal papilloma: flexible endoscopic ablation by radiofrequency," *World Journal of Gastrointestinal Endoscopy*, vol. 7, no. 3, pp. 290–294, 2015.

[14] S. Tanimu, Rafiullah, J. Resnick, and A. A. Onitilo, "Oesophageal papillomatosis, not amenable to endoscopic therapies, treated with oesophagectomy," *BMJ Case Reports*, vol. 2014, 2014.

52

A Rare Case of Metastatic Hepatocellular Carcinoma Masquerading as a Forehead Hematoma

Kimberly Sanders,[1] Ashley Thomas,[1] Carmen Isache,[1] and Anwer Siddiqi[2]

[1]*Department of Internal Medicine, University of Florida College of Medicine Jacksonville, Jacksonville, FL, USA*
[2]*Department of Pathology, University of Florida College of Medicine Jacksonville, Jacksonville, FL, USA*

Correspondence should be addressed to Kimberly Sanders; kimberly.sanders2@jax.ufl.edu

Academic Editor: Olga I. Giouleme

Hepatocellular carcinoma (HCC) is the most common primary liver cancer and can arise from any form of chronic liver disease or cirrhosis. With increasing rates of metabolic syndrome and obesity, it is not surprising that NASH is quickly becoming a leading cause of chronic liver disease and HCC in the western hemisphere (Wang and Malhi, 2018). Metastasis is usually found in advanced stages of the disease, owing to its poor prognosis. The lung, bone, and lymph nodes are the most frequent sites of metastasis (Balogh et al., 2016, and Becker et al., 2014). On the other hand, metastasis to the skin and cranium is relatively rare. Literature review reveals less than 10 reported cases in the last 10 years. Herein, we report an unusual case of a "forehead hematoma" leading to the formal diagnosis of metastatic HCC.

1. Introduction

Hepatocellular carcinoma (HCC) is a leading cause of morbidity and mortality with increasing incidence worldwide [1]. What was formerly thought of as a malignancy predominantly affecting Eastern Asians [2] has broken racial barriers and border lines to affect almost all ethnicities and countries alike. Men in their fourth to fifth decades are more commonly affected than women. Its incidence has been increasing in the US and Western Hemisphere, quickly becoming one of the highest causes of death and ultimately increasing the economic healthcare burden [2, 3]. Therefore, it is imperative for primary care physicians, gastroenterologists, and internists to screen for HCC in at-risk populations. The majority of HCC cases are due to cirrhosis or chronic liver disease from alcohol abuse or viral infection from hepatitis B or hepatitis C [3]. Hepatitis B accounts for 44% of HCC cases, the majority of which arise in Asia, while hepatitis C accounts for 21% of cases worldwide [4]. As expected with increasing rates of diabetes and obesity, nonalcoholic steatohepatitis (NASH) is starting to account for a large percentage of HCC cases in the US, with an annual incidence of 2.6% and rising [5]. Diabetes and metabolic syndrome alone increase the risk for HCC by up to 2 fold [5], reflecting the importance of patient counseling and screening.

Early stages of HCC are largely asymptomatic, leading to a delay in presentation. As a result, HCC is usually diagnosed at advanced stages, owing to its poor prognosis and median survival <20 months [5]. The presence of metastasis at the time of diagnosis is even more dismal. Approximately 5–15% of patients have evidence of metastasis at the time of diagnosis and 30–50% of patients develop metastasis at some point in the disease process, owing to the aggressive nature of this cancer [6]. The lung is the most common site of metastasis, followed by lymph nodes and bone [7]. Bony metastases have a predilection to the spine, pelvis, and ribs [8]. However, metastases to the skull, as well as skin and soft tissue, are relatively rare.

2. Case Presentation

A 77-year-old female with a past medical history of hypertension was admitted for new onset ascites and decompensated cirrhosis. She presented to the emergency room for progressively worsening shortness of breath, abdominal distention, and 10-pound weight loss over 4 weeks. Incidentally, the patient was also noted to have a painless soft tissue mass on her forehead. She reported that the lesion had been enlarging over 4 months which she thought to be secondary to a hematoma that developed after hitting her head on a door. She denied prior history of alcohol abuse. There was no personal or family history of liver disease, cancer, or autoimmune diseases. Vital signs were stable, with a BMI of 26. Physical exam was notable for significant abdominal distention, palpable hepatosplenomegaly, and a fixed nontender firm mass on her forehead. No encephalopathy, asterixis, or stigmata of liver disease was appreciated. Cardiopulmonary exam was unremarkable without crackles or peripheral edema. Initial labs demonstrated thrombocytopenia and a mild transaminitis. INR and bilirubin were within normal limits. Computed tomography (CT) of the abdomen and pelvis revealed large-volume ascites, splenomegaly, and cirrhotic liver morphology with multifocal hyperattenuating liver lesions, the largest measuring 6 cm × 5 cm × 5 cm involving segments II-II with extracapsular extension, associated with porta hepatis and both mesenteric and anterior mediastinal lymphadenopathy. Findings were highly suspicious for metastatic hepatocellular carcinoma (Figure 1). CT head revealed a 3.1 cm mass eroding through the frontal calvarium (Figure 2). Further investigations were significant for hemoglobin A1c (7.4%) and hypertriglyceridemia (201 mg/dL). Chronic liver disease workup was otherwise unremarkable including viral hepatitis serologies (HAV, HBcAb, HBcAg, and HCV Ab), ceruloplasmin, ferritin and transferrin, ANA, C-ANCA, P-ANCA, mitochondrial antibody, anti-smooth muscle antibody, and IgG. Serum alpha feto protein (AFP) was elevated at 97.9 ng/ml. Transthoracic echocardiogram was not performed. Diagnostic paracentesis revealed SAAG (serum to ascites albumin gradient) >1.1 and low total protein, consistent with portal hypertension. Fluid cytology was negative for malignant cells.

CT liver mass protocol demonstrated ill-defined infiltrative mass in left hepatic lobe (segments 2 and 3 extending to segments 4A and 4B) and multiple hypoattenuating lesions in the right hepatic lobe concerning for multifocal HCC but no significant arterial phase enhancement or delayed venous washout. Due to poorly delineated margins, the masses were unable to be measured accordingly. As imaging was indeterminate and there was a high clinical suspicion for HCC, a biopsy was necessary to confirm the diagnosis. Given the location and accessibility, a core needle biopsy of the forehead lesion was performed to provide pathologic diagnosis and identify the presence of metastasis, which would ultimately determine treatment. Pathology revealed a well to moderately differentiated tumor with trabecular pattern. Morphologically, these tumor cells resemble hepatocytic cells with slight atypia (Figures 3 and 4). No bile production was noted on the limited biopsy. A positive Hep Par-1 staining confirmed the lineage of these cells to be hepatocellular in origin (Figure 5). Polyclonal CEA staining (Figure 6) demonstrated a diffuse canalicular pattern, highly suggestive of HCC, rather than cytoplasmic staining as seen in cholangiocarcinoma and many other cancers. AFP staining was negative. Other types of immunohistochemistry with arginase or keratin 7 or 20 were not performed. At our institution, these stains are reserved for situations in which the metastatic tumor cells are poorly differentiated or if Hep Par-1 is negative.

The patient was classified as Child-Pugh class B, given her large volume ascites, absence of encephalopathy, total bilirubin <2 mg/dL, albumin 3 g/dL, and INR <1.7. However, due to evidence of metastasis on imaging, she was deemed a poor liver transplant candidate-based Milan and USCF criteria. She was managed medically with diuretics for ascites and was discharged home to follow-up with oncology for palliative chemotherapy. Unfortunately, the patient succumbed to her disease before the initiation of any treatment and passed away 2 months later.

3. Discussion

Hepatocellular carcinoma (HCC) is one of the few cancers that can be diagnosed without tissue biopsy [1] but by multiphase contrast-enhanced CT or MRI. In cirrhotic or high-risk patients, the diagnostic criteria includes size ≥1 cm, arterial phase enhancement, and a combination of washout, capsule enhancement, or a 50% interval increase in size ≤6 months [9]. If imaging is inconclusive, a tissue biopsy can be pursued. In noncirrhotic patients or in cases in which the primary tumor is unknown, a liver biopsy is necessary to diagnose HCC. Characteristic histological features include wide trabeculae of more than 3 cells, increased nuclear-cytoplasmic ratio, unpaired arteries, and loss of reticulin network [9]. However, histopathology alone is insufficient to establish the diagnosis as a number of tumors can mimic the morphologic features of HCC, especially in metastasis. Immunohistochemistry with Hep Par-1, heat-shock protein 70 (HSP70), arginase-1, and glypican-3, among many others, aids in the differentiation of these tumors and improves the diagnostic yield. For example, glypican-3, HSP70, and glutamine synthetase staining can distinguish HCC from high-grade dysplastic nodules in the liver [10]. However, these particular staining methods were not performed in our patient as the biopsy was obtained from an extrahepatic site and, therefore, the differentiation of HCC from a high-grade dysplastic nodule was not warranted. This patient's biopsy revealed well-differentiated tumor cells resembling hepatocytes with atypia, and its lineage was confirmed with positive Hep Par-1 staining. Furthermore, polyclonal CEA staining of this cranial lesion showed a diffuse canalicular pattern, highly suggestive of HCC. In contrast, cholangiocarcinoma and many other cancers demonstrate a cytoplasmic pattern on polyclonal CEA staining. At our institution, arginase and keratin 7 and 20 are reserved for poorly differentiated metastatic tumor cells or negative Hep Par-1 staining.

Early screening and recognition for HCC allows for multiple treatment options and therefore improved survival outcomes. Management involves a multidisciplinary approach, and selection is based on tumor size, location, liver

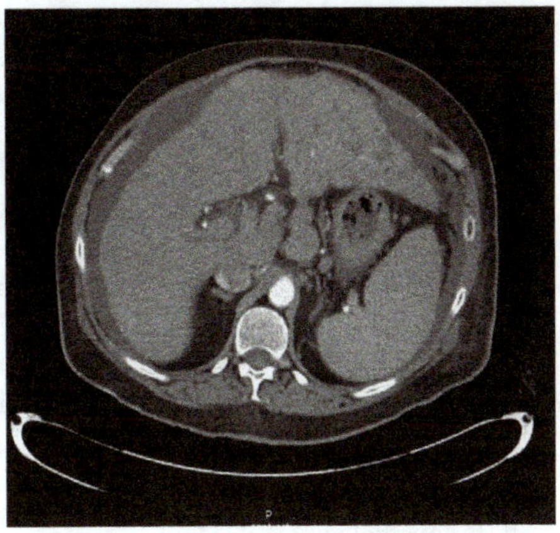

Figure 1: CT liver mass protocol with IV contrast showing evidence of cirrhosis with features of portal hypertension, an ill-defined infiltrative mass in left hepatic lobe suggestive of infiltrative HCC, hypoattenuating lesions in the right hepatic lobe, and periportal lymphadenopathy.

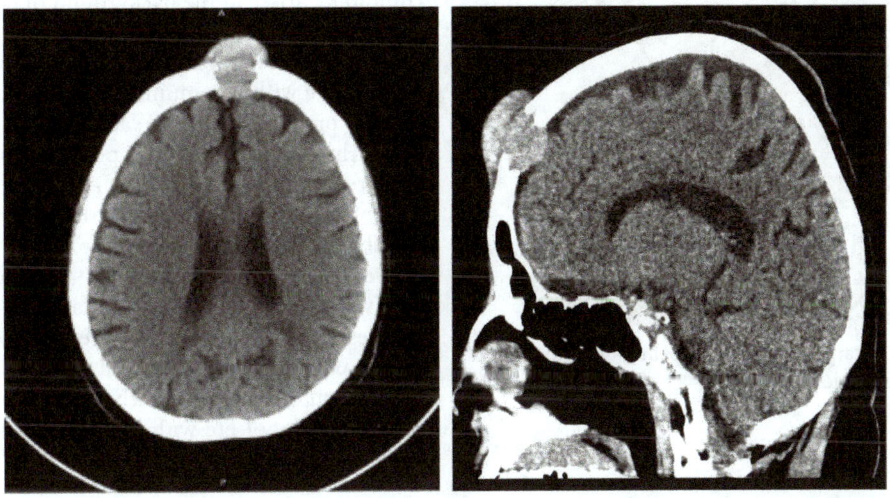

Figure 2: Cross-sectional and sagittal images of CT head (with and without contrast) demonstrating a 3.1 cm × 3 cm × 3 cm enhancing soft tissue mass eroding through the frontal calvarium and extending into the anterior soft tissues of the scalp in the epidural space overlying the left frontal lobe.

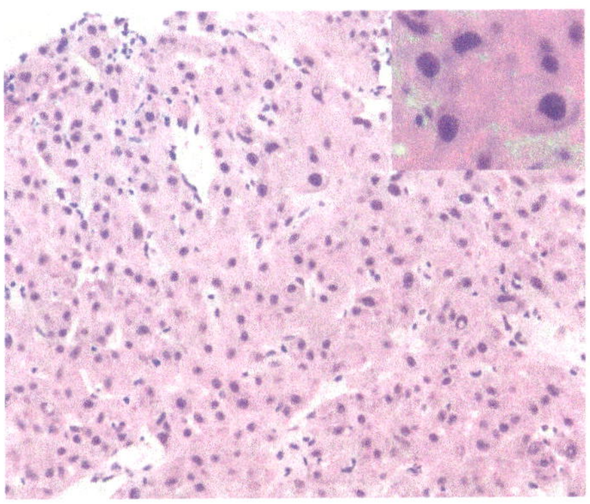

Figure 3: H&E 10× section shows well to moderately differentiated HCC with trabecular pattern. The inset (H&E 20×) shows large pleomorphic nuclei with nucleoli (histopathology of forehead lesion).

function, and presence of extrahepatic spread. Orthotopic liver transplantation (OLT) is the definitive treatment of HCC. Unfortunately, as earlier stages of HCC are largely asymptomatic, most patients present with advanced disease and, therefore, are not candidates for OLT based on the Milan criteria (up to three liver lesions ≤3 cm or a single lesion ≤5 cm, in the absence of macrovascular invasion or extrahepatic metastasis) [11]. Metastatic disease, although limited in its therapeutic options, can be treated with sorafenib, an oral tyrosine kinase inhibitor. Sorafenib works on a variety of different receptors and mechanisms to inhibit tumor angiogenesis and proliferation [12]. It is reserved for advanced HCC with preserved liver function in those who are not surgical candidates or have failed other locoregional therapies. For years, sorafenib was the only treatment option for these patients with a median survival of less than three months [13]. Since 2017, advances have been made in targeted immunotherapy with several new drugs demonstrating noninferiority to sorafenib and a median survival of one year [13]. And most recently, immunotherapy with checkpoint inhibitors (CPIs) have demonstrated promising

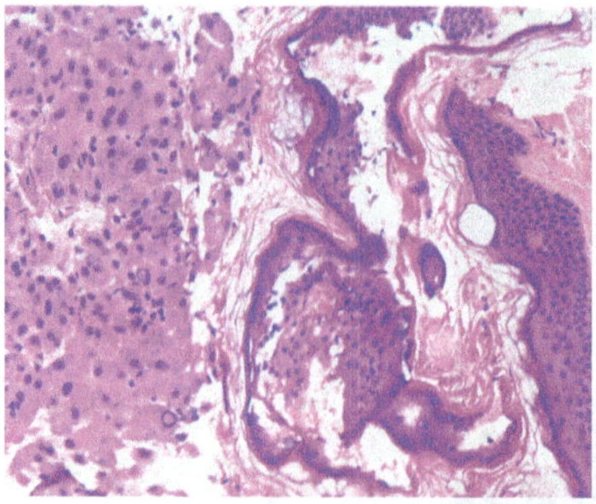

Figure 4: H&E 10× showing the forehead skin fragment as a contaminant on the right and the tumor on the left (histopathology of forehead lesion).

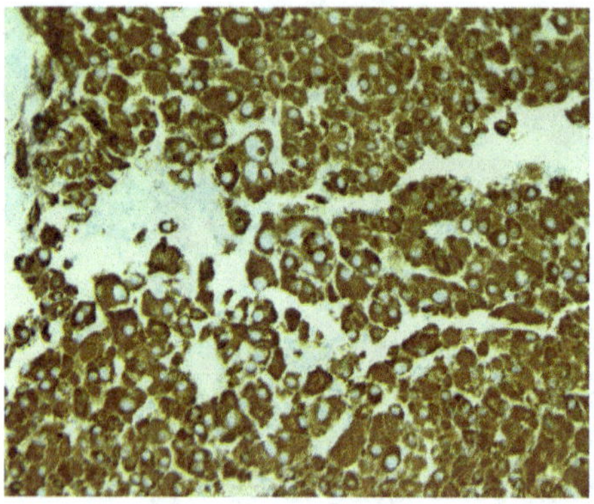

Figure 5: Hep Par-1 stain positive (histopathology and immunostaining of forehead lesion).

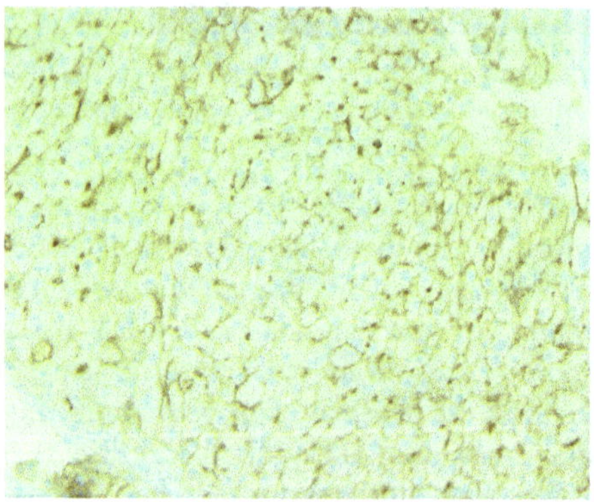

Figure 6: Positive polyclonal CEA staining, diffuse canalicular pattern (histopathology and immunostaining of forehead lesion).

results in treatment responses in patients with advanced HCC, prompting a number of clinical trials to evaluate this potential therapeutic benefit [14].

Cranial and cutaneous metastases of HCC are relatively rare and even more unusual to be the primary presentation of HCC. This patient exhibited evidence of metastasis on her forehead several months before developing any features of cirrhosis. In the absence of significant alcohol consumption and after exclusion of other causes, the etiology of her cirrhosis is presumed to be from NASH in the setting of unrecognized diabetes mellitus and hyperlipidemia. However, without proper histopathological examination of the liver, NASH is indistinguishable from cryptogenic cirrhosis (which includes the progression of NASH to "burnt out NASH"). This case illustrates the rare locations HCC can metastasize to but, also, reflects the importance of a thorough history and physical examination, keeping a vigilant eye for abnormal lesions that should be investigated to rule out malignancy. Early recognition of this patient's enlarging forehead mass could have lead an earlier diagnosis, which may not have changed her overall poor prognosis but may have allowed for improved quality of life by preventing decompensation with early palliation.

4. Conclusion

Hepatocellular carcinoma is an aggressive tumor that most commonly arises in the background of chronic liver disease and cirrhosis from alcohol abuse, viral hepatitis, NASH, or several other conditions that affect the liver. It can be largely preventable with community education on minimizing risk factors, proper screening, vaccination against hepatitis B, and early treatment of at-risk populations, i.e., screening for and treating hepatitis C or NASH, for example. Routine screening for HCC in liver cirrhosis patients has made it possible to identify and treat the tumor in its early stages. However, many are diagnosed at advanced stages, with low survival rates at two years of diagnosis. Extrahepatic metastases are rarely the primary presentation of HCC, but it is important to hold high clinical suspicion of an underlying primary malignancy, as early diagnosis may lead to improved quality of life with early treatment or palliation.

Disclosure

The abstract of the manuscript was presented in AFMR Meeting Abstracts in February 2019.

References

[1] X. J. Wang and H. Malhi, "Nonalcoholic fatty liver disease," *Annals of Internal Medicine*, vol. 169, no. 9, pp. ITC65–ITC80, 2018.

[2] J. Balogh, D. Victor, E. H. Asham et al., "Hepatocellular carcinoma: a review," *Journal of Hepatocellular Carcinoma*, vol. 3, pp. 41–53, 2016.

[3] A. K. Becker, D. K. Tso, A. C. Harris, D. Malfair, and S. D. Chang, "Extrahepatic metastases of hepatocellular carcinoma: a spectrum of imaging findings," *Canadian Association of Radiologists Journal*, vol. 65, no. 1, pp. 60–66, 2014.

[4] A. Baecker, X. Liu, C. La Vecchia, and Z. F. Zhang, "Worldwide incidence of hepatocellular carcinoma cases attributable to major risk factors," *European Journal of Cancer Prevention*, vol. 27, no. 3, pp. 205–212, 2018.

[5] R. Dhanasekaran, S. Bandoh, and L. R. Roberts, "Molecular pathogenesis of hepatocellular carcinoma and impact of therapeutic advances," *F1000 Research*, vol. 5, p. 879, 2016.

[6] D. Subasinghe, C. T. Keppetiyagama, H. Sudasinghe, S. Wadanamby, N. Perera, and S. Sivaganesh, "Solitary scalp metastasis-a rare presentation of hepatocellular carcinoma," *Annals of Surgical Innovation and Research*, vol. 9, p. 4, 2015.

[7] S. Y. Bae, H. J. Kim, H. H. Oh et al., "Multiple bone metastases as the first manifestation of hepatocellular carcinoma in patient with noncirrhotic liver," *Case Reports in Oncological Medicine*, vol. 2015, Article ID 512849, 2015.

[8] X. Guo, J. Yin, and Y. Jiang, "Solitary skull metastasis as the first symptom of hepatocellular carcinoma: case report and literature review," *Neuropsychiatric Disease and Treatment*, vol. 10, pp. 681–686, 2014.

[9] D. Chen, Z. Li, Q. Song, L. Qian, B. Xie, and J. Zhu, "Clinicopathological features and differential diagnosis of hepatocellular carcinoma in extrahepatic metastases," *Medicine (Baltimore)*, vol. 97, no. 50, Article ID e13356, 2018.

[10] J. A. Marrero, L. M. Kulik, C. B. Sirlin et al., "Diagnosis, staging, and management of hepatocellular carcinoma: 2018 practice guidance by the American association for the study of liver diseases," *Hepatology*, vol. 68, no. 2, pp. 723–750, 2018.

[11] S. Daher, M. Massarwa, A. A. Benson, and T. Khoury, "Current and future treatment of hepatocellular carcinoma: an updated comprehensive review," *Journal of Clinical and Translational Hepatology*, vol. 6, no. 1, pp. 69–78, 2018.

[12] Z. Y. Tang, "Hepatocellular carcinoma-cause, treatment and metastasis," *World Journal of Gastroenterology*, vol. 7, no. 4, pp. 445–454, 2001.

[13] H. Cheng, G. Sun, H. Chen et al., "Trends in the treatment of advanced hepatocellular carcinoma: immune checkpoint blockade immunotherapy and related combination therapies," *American Journal of Cancer Research*, vol. 9, no. 8, pp. 1536–1545, 2019.

[14] L. A. Huppert, J. D. Gordan, and R. K. Kelley, "Checkpoint inhibitors for the treatment of advanced hepatocellular carcinoma," *Clinical Liver Disease (Hoboken)*, vol. 15, no. 2, pp. 53–58, 2020.

53

A Case of Ulcerated Gastric Mass and Anemia due to Strongyloidiasis

Monjur Ahmed, Kristen Singer, Cecilia Kelly, Brian O'hara, and Curtis Alloy

Thomas Jefferson University, Philadelphia, PA, USA

Correspondence should be addressed to Monjur Ahmed; monjurahmedmd@gmail.com

Academic Editor: Tetsuo Hirata

Strongyloidiasis is an intestinal infection caused by the nematode *Strongyloides*, and it is rarely seen in our clinical practice in the United States. Although it remains localized to the gastrointestinal tract most of the time, it can disseminate to other organs when it causes autoinfection in the setting of immunosuppression. The clinical manifestations vary depending on the involved organ. A case of disseminated strongyloidiasis presenting as a case of ulcerated gastric mass and anemia is described here along with a review of the literature on this condition.

1. Introduction

Strongyloides stercoralis infection is a rare, soil-transmitted, neglected tropical disease. About 50% of patients infected with *Strongyloides* are asymptomatic. As the larvae of *Strongyloides* penetrate the human skin and, then, migrate to the lungs via bloodstream and lymphatics and are, then, swallowed to be transported to the small bowel, patients may present with various cutaneous, pulmonary, and gastrointestinal symptoms during their journey. Patients may notice a mildly itchy skin rash at the site of larval penetration and may develop cough and wheezing during larval migration through the pulmonary parenchyma. But, most commonly, patients generally present with abdominal pain, diarrhea, and occasionally, anorexia, nausea, and vomiting due to congestion, thickening, and ulceration of small intestinal and colonic mucosa. We present here a case of *Strongyloides* infection in an Asian man who not only had abdominal pain but also an ulcerated gastric mass and iron deficiency anemia.

2. Key Words

Strongyloidiasis, disseminated strongyloidiasis, gastric mass and strongyloidiasis, anemia and strongyloidiasis, and diagnosis of strongyloidiasis.

3. Case

A 68-year-old Lao-speaking male presented with generalized weakness, postprandial dull aching, nonradiating epigastric pain, early satiety, and bloating for about 2 months. He denied any weight loss, fever, or night sweats. He did not have any history of taking nonsteroidal anti-inflammatory drugs, and there was no history of overt gastrointestinal bleeding. He was known to have hyperlipidemia and ascending aortic aneurysm. He was an everyday cigarette-smoker (1/2 pack per day for 25 years) and was a social alcohol drinker. In 1980, he moved from Laos to the United States and worked as a farmer. He had no significant family history of any illness. He was taking aspirin 81 mg daily, atorvastatin 40 mg daily, and multivitamin 1 capsule daily. On examination, he appeared thin built. Vital signs revealed a pulse of 84/minute, blood pressure 121/82 mm Hg, and temperature 98.4°F. Physical examination showed pale conjunctiva, no pedal edema, heart: S1 and S2 regular, no murmur, and breath sounds vesicular, and few crackles at the lung bases. The abdomen was soft and nontender without a palpable mass, and rectal examination was notable for heme-negative stool. Remainder of the examination was unremarkable.

Laboratory studies showed a hemoglobin of 4.7 gm/dl, WBC 10,600/cmm, platelet count 509,000/cmm, MCV 68, serum iron 11 microgram/dl, TIBC 275, iron saturation 4%, and ferritin 10 ng/dl. He was admitted as a case of severe iron deficiency anemia due to chronic occult gastrointestinal blood loss. He was transfused a few units of packed red blood cells with subsequent improvement of his hemoglobin to 8.4 gm/dl. A CT scan showed gastric wall thickening. Upper endoscopy revealed an ulcerated friable mass in the gastric antrum extending proximally to the incisura angularis (Figure 1). Multiple biopsies were taken from the mass, and histopathology showed chronic active gastritis with mucosal necrosis, granulation tissue, and necroinflammatory exudate, negative for *Helicobacter pylori* infection. He was started on ferrous sulfate 325 mg daily and pantoprazole 40 mg daily and was discharged.

Three months later, the patient was readmitted with epigastric pain, anorexia, nausea, and vomiting. His physical examination was unchanged except for worsened pallor. His hemoglobin was 5.8 gm/dl. He was again transfused 3 units of packed red blood cells, and his hemoglobin increased to 7.9 gm/dl. Upper endoscopy again showed an ulcerated antral mass, with repeat biopsies demonstrating similar histopathology as before. There was no evidence of malignancy. He was discharged home. Two weeks following discharge, he represented to the hospital with generalized weakness and fatigue. His hemoglobin was found to be 4.7 gm/dl, and upper endoscopy demonstrated the same ulcerated mass. Surgery was, then, consulted, and the patient underwent laparoscopic subtotal gastrectomy with Roux-en-Y reconstruction with vagotomy. Histopathology of the ulcerated mass showed ulceration, inflammation, granulation tissue, fibrosis, reactive changes, focal gastritis with intestinal metaplasia, and scattered microscopic foci with morphology consistent with a nematode favoring strongyloides (Figure 2). Postoperatively, stool assay by wet mount after concentration showed strongyloides stercoralis larvae. Serum strongyloides IgG ELISA resulted positive. The patient was discharged home and seen in consultation by infectious diseases, with a plan to start antihelminthic treatment. However, prior to initiating treatment, he developed sepsis and was admitted to an outside hospital, where he unfortunately clinically deteriorated and expired.

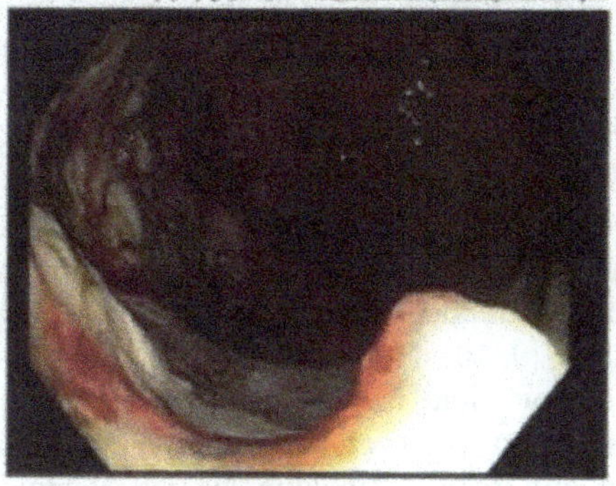

FIGURE 1: Ulcerated gastric antral mass.

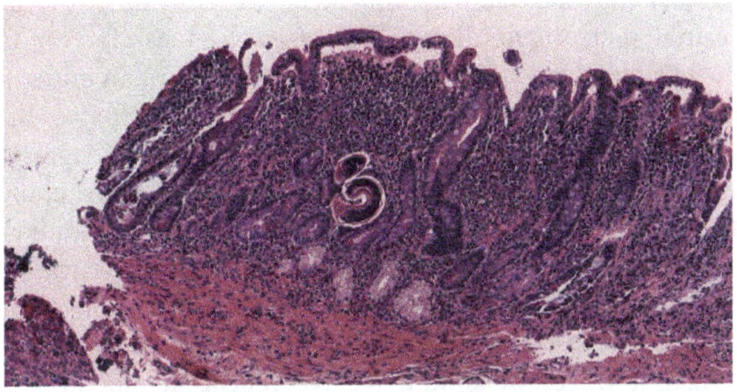

FIGURE 2: H&E stain of gastric mass showing the nematode and inflammatory cells.

4. Discussion and Conclusions

Strongyloidiasis is a global infection more commonly seen in Southeast Asia, sub-Saharan Africa, Latin America, Caribbean islands, and Eastern, Southern, and Central Europe [1]. Worldwide, there are 30 to 100 million people infected with *Strongyloides stercoralis* [2]. In the United States, strongyloidiasis is mostly seen in eastern Kentucky and rural Tennessee. But, sporadically, the infection is seen in immigrants from the endemic area, world war II veterans, and residents of mental institutions [3]. *Strongyloides stercoralis* is a potentially lethal cosmopolitan nematode or roundworm also known as human threadworm. It has complex stages of life consisting of a free-living cycle, parasitic cycle, and autoinfection cycle. In the autoinfection cycle, the rhabditiform larvae transform inside the gastrointestinal tract into the infective filariform larvae which can penetrate the intestinal mucosa (internal autoinfection) or perianal skin (external autoinfection) to complete the life cycle. A pathognomonic feature of strongyloides external autoinfection is larva currens in which larvae can be seen creeping under the skin. Once internal autoinfection occurs, the filariform larvae can migrate to the lungs, tracheobronchial tree, and small intestine. If untreated, the autoinfection cycle can result in persistent infection in an individual even after many years of residence in a nonendemic area. Patients with chronic infection may remain asymptomatic for many years except occasional abdominal pain, diarrhea, constipation, and skin rash. Autoinfection may lead to hyperinfection syndrome or disseminated strongyloidiasis if the body's defense mechanism is compromised by different factors, including the use of corticosteroids, immunosuppressive agents or chemotherapy, diabetes mellitus, cirrhosis, malignancy, alcoholism, malnutrition, solid organ transplantation, hematopoietic stem cell transplantation, and HTLV-1 (human T-lymphotropic virus type 1) and HIV (human immunodeficiency virus) infection [4]. In hyperinfection syndrome, the worm burden in the small intestine is excessive due to accelerated normal life cycle of the worm. In disseminated strongyloidiasis, plenty of autoinfective larvae migrate through different organs (the central nervous system, heart, and urinary tract) that are not part of their normal life cycle, and many of them carry enteric organisms from the intestine [5], leading to pneumonia [6], meningitis [7], and sepsis [8]. The case we described had gastric strongyloidiasis as part of his disseminated strongyloidiasis. Cases of disseminated strongyloidiasis with gastroduodenal involvement, including multiple granular lesions, ulcerations, and even duodenal obstruction, have been reported in the literature [9, 10]. However, this is the first case of disseminated strongyloidiasis in which a patient presented with an ulcerated gastric mass and iron deficiency anemia. Intake of aspirin and regular smoking cigarettes could lead to gastric ulcer formation, and the presence of the *Strongyloides* nematode could be a chance finding. But, positive serology, positive stool test, and inflammatory gastric mass with the *Strongyloides* nematode confirmed the diagnosis of disseminated strongyloidiasis. The patient had risk factors for developing strongyloidiasis as he was a native of an endemic area and also worked as a farmer in the United States. But, the obvious reason for developing disseminated strongyloidiasis is unknown. Ivermectin is the treatment of choice for both uncomplicated and complicated strongyloidiasis [11]. Patients should be followed up to confirm eradication, typically with stool testing for the presence of *Strongyloides* larvae 2 to 4 weeks after completing treatment. Patients with persistent infection should receive repeat dosing of ivermectin. Ivermectin was found to be more effective than albendazole or thiabendazole for treatment of strongyloidiasis [11, 12]. In the case of severe disease (hyperinfection syndrome and disseminated strongyloidiasis), ivermectin plus antibiotics against Gram-negative organisms should be initiated and continued for at least 2 weeks. Ideally, treatment should be continued until patients become asymptomatic and daily stool tests for *Strongyloides* larvae remain negative for at least 2 weeks. Successful treatment of disseminated strongyloidiasis with a combination of ivermectin and thiabendazole for 2 weeks has been reported [13]. Suppressive treatment with ivermectin should be given once a month for at least 6 months to patients with persistent immunosuppression who have become asymptomatic after initial treatment [14]. It is also recommended that if patients with hyperinfection/desseminated infection do not respond to initial treatment, they should be tested for underlying immunosuppression such as HIV or HTLV-1 infection. The mortality of patients with hyperinfection syndrome and disseminated strongyloidiasis can be as high as 70 to 90% despite aggressive supportive therapy [15]. In conclusion, strongyloidiasis should be considered in high-risk individuals with inflammatory gastric mass and iron deficiency anemia.

References

[1] S. Puthiyakunnon, S. Boddu, Y. Li et al., "Strongyloidiasis-an insight into its global prevalence and management," *PLoS Neglected Tropical Diseases*, vol. 8, no. 8, Article ID e3018, 2014.

[2] Strongyloides-epidemiology & risk factors-CDC," https://www.cdc.gov/parasites/strongyloides/epi.html.

[3] A. A. F. Mahmoud, "Strongyloidiasis," *Clinical Infectious Diseases*, vol. 23, no. 5, pp. 949–953, 1996.

[4] M. Mukaigawara, M. Narita, S. Shiiki et al., "Clinical characteristics of disseminated strongyloidiasis, Japan, 1975–2017," *Emerging Infectious Diseases*, vol. 26, no. 3, pp. 401-408, 2020.

[5] R. Pukkila-Worley, V. Nardi, and J. A. Branda, "Case 28-2014," *New England Journal of Medicine*, vol. 371, no. 11, pp. 1051–1060, 2014.

[6] E. Chu, W. L. Whitlock, and R. A. Dietrich, "Pulmonary hyperinfection syndrome with *Strongyloides stercoralis*," *Chest*, vol. 97, no. 6, pp. 1475–1477, 1990.

[7] T. Shimasaki, S. Shiiki, and H. Chung, "Five cases of recurrent meningitis associated with chronic strongyloidiasis," *The American Journal of Tropical Medicine and Hygiene*, vol. 92, no. 3, pp. 601–604, 2015.

[8] A. K. Jain, S. K. Agarwal, and W. el-Sadr, "Streptococcus bovis bacteremia and meningitis associated with *Strongyloides stercoralis* colitis in a patient infected with human immunodeficiency virus," *Clinical Infectious Diseases*, vol. 18, no. 2, pp. 253-254, 1994.

[9] T. Minamide, M. Fukushima, and T. Inokuma, "Gastroduodenal involvement in disseminated strongyloidiasis," *JGH Open*, vol. 2, no. 2, pp. 75-76, 2018.

[10] F. Yazdanpanah, H. Saba, R. Rahmani, Z. J. Schreiber, and P. Hindy, "*Strongyloides* hyperinfection presenting as a gastric outlet obstruction," *Cureus*, vol. 12, no. 1, Article ID e6603, 2020.

[11] C. Henriquez-Camacho, E. Gotuzzo, J. Echevarria et al., "Ivermectin versus albendazole or thiabendazole for *Strongyloides stercoralis* infection. version 2," *Cochrane Database of Systematic Reviews*, vol. 2016, no. 1, Article ID CD007745, 2016.

[12] Y. Suputtamongkol, N. Premasathian, K. Bhumimuang et al., "Efficacy and safety of single and double doses of ivermectin versus 7-day high dose albendazole for chronic strongyloidiasis," *PLoS Neglected Tropical Diseases*, vol. 5, no. 5, Article ID e1044, 2011.

[13] P. Pornsuriyasak, K. Niticharoenpong, and A. Sakapibunnan, "Disseminated strongyloidiasis successfully treated with extended duration ivermectin combined with albendazole: a case report of intractable strongyloidiasis," *The Southeast Asian Journal of Tropical Medicine and Public Health*, vol. 35, no. 3, pp. 531–534, 2004.

[14] M. Segarra-Newnham, "Manifestations, diagnosis, and treatment of Strongyloides stercoralis infection," *Annals of Pharmacotherapy*, vol. 41, no. 12, pp. 1992–2001, 2007.

[15] C. S. Lam, M. K. H. Tong, K. M. Chan, and Y. P. Siu, "Disseminated strongyloidiasis: a retrospective study of clinical course and outcome," *European Journal of Clinical Microbiology & Infectious Diseases*, vol. 25, no. 1, pp. 14–18, 2006.

Permissions

All chapters in this book were first published by Hindawi Publishing Corporation; hereby published with permission under the Creative Commons Attribution License or equivalent. Every chapter published in this book has been scrutinized by our experts. Their significance has been extensively debated. The topics covered herein carry significant findings which will fuel the growth of the discipline. They may even be implemented as practical applications or may be referred to as a beginning point for another development.

The contributors of this book come from diverse backgrounds, making this book a truly international effort. This book will bring forth new frontiers with its revolutionizing research information and detailed analysis of the nascent developments around the world.

We would like to thank all the contributing authors for lending their expertise to make the book truly unique. They have played a crucial role in the development of this book. Without their invaluable contributions this book wouldn't have been possible. They have made vital efforts to compile up to date information on the varied aspects of this subject to make this book a valuable addition to the collection of many professionals and students.

This book was conceptualized with the vision of imparting up-to-date information and advanced data in this field. To ensure the same, a matchless editorial board was set up. Every individual on the board went through rigorous rounds of assessment to prove their worth. After which they invested a large part of their time researching and compiling the most relevant data for our readers.

The editorial board has been involved in producing this book since its inception. They have spent rigorous hours researching and exploring the diverse topics which have resulted in the successful publishing of this book. They have passed on their knowledge of decades through this book. To expedite this challenging task, the publisher supported the team at every step. A small team of assistant editors was also appointed to further simplify the editing procedure and attain best results for the readers.

Apart from the editorial board, the designing team has also invested a significant amount of their time in understanding the subject and creating the most relevant covers. They scrutinized every image to scout for the most suitable representation of the subject and create an appropriate cover for the book.

The publishing team has been an ardent support to the editorial, designing and production team. Their endless efforts to recruit the best for this project, has resulted in the accomplishment of this book. They are a veteran in the field of academics and their pool of knowledge is as vast as their experience in printing. Their expertise and guidance has proved useful at every step. Their uncompromising quality standards have made this book an exceptional effort. Their encouragement from time to time has been an inspiration for everyone.

The publisher and the editorial board hope that this book will prove to be a valuable piece of knowledge for researchers, students, practitioners and scholars across the globe.

List of Contributors

Michael Coles, Victoria Madray and Pearl Uy
Augusta University, 1120 15th Street, Augusta, Georgia 30912, USA

Margaret R. Paulson
Division of Hospital Internal Medicine, Mayo Clinic Health Systems, Eau Claire, Wisconsin 2321 Stout Road, Menomonie, Wisconsin 54751, USA

Abdullah S. Eldaly, Francisco R. Avila, Ricardo A. Torres-Guzman, Karla C. Maita, John P. Garcia, Luiza Palmieri Serrano, Omar S. Emam and Antonio J. Forte
Division of Plastic Surgery, Mayo Clinic, 4500 San Pablo Road, Jacksonville, Florida 32224, USA

Michael J. Maniaci
Division of Hospital Internal Medicine, Mayo Clinic, 4500 San Pablo Road, Jacksonville, Florida 32224, USA

Neha Mehta, Man Bahadur Paudyal, Rajan Chamlagain and Moon Shrestha
Tribhuvan University Teaching Hospital, Maharajgunj 44600, Nepal

Sangam Shah
Maharajgunj Medical Campus, Institute of Medicine, Tribhuvan University, Maharajgunj 44600, Nepal

Ashish Mehta
BP Koirala Institute of Health Sciences, Dharan 56700, Nepal

Prabin Bhattarai
Department of Internal Medicine, Maharajgunj Medical Campus, Institute of Medicine, Tribhuvan University, Maharajgunj 44600, Nepal

Donald Ewing and Ava Brozovich
Texas A&M University College of Medicine, 8447 Bryan Rd., Bryan, TX 77807, USA

Bincy Abraham
Texas A&M University College of Medicine, 8447 Bryan Rd., Bryan, TX 77807, USA
Houston Methodist Hospital, Department of Gastroenterology, 6550 Fannin St., Houston, TX 77096, USA

Ethan Burns, Gonzalo Acosta and Courtney Hatcher
Houston Methodist Hospital, Department of Medicine, 6550 Fannin St., Houston, TX 77096, USA

Pragnesh Patel
Houston Methodist Hospital, Department of Gastroenterology, 6550 Fannin St., Houston, TX 77096, USA

Leena Samuel and Rose Anton
Houston Methodist Hospital, Department of Pathology and Genomic Medicine, 6550 Fannin St., Houston, TX 77030, USA

M. B. Gilani, T. Akcan and M. Peterson
Department of Internal Medicine, Marshfield Clinic Health System—Marshfield, Marshfield, WI 54449, USA

A. Zahid
Department of Hospital Medicine, Marshfield Clinic Health System—Marshfield, Marshfield, WI 54449, USA

Khin San Aye and Than Than Aye
Department of Gastroenterology, University of Medicine 2, Yangon, Myanmar

Aung Khine Zan
Yangon General Hospital, Myanmar

Myo Thet Tin
Nay Pyi Taw General Hospital (1000-bedded),Myanmar

Mohammad Hossein Bagheripour
Department of General Surgery, Faculty of Medicine, Rafsanjan University of Medical Sciences, Rafsanjan, Iran

Mohammad Ali Zakeri
Social Determinants of Health Research Centre, Rafsanjan University of Medical Sciences, Rafsanjan, Iran
Non-Communicable Diseases Research Center, Rafsanjan University of Medical Sciences, Rafsanjan, Iran

Anoush Calikyan
Frank H. Netter School of Medicine at Quinnipiac University, North Haven, CT, USA

Agedi N. Boto
St. Vincent's Medical Center, Department of Pathology, Bridgeport, CT, USA

Valeriia Klymenko
St. Vincent's Medical Center, Department of Medical Oncology, Bridgeport, CT, USA

Imran M. Siddiqui
St. Vincent's Medical Center, Department of Surgical Oncology, Bridgeport, CT, USA

Yuichi Takano, Fumitaka Niiya, Takahiro Kobayashi, Eiichi Yamamura, Naotaka Maruoka and Masatsugu Nagahama
Division of Gastroenterology, Department of Internal Medicine, Showa University Fujigaoka Hospital, Yokohama, Kanagawa, Japan

Tomoko Norose and Nobuyuki Ohike
Department of Diagnostic Pathology, Showa University Fujigaoka Hospital, Yokohama, Kanagawa, Japan

Mohammad Nabil Rayad and Noreen Mirza
Department of Internal Medicine, St Michael's Medical Center, 111 Central Ave, Newark, NJ 07102, USA

Maria Bernardeth Herrera-Gonzalez
Division of Health Sciences, University of Monterrey, Avenida Ignacio Morones Prieto 4500-Pte, San Pedro Garza Garcia, Nuevo Leon 66238, Mexico

Yatinder Bains and Sarahi Herrera-Gonzalez
Department of Gastroenterology, St Michael's Medical Center, 111 Central Ave, Newark, NJ 07102, USA

Roberto Castiglione, Aldo E. Calogero and Enzo Vicari
Department of Clinical and Experimental Medicine, University of Catania, Catania, Italy

Giovanna Calabrini and Anna Cosentino
Pathology Unit, Gravina Hospital, Caltagirone, Italy

Placido D'Agati
Department "GF Ingrassia" Hygiene and Public Health, University of Catania, Catania, Italy

Filippo Fraggetta
Pathology Unit, Cannizzaro Hospital, Catania, Italy

Michele Salemi
Oasi Research Institute-IRCCS, Troina, EN, Italy

Samar Said, Rondell P. Graham, Tsung-Teh Wu, Saba Yasir, Lizhi Zhang and Andrew L. Folpe
Department of Laboratory Medicine and Pathology, Mayo Clinic, Rochester, MN, USA

Mateusz Jagielski, Michał Zieliński, Jacek Piątkowski and Marek Jackowski
Department of General, Gastroenterological and Oncological Surgery, Collegium Medicum Nicolaus Copernicus University, Torún, Poland

Maarij Baig
Internal Medicine Residency Program, Inspira Medical Center in Vineland, Vineland, NJ 08360, USA

Lin Zheng and Alka Farmer
Division of Hospital Medicine, Department of Medicine, Cooper Medical School of Rowan University, Camden, NJ 08103, USA

Mariana Aşchie
Department of Clinical Pathology, "St. Apostle Andrew" Emergency County Hospital, Constanta, Romania
Center for Research and Development of the Morphological and Genetic Studies of Malignant Pathology-CEDMOG, "Ovidius" University of Constanta, Constanța, Romania
Academy of Medical Sciences, Bucharest, Romania

Mădălina Boşoteanu
Department of Clinical Pathology, "St. Apostle Andrew" Emergency County Hospital, Constanta, Romania
Faculty of Medicine, "Ovidius" University of Constanta, Constanța, Romania

Cătălin Adrian Boşoteanu
Department of Clinical Pathology, "St. Apostle Andrew" Emergency County Hospital, Constanta, Romania

Gabriela Izabela Bălțătescu and Miruna Cristian
Department of Clinical Pathology, "St. Apostle Andrew" Emergency County Hospital, Constanta, Romania
Center for Research and Development of the Morphological and Genetic Studies of Malignant Pathology-CEDMOG, "Ovidius" University of Constanta, Constanța, Romania

Angelica Potamian
Department of Radiology, Clinical Pneumophthisiology Hospital, Constanta, Romania

Mohamed Abdallah, Ahmad Gohar, Smitha Naryana Gowda, Hafez M. Abdullah and Ali Al-hajjaj
Internal Medicine, University of South Dakota Sanford School of Medicine, Vermillion, SD 57069, USA

Bilal Niazi and Sameh Elias
Department of Internal Medicine, HMH-Palisades Medical Center, North Bergen, NJ, USA

Michael Sciarra and Saad Ali
Department of Gastroenterology, HMH-Palisades Medical Center, North Bergen, NJ, USA

Yoshitsugu Misumi and Kouichi Nonaka
Department of Digestive Endoscopy, Tokyo Women's Medical University Hospital, 8-1, Kawada-cho, Shinjuku-ku, Tokyo 162-8666, Japan

Shin Ichihara
Department of Surgical Pathology, Sapporo-Kosei General Hospital, 8-5, Kita 3 Jouhigashi, Chu-o-ku, Sapporo, Hokkaido 060-0033, Japan

Hiromi Onizuka and Yoji Nagashima
Department of Surgical Pathology, Tokyo Women's Medical University Hospital, 8-1, Kawada-cho, Shinjuku-ku, Tokyo 162-8666, Japan

Hakon Blomstrand
Department of Clinical Pathology and Department of Clinical and Experimental Medicine, Linköping University, 58183 Linköping, Sweden

Karin Adolfsson
Department of Oncology, Ryhov County Hospital, 55305 Jönköping, Sweden

Per Sandström and Bergthor Björnsson
Department of Surgery and Department of Clinical and Experimental Medicine, Linköping University, 58183 Linköping, Sweden

Seyed Mostafa Meshkati Yazd
Department of Surgery, Tehran University of Medical Sciences, Tehran, Iran

Hamidreza Bayati
Department of Surgery, Iran University of Medical Sciences, Tehran, Iran

Sara Sadat Nabavizadeh
Student Research Committee, Shiraz University of Medical Sciences, Shiraz, Iran

Reza Shahriarirad
Thoracic and Vascular Surgery Research Center, Shiraz University of Medical Science, Shiraz, Iran

Zaid Imam
Department of Internal Medicine, William Beaumont Hospital, Royal Oak, MI, USA

C. Roberto Simons-Linares
Gastroenterology and Hepatology Department, Digestive Diseases Institute, Cleveland Clinic, Cleveland, OH, USA

Chukwunonso Chime and Harish Patel
Division of Gastroenterology, BronxCare Hospital Center a Clinical Aliate of Mt Sinai Health Systems and Academic Aliate of Icahn School of Medicine, Bronx, NY 10457, USA
Department of Medicine, BronxCare Hospital Center a Clinical Aliate of Mt Sinai Health Systems and Academic Aliate of Icahn School of Medicine, Bronx, NY 10457, USA

Peter Bhandari
Department of Medicine, BronxCare Hospital Center a Clinical Aliate of Mt Sinai Health Systems and Academic Aliate of Icahn School of Medicine, Bronx, NY 10457, USA

Masooma Niazi
Department of Pathology, BronxCare Hospital Center a Clinical Aliate of Mt Sinai Health Systems and Academic Aliate of Icahn School of Medicine, Bronx, NY 10457, USA

Filipe Bessa, Pedro Gaspar, Pedro Antunes Meireles, Maria Inês Parreira, Juliana Serrazina Pedro, Marisa Teixeira da Silva, João Meneses, Rui Victorino and Catarina Mota
Clínica Universitária de Medicina II, CHLN-Hospital de Santa Maria, Lisbon, Portugal

Amir Mohammad Salehi
School of Medicine, Hamadan University of Medical Sciences, Hamadan, Iran

Hossain Salehi
Gastroenterology Ward, Farhikhtegan Hospital, Azad University of Medical Sciences, Tehran, Iran

Maryam Hasanzarrini
Hepatology of Hamadan University of Medical School, Hamadan, Iran

Elham Khanlarzadeh
Department of Community Medicine, School of Medicine Hamadan University of Medical Sciences, Hamadan, Iran

Michihiro Kamigaki, Satoko Kunita, Makoto Nakano, Miwako Tanaka, Shinya Aoki, Katsutoshi Tsuga, Hiroyuki Ito and Hideo Matsuura
Department of Internal Medicine, Saiseikai Kure Hospital, 2-1-13 Sanjo, Kure City, Hiroshima Prefecture 737-0821, Japan

Jong Soo Lee, Eun Hee Kim and Hye Won Park
Division of Gastroenterology, Health Screening and Promotion Center, Asan Medical Center, University of Ulsan College of Medicine, Seoul, Republic of Korea

Dong-Hoon Yang and Jin Hwa Park
Department of Gastroenterology, Asan Medical Center, University of Ulsan College of Medicine, Seoul, Republic of Korea

Sungwon Park
Division of Radiology, Health Screening and Promotion Center, Asan Medical Center, University of Ulsan College of Medicine, Seoul, Republic of Korea

Jeonghun Lee
Department of Internal Medicine, Ye Hospital, Anyang, Republic of Korea

Younghye Kim
Green Cross Reference Laboratory, Yongin, Republic of Korea

Christopher Hakim
Department of Internal Medicine, Ascension Providence Hospital, Michigan State University College of Human Medicine, Southfield, USA

Constantine Melitas and Kha Ngo
Department of Gastroenterology, Ascension Providence Hospital, Michigan State University College of Human Medicine, Southfield, USA

Eric Nguyen
American University of the Caribbean School of Medicine, Coral Gables, USA

Samuel Galante Romanini, Juan Pablo Román Serrano, Juliana Silveira Lima de Castro, Isabela Trindade Torres, Alex Ingold, André Lucchiari Borini, Luiz Augusto Sanches Zulske and Maria Bruna Feitosa Matias
Gastrointestinal Endoscopy, Department of Gastrointestinal Endoscopy, Hospital 9 de Julho, São Paulo, Brazil

José Celso Ardengh
Gastrointestinal Endoscopy, Department of Gastrointestinal Endoscopy, Hospital 9 de Julho, São Paulo, Brazil
Department of Radiology, Irmandade da Santa Casa de Misericórdia de São Paulo, São Paulo, Brazil
Hospital do Servidor P´ublico Municipal, São Paulo, Brazil
Gastrointestinal Endoscopy Service, Department of Gastrointestinal Endoscopy, Hospital das Clinicas, University of São Paulo Riberão Preto, São Paulo, Brazil

Jéssica Said de Marchi
Department of Radiology, Irmandade da Santa Casa de Misericórdia de São Paulo, São Paulo, Brazil

José Andrés Sanchez Pulla
Hospital do Servidor P´ublico Municipal, São Paulo, Brazil

Daniela Jaqueline Rivadeneira and Hesheng Luo
Department of Gastroenterology, Renmin Hospital ofWuhan University,Wuhan 430060, China

D. Guinan
West Virginia University Department of Behavioral Medicine and Psychiatry, General Psychiatry Resident PGY-2, USA

T. Drvar
West Virginia University, USA

D. Brubaker
West Virginia University School of Medicine, MS-4, USA

M. Ang-Rabanes
West Virginia University Department of Behavioral Medicine and Psychiatry, Assistant Professor, USA

J. Kupec
West Virginia University Department of Medicine Section of Digestive Diseases, Assistant Professor, USA

P.Marshalek
West Virginia University Department of Behavioral Medicine and Psychiatry, Medical Director, USA

Maria Mironova, Mohammed K. Mahdi and Rosemarie C. Nielson
Department of Medicine, Capital Health Regional Medical Center, 750 Brunswick Ave, Trenton, NJ 08638, USA

Jyoti Bhatia
Department of Gastroenterology, Capital Health Hopewell, One Capital Way, Pennington, NJ 08534, USA

Cataldo Doria
Cancer Center, Capital Health Hopewell, Two Capital Way, Pennington, NJ 08534, USA

Ali Zakaria and Michael Raphael
Division of Gastroenterology, Providence-Providence Park Hospital and Medical Center, Michigan State University/College of Human Medicine, Southfield, Michigan, USA

Nour Hammad
Department of Internal Medicine, Providence-Providence Park Hospital and Medical Center, Michigan State University/College of Human Medicine, Southfield, Michigan, USA

Cynthia Vakhariya
Division of Hematology & Oncology, Providence-Providence Park Hospital and Medical Center, Michigan State University/College of Human Medicine, Southfield, Michigan, USA

Inayat Gill and Ahmed Edhi
Division of Gastroenterology, Department of Internal Medicine, William Beaumont Hospital at Royal Oak, 3535 W. #irteen Mile Rd, Royal Oak, MI 48073, USA

Mitual Amin
Department of Pathology, William Beaumont Hospital at Royal Oak, 3600 W. #irteen Mile Rd, Royal Oak, MI 48073, USA
Department of Pathology, Oakland University William Beaumont School of Medicine, 3600 W. #irteen Mile Rd, Royal Oak, MI 48073, USA

Mitchell S. Cappell
Division of Gastroenterology, Department of Medicine, Building 1, Room 3210, Aleda E. Lutz VA Medical Center, 1500 Weiss St, Saginaw, MI 48602, USA

Koki Yamada
Department of Gastroenterology, Okinawa Chubu Hospital, 271 Miyazato, Uruma 904-2293, Japan

Susumu Shinoura
School of Psychology and Healthcare Management at Akasaka, Department of Healthcare Management, International University of Health and Welfare, 4-1-26 Akasaka, Minato, Tokyo 107-8402, Japan

Kaoru Kikuchi
Division of Gastroenterology, Yaeyama Hospital, 584-1 Maezato, Ishigaki 907-0002, Okinawa, Japan

Ikponmwosa Enofe, Jacob Burch and Manoj Rai
Internal Medicine Resident, Michigan State University, Sparrow Hospital, East Lansing, MI, USA

Julie Yam
Gastroenterology Fellow, Michigan State University, East Lansing, MI, USA

Rajarajeshwari Ramachandran and Denzil Etienne
Department of Gastroenterology, Brooklyn Hospital Center, Brooklyn, NY, USA

Vikash Kumar and Giovannie Isaac-Coss
Department of Internal Medicine, Brooklyn Hospital Center, Brooklyn, NY, USA

Elias Estifan
Department of Internal Medicine, St. Joseph's University Medical Center-New York Medical College, Paterson, NJ 07503, USA

Varun Patel and Matthew Grossman
Division of Gastroenterology, St. Joseph's University Medical Center-New York Medical College, Paterson, NJ 07503, USA

Joyce J. Kim
Department of Medicine, Emory University School of Medicine, Atlanta, Georgia

Ramzi H. Mulki and Kavya M. Sebastian
Department of Medicine, Division of Digestive Diseases, Emory University School of Medicine, Atlanta, Georgia

Elias Estifan
Department of Internal Medicine, St. Joseph's University Medical Center, New York Medical College, USA

Varun Patel and Matthew Grossman
Division of Gastroenterology, St. Joseph's University Medical Center, New York Medical College, USA

Andrew Spiel, Ravi Patel, Antonio Bosch and Deepak Gopal
Division of Gastroenterology & Hepatology, Department of Medicine, Univeristy of WIsconsin School of Medicine and Public Health, Madison, WI, USA

Rebecca Minter and Amir Ali Rahnemai Azar
Division of Surgical Oncology, Department of Surgery, University of Wisconsin School of Medicine and Public Health, Madison, WI, USA

Rashmi Agni
Department of Pathology & Laboratory Medicine, University of Wisconsin School of Medicine and Public Health, Madison, WI, USA

Osayande Osagiede and Dorin Colibaseanu
Mayo Clinic, Department of Surgery, Jacksonville, FL, USA

Paula Pacurari
West Virginia University School of Medicine, Morgantown, WV, USA

Nezar Jrebi
West Virginia University, Department of Surgery, Morgantown, WV, USA

Shireen Samargandy, Hani Marzouki, Talal Al-Khatib and Mazin Merdad
Department of Otolaryngology-Head and Neck Surgery, King Abdulaziz University, Jeddah, Saudi Arabia

Eoghan P Burke
Royal College of Surgeons Ireland, Dublin, Ireland

M. Sava
Western University of Health Sciences, Ventura, CA, USA
Community Memorial Health Systems, Graduate Medical Education, Ventura, CA, USA

A. Frugoli and T. Huynh
Community Memorial Health Systems, Graduate Medical Education, Department of Internal Medicine, Ventura, CA, USA

L. Kong
Community Memorial Health Systems, Graduate Medical Educations, Department of Hematology Oncology, Ventura, CA, USA

M. Salehpour
Community Memorial Hospital, Department of General Surgery, Ventura, CA, USA

B. Barrows
Community Memorial Hospital, Department of Pathology, Ventura, CA, USA

José Carvalho, Francisco Teixeira Silva, Alexandra Esteves, Carlos Ribeiro and Diana Guerra
Serviço de Medicina Interna, ULSAM—Hospital de Santa Luzia, Viana Do Castelo, Portugal

Margarida Teixeira
Serviço de Anatomia Patológica, Hospital de Braga, Braga, Portugal

Akwe Nyabera, Mohanad Elfishawi, Francisco Cuevas, Fahad Riaz and Adriana Abrudescu
NYC Health + Hospitals/ Queens, Jamaica, NY, USA

Fahad Malik, Manuel Gonzalez and Wahib Zafar
Internal Medicine, Richmond University Medical Center, Staten Island, NY 10310, USA

Thomas Enke
The University of Nebraska Medical Center, NE, USA

Wuttiporn Manatsathit
Division of Gastroenterology and Hepatology, University of Nebraska Medical Center, Omaha, NE, USA

Shaheed Merani
Department of Transplant Surgery, University of Nebraska Medical Center, Omaha, NE, USA

Kurt Fisher
Department of Pathology, University of Nebraska Medical Center, Omaha, NE, USA

Evangelia Pliakou, Dimitra-Ioanna Lampropoulou, Nikolaos Soupos and Gerasimos Aravantinos
Second Department of Medical Oncology, General Oncology Hospital of Kissia "Agioi Anargiroi", Athens, Nea Kissia 14564, Greece

Dustin J. Uhlenhopp
Department of Internal Medicine, MercyOne Des Moines Medical Center, Des Moines, IA, USA

Kristin M. Olson
Division of Gastroenterology and Hepatology, University of Nebraska Medical Center, Omaha, NE, USA

Tagore Sunkara
Department of Gastroenterology and Hepatology, MercyOne Des Moines Medical Center, Des Moines, IA, USA

Kimberly Sanders, Ashley Thomas and Carmen Isache
Department of Internal Medicine, University of Florida College of Medicine Jacksonville, Jacksonville, FL, USA

Anwer Siddiqi
Department of Pathology, University of Florida College of Medicine Jacksonville, Jacksonville, FL, USA

Monjur Ahmed, Kristen Singer, Cecilia Kelly, Brian O'hara and Curtis Alloy
Thomas Jefferson University, Philadelphia, PA, USA

Index

www.ingramcontent.com/pod-product-compliance
Lightning Source LLC
LaVergne TN
LVHW082145200926
848484LV00008B/2107